Saunders Nursing Survival Guide:

Critical Care & Emergency Nursing

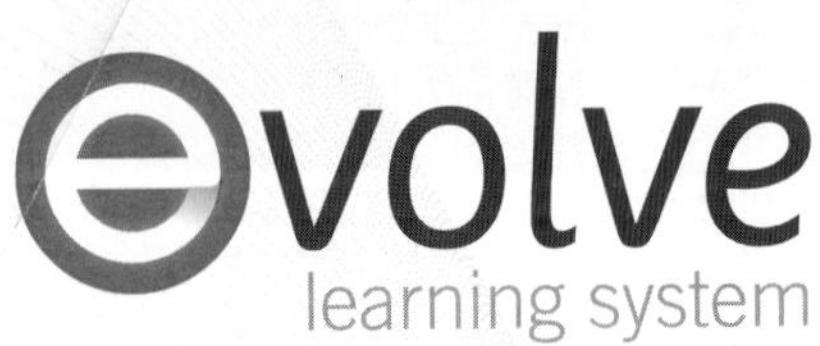

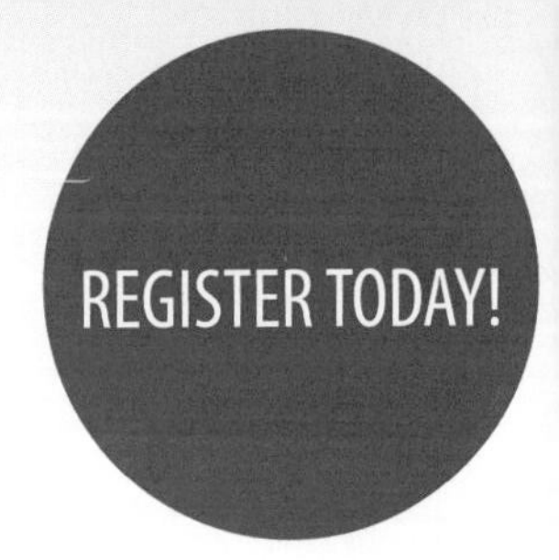

To access your Student Resources, visit:

http://evolve.elsevier.com/Schumacher/criticalcare/

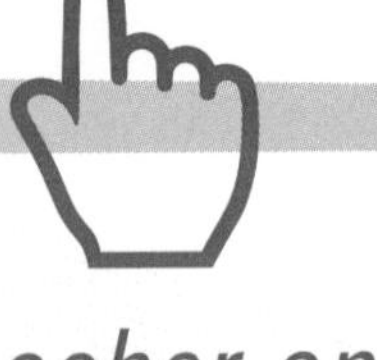

Evolve® Student Resources for *Schumacher and Chernecky: Saunders Nursing Survival Guide: Critical Care & Emergency Nursing*, **Second Edition**, offer the following feature:

Student Resources

- **NCLEX® Review questions**
  Interactive NCLEX® examination-style review questions test your understanding of content and help you practice for the Boards.

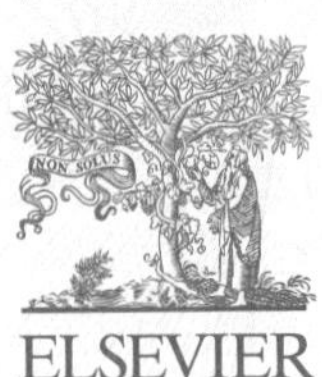

Saunders Nursing Survival Guide: Critical Care & Emergency Nursing

Second Edition

Lori Schumacher, PhD, RN, CCRN
Associate Professor and Associate Dean
Medical College of Georgia, School of Nursing
Augusta, Georgia

Cynthia Chernecky, PhD, RN, CNS, AOCN, FAAN
Professor
Medical College of Georgia, School of Nursing
Augusta, Georgia

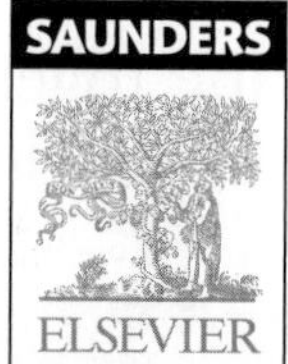

SAUNDERS
ELSEVIER

11830 Westline Industrial Drive
St. Louis, Missouri 63146

SAUNDERS NURSING SURVIVAL GUIDE:
CRITICAL CARE & EMERGENCY NURSING ISBN-13: 978-1-4160-6169-4

Copyright © 2010 by Saunders, an imprint of Elsevier Inc.
NCLEX, NCLEX-RN, and NCLEX-PN are federally registered trademarks and service marks of the National Council of State Boards of Nursing, Inc.

All rights reserved. No part of this publication may be reproduced or transmitted in any form or by any means, electronic or mechanical, including photocopying, recording, or any information storage and retrieval system, without permission in writing from the publisher. Permissions may be sought directly from Elsevier's Rights Department: phone: (+1) 215 239 3804 (US) or (+44) 1865 843830 (UK); fax: (+44) 1865 853333; e-mail: healthpermissions@elsevier.com. You may also complete your request on-line via the Elsevier website at http://www.elsevier.com/permissions.

Notice

Knowledge and best practice in this field are constantly changing. As new research and experience broaden our knowledge, changes in practice, treatment and drug therapy may become necessary or appropriate. Readers are advised to check the most current information provided (i) on procedures featured or (ii) by the manufacturer of each product to be administered, to verify the recommended dose or formula, the method and duration of administration, and contraindications. It is the responsibility of the practitioner, relying on their own experience and knowledge of the patient, to make diagnoses, to determine dosages and the best treatment for each individual patient, and to take all appropriate safety precautions. To the fullest extent of the law, neither the Publisher nor the Authors assumes any liability for any injury and/or damage to persons or property arising out of or related to any use of the material contained in this book.

The Publisher

Previous edition copyrighted 2005

Library of Congress Cataloging-in-Publication Data
Schumacher, Lori.
Critical care & emergency nursing / Lori Schumacher, Cynthia Chernecky. — 2nd ed.
p. ; cm. — (Saunders nursing survival guide)
Includes bibliographical references and index.
ISBN 978-1-4160-6169-4 (pbk. : alk. paper) 1. Emergency nursing. 2. Intensive care nursing. I. Chernecky, Cynthia C. II. Title. III. Title: Critical care and emergency nursing. IV. Series.
[DNLM: 1. Emergency Nursing. 2. Critical Care. WY 154 S392c 2010]
RT120.E4S355 2010
616.02'5—dc22

2008045853

Acquisitions Editor: Michele Hayden
Developmental Editor: Heather Bays
Publishing Services Manager: Deborah Vogel
Project Manager: Brandilyn Tidwell
Designer: Teresa McBryan

Printed in the United States of America

Last digit is the print number: 9 8 7 6 5 4

Working together to grow
libraries in developing countries

www.elsevier.com | www.bookaid.org | www.sabre.org

ELSEVIER BOOK AID International Sabre Foundation

About The Authors

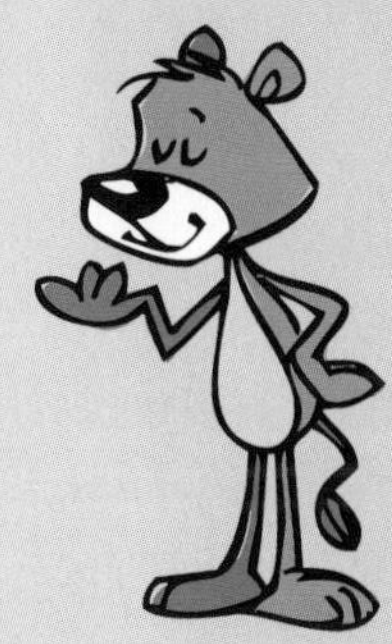

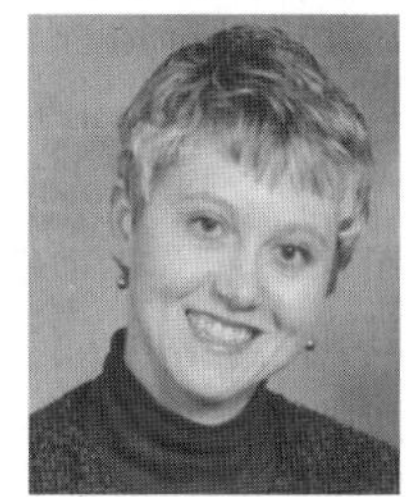

Lori Schumacher earned her degrees at Duquesne University (PhD), the University of Minnesota (MS), and Creighton University (BSN). She has over 15 years of experience in critical care and neuroscience nursing, and maintains CCRN certification. She is active in her church, and is an accomplished flutist. Lori enjoys giving flute lessons and spending time with her family, friends, and four cats.

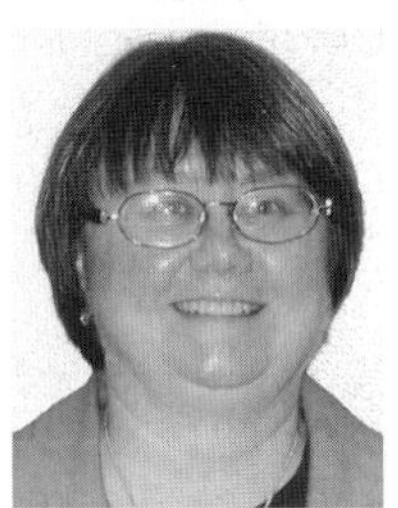

Dr. Cynthia Chernecky earned her degrees at the Case Western Reserve University (PhD), the University of Pittsburgh (MN), and the University of Connecticut (BSN). She also earned an NCI fellowship at Yale University and a postdoctorate visiting scholarship at UCLA. Her clinical areas of expertise are critical care oncology and vascular access. She has more than 30 published books as editor and author with five having won prestigious awards, among them *Laboratory Tests and Diagnostic Procedures* (fifth edition), *Advanced and Critical Care Oncology Nursing: Managing Primary Complications, ECG & the Heart, Fluid and Electrolytes, IV Therapy and Acute Care Oncology Nursing.* She is a national and international speaker, researcher, and published scholar. She is also active in the Orthodox Church, is supportive of Saints Mary & Martha Orthodox Monastery, and enjoys life with family, friends, colleagues, and a West Highland white terrier.

Contributors to the First Edition

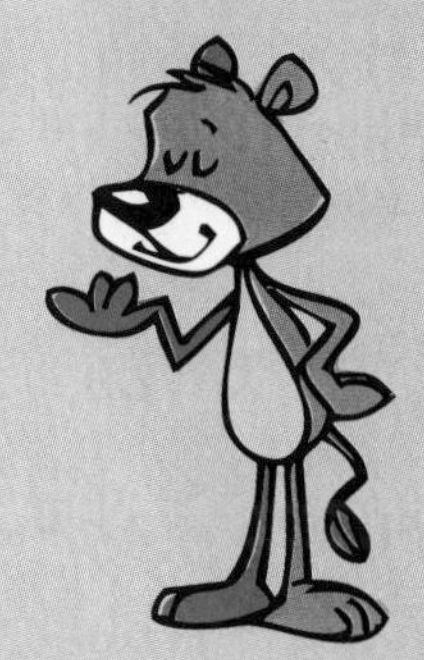

John Aiken, RN, BSN

Robert Dee Bledsoe, MSN, RN, CDE, CWOCN

Julie M. Brown, MSN, CRNA, BSN, RN

James A. Cleveland, BSN, MSN, RN

Kimberly D. Davis, MN, CRNA

Juanita L. Derouen, BSN, RN

Lillian Fogarty, BSN, RN, MN, CRNA

Brenda L. Garman, RN, BSN, MEd

Kitty M. Garrett, RN, MSN, CCRN

Renee B. Guidry, MN, MSN, CRNA, CCRN, APRN

Kathleen M. Hall, MN, MSN, ATCN, CPAN, CRNA

Walter H. Harwood, III, RN

Rebecca K. Hodges, MSN, RN, CCRN

Robin Foell Johns, MSN, RN

Thomas B. Johnson, CRNA

Rosalind Gail Jones, DNP, APRN

Matthew W. Kervin, MN, CRNA

Jane E. Kwilecki, MSN, ARNP, CCRN

Christine Langer, CRNA

Nancy J. Newton, RN, BSN

Lyza Reddick, MSN, CRNA

Carl A. Ross, PhD, RN, CRNP

Jeanne R. Russell, RN, BSN, SNP

Brenda K. Shelton, RN, MS, CCRN, AOCN

Lynn C. Simko, PhD, RN, CCRN

Nancy Stark, DNP, RN

Kathryn Thornton Tinkelenberg, MS, RN

Kathleen R. Wren, PhD, CRNA

Timothy L. Wren, RN, DNP

Diane Salentiny Wrobleski, PhD, RN, APRN, BC, CEN

Contributors

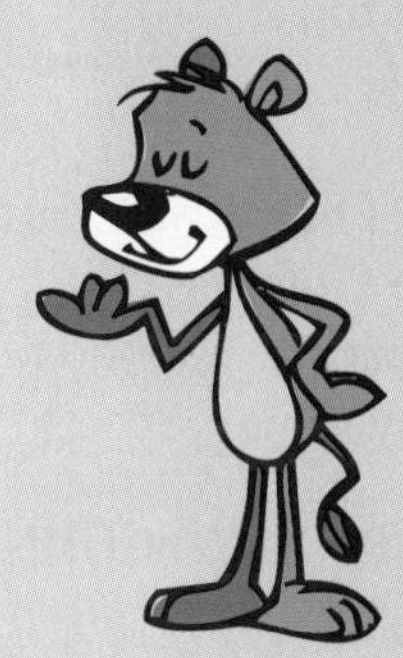

John P. Beilman, MSN, APRN-BC
Clinical Instructor
School of Nursing
Medical College of Georgia
Augusta, Georgia

Annette M. Bourgault, RN, MSc, CNCC[C]
Instructor
Department of Physiological and Technological Nursing
Medical College of Georgia
Augusta, Georgia

James A. Cleveland, AN, RN, MSN, CNS
Chief of Emergency Nursing Sevices
Department of Emergency Medicine
Brooke Army Medical Center
Fort Sam Houston, Texas;
Consultant to the Office of the Surgeon General
Emergency Trauma Nursing
Fort Sam Houston, Texas

Kitty M. Garrett, MSN, RN, CCRN
Instructor
Department of Physiological and Technological Nursing
Medical College of Georgia
Augusta, Georgia

Becki V. Hodges, RN, MSN, CCRN
Critical Care Clinical Nurse Specialist
Trinity Hospital
Augusta, Georgia

Rosalind Jones, DNP, APRN-BC
Assistant Professor
Health Environments & Systems
Medical College of Georgia
Augusta, Georgia

James I. Masiongale, CRNA, MHS
Instructor and Assistant Program Director
Nursing Anesthesia Program
School of Nursing
Medical College of Georgia
Augusta, Georgia

Amy J. Masiongale, CRNA, MSNA
Assistant Director for Didactic Instruction/Instructor
Nursing Anesthesia Program
Medical College of Georgia School of Nursing
Augusta, Georgia

Stacy Sakata-Delph, RN, MSN, CCNL
Joseph M. Still Burn Center
Augusta, Georgia

Lynn M. Simko, PhD, RN, CCRN
Clinical Associate Professor
Duquesne University
Pittsburgh, Pennsylvania

Susan A. Walsh, RN, MN, CCRN
Assistant Professor
School of Nursing
Clayton State University
Morrow, Georgia

Peter Way, APRN, MN, FNP-C, PNP-C
Instructor
Department of Physiological and Technological Nursing
Medical College of Georgia
Augusta, Georgia

Faculty and Practitioner Reviewers

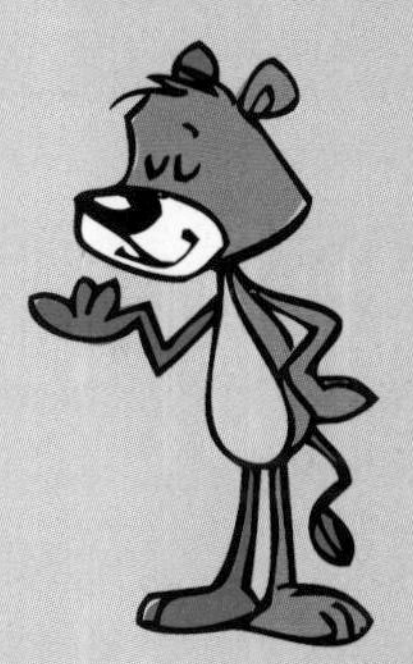

Jane L. Echols, RN, BSN, CCRN
Burn Center
Doctors Hospital
Joseph M. Still Burn Center
Augusta, Georgia

Stephanie C. Greer, RN, MSN
Associate Degree Nursing Instructor
Southwest Mississippi Community College,
Summit, Mississippi

Linda L. Hutchinson, MSN, RN, APRN-BC
Critical Care CNS/Educator
Staff Development Department
Toledo Hospital
Toledo, Ohio

Preface

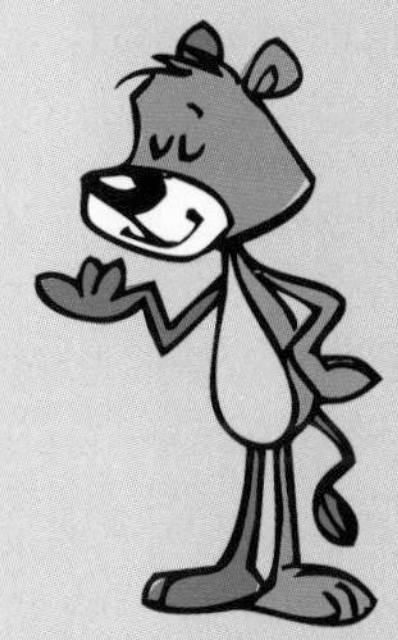

The Saunders Nursing Survival Guide series was created with your input. Nursing students told us about topics they found difficult to master, such as critical care and emergency and hemodynamics. Based on information from focus groups at the National Student Nurses Association meeting, this series was developed on your recommendations. You said to keep the text to a minimum; to use an engaging, fun approach; to provide enough space to write on the pages; to include a variety of activities to appeal to the different learning styles of students; to make the content visually appealing; and to provide NCLEX review questions so you could check your understanding of key topics and review as necessary. This series is a result of your ideas!

Understanding the concepts and principles of critical care and emergency nursing provides a solid foundation for the nurse who works with critically ill patients to guide drug therapy, who monitors hemodynamic parameters, and who is expected to make sound clinical decisions. It is essential for any nurse working in critical care and emergency nursing to be aware of the assessment and technical skills and nursing knowledge associated with the nursing management for these types of patients.

Critical Care & Emergency Nursing in the *Saunders Nursing Survival Guide Series* was developed to explain difficult concepts in an easy-to-understand manner and to assist nursing students in the mastery of these concepts. A basic understanding of pathophysiology, anatomy, and physiology is assumed because the content in this text builds on previous nursing knowledge and provides the fundamental introduction to critical care and emergency nursing. *Critical Care & Emergency Nursing* can also serve as a valuable guide and resource for the novice and the experienced nurse who want to review concepts and principles of critical care and emergency nursing.

We include many features in the margins to help you focus on the vital information you will need to succeed in the classroom and in the clinical setting. **TAKE HOME POINTS** are made up of both study tips for classroom tests and "pearls of wisdom" to assist you in caring for patients. Both are drawn from our many years of combined academic and clinical experience. Content marked with a **Caution icon** is vital and usually involves nursing actions that may have life-threatening consequences or may significantly affect patient outcomes. The **Lifespan icon** and the **Culture icon** highlight variations in treatment that may be necessary for specific age or ethnic groups. A **Calculator icon** will draw your eye to important formulas. A **Web Links icon** will direct you to sites on the Internet that will give more detailed information on a given topic. Each of these icons is designed to help you focus on real-world patient care, the nursing process, and positive patient outcomes.

We also use consistent headings that emphasize specific nursing actions. **What It IS** provides a definition of a topic. **What You NEED TO KNOW** provides the explanation of the topic. **What You DO** explains what you do as a practicing nurse. **Do You UNDERSTAND?** provides questions and exercises that are both entertaining and useful to reinforce the topic's concepts. This four-step approach provides you with information and helps you learn how to apply it to the clinical setting.

Our inspirations and goals for *Critical Care & Emergency Nursing* were to make difficult topics easier. We have used real-world clinical experiences and expertise to bring you a text that will help you understand critical care and emergency nursing to facilitate better patient care. The art and science of nursing is based on understanding, which is the key to critical thinking and clinical decision making. Our hope is for you to share your new insights and understanding with others and apply this information to affect nursing care positively.

Lori Schumacher, PhD, RN, CCRN
Cynthia C. Chernecky, PhD, RN, CNS, AOCN, FAAN

Acknowledgments

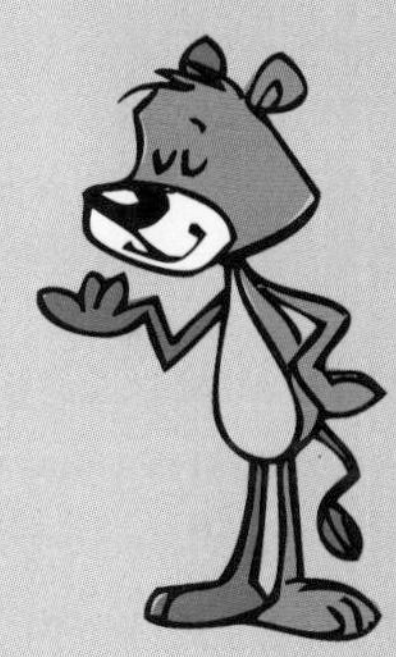

I would like to extend grateful appreciation to my family, colleagues, and students who have provided me with continuous support and encouragement through this endeavor. To my students, who, without them and their desire to learn critical care nursing, none of this would have been possible. I also want to express special thanks to the doctoral faculty at Duquesne University, especially Dr. Joannie Lockhart and Dr. Gladys Husted, for their inspiration and encouragement through my doctoral studies and the publishing of this book. I especially wish to extend my deepest gratitude to my family. To my sister, Julie, and my father and mother, Stan and Sandy, who have continually inspired me in all my nursing endeavors. I wish to dedicate this book to them. Thank you to all the critical care and emergency nurses at Buffalo General Hospital, Medical College of Georgia Health Inc., and WCA Hospital for your diligence and care that you provided to my father during his numerous visits to your nursing units—without you, great things would not be possible! I appreciate and will never forget all the encouragement that Dad gave me through the writing and editing process of this book, although he was ill and not feeling his best. Through his illness, he always strived and was determined to make life better and to live to the best of his abilities.

Dad, it is your determination, strength, love, wisdom, and encouragement that I will always cherish and will attempt to foster in my nursing endeavors and those of my students.

Lori Schumacher

The added strengths of this edition could not have been accomplished without the true professionalism of editors, contributors, reviewers, students, and publication team. Vision and unselfishness are qualities of all of these professionals. We could not have completed this book from idea to present edition without a professional environment that encouraged and supported us in our educational efforts, both in our jobs and from the many experts at Elsevier.

Special thanks for the support and continuous encouragement of my mother, Olga, the nuns of Saints Mary and Martha Orthodox Monastery, and Peter and Katya McNeill. Professional thanks to Drs. Linda Sarna, Ann Kolanowski, Jean Brown, Geri Padilla, Mary Cooley, Leda Danao, Rich Haas, Fred Lupien, Georgia Narsavage, and to Denise Macklin, Paula T. Rieger, Jennifer Edmunds, Kitty Garrett, Becki Hodges, Nancy Stark, Rebecca Rule, and Ingrid Porter for their support and encouragement.

And, finally, to my dog, who gave up long walks and play time so I could write and edit.

Cynthia (Cinda) Chernecky

Contents

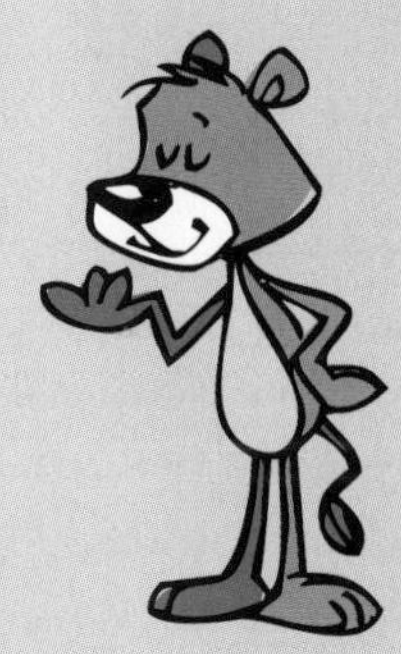

Review of Hemodynamics

Chapter 1

What You WILL LEARN

After reading this chapter, you will know how to do the following:

- ✔ Describe the physiologic basis for hemodynamic monitoring in critically ill patients.
- ✔ Discuss factors that influence cardiac performance and hemodynamic values.
- ✔ Identify normal values for intraarterial, right atrial, left atrial, and pulmonary artery pressure monitoring.
- ✔ Identify appropriate nursing interventions when caring for a patient with hemodynamic monitoring.

What IS Hemodynamics?

Hemodynamics is the study of forces involved in the flow of blood through the cardiovascular and circulatory systems. Components of hemodynamics are blood pressure (BP) or cardiac output (CO) × systemic vascular resistance (SVR), central venous pressure (CVP), and right and left heart pressures.

The physiologic principles of hemodynamics include factors that affect myocardial function, regulate BP, and determine cardiac performance and CO. Understanding the basic concepts of pressure, flow, and resistance provides an insight into the understanding of hemodynamic values. Assessing ventricular function through the evaluation of hemodynamic variables enables the nurse to identify cardiovascular problems and to determine appropriate interventions. This chapter provides a basis for the interpretation of hemodynamic values and clinical application.

What IS the Circulatory System?

The body has a complex network of veins and arteries within a continuous circuit that makes up the *circulatory system.* The heart pumps a constant volume of blood through this system to maintain balance between oxygen delivery and demand.

What You NEED TO KNOW

Several mechanisms regulate the flow of blood through the system. When the body's metabolic demands increase, the blood vessels constrict in an attempt to force blood back to the heart. When the metabolic demand decreases, the veins dilate. This dilation causes pooling of blood in the periphery and reduces venous return to the heart. Other mechanisms that control flow are the result of the ability of the heart to increase or decrease heart rate (HR) and strength of contraction.

How Does the Heart Work?

The function of the heart is to pump blood through the body. The heart is composed of two upper chambers called the *atria* and two lower chambers called the *ventricles.* The atria serve as reservoirs for incoming blood, and the ventricles are the main pumping chambers of the heart. The atria are separated from the ventricles by **atrioventricular valves (AV valves)**. The tricuspid valve separates the right atrium from the right ventricle, and the mitral valve separates the left atrium from the left ventricle. Two other valves, the **pulmonic** semilunar and the **aortic** semilunar, help control the flow of blood from the ventricles to the lungs and systemic circulation. The pulmonic semilunar valve controls the flow of blood from the right ventricle to the lungs, and the aortic semilunar valve controls the flow of blood from the left ventricle to the aorta.

The electrical conduction system is specialized tissue that allows electrical impulses to travel very efficiently from the atria to the ventricles. **Depolarization** is the electrical activation of the muscle cells of the heart and stimulates cellular contraction. Once the cells are depolarized, they return to their original state of electrolyte balance, which is called **repolarization**.

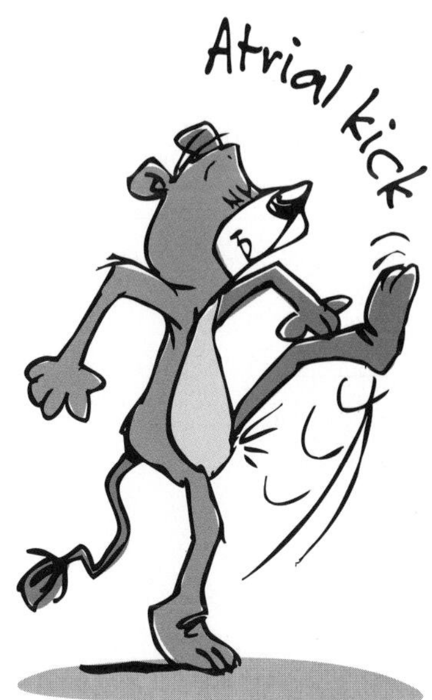

Atria contract.

Cardiac Cycle

The right atrium receives venous blood from the systemic circulation while the left atrium receives reoxygenated blood from the lungs. While both atria are filling with blood, the sinoatrial (SA) node in the electrical conduction system fires and starts the process of depolarization. As the atria fill with blood, the pressure within the atria increases, forcing the AV valves to open. The majority of ventricular filling **(diastole)** passively occurs when the AV valves open. After atrial depolarization, the atria contract, forcing the remaining atrial blood into the ventricles. This contraction is referred to as the **atrial kick** and is responsible for as much as a 30% contribution to CO.

After atrial contraction, the atria begin to relax and atrial pressure decreases. The electrical impulses from the atria now travel through the remainder of the conduction system and cause ventricular depolarization, which is the beginning of ventricular contraction. Ventricular pressure now exceeds atrial pressure, and the AV valves close and the semilunar valves open. Desaturated blood is ejected from the right ventricle into the lungs, where it drops off carbon dioxide and picks up oxygen. Oxygenated blood from the left ventricle is ejected into the systemic circulation via the aorta. The ejection of blood from the ventricles is referred to as **systole**.

Stroke volume (SV) is the volume of blood that is ejected during systole. Left ventricular end *systolic* volume (LVESV) is the amount of blood that remains in the left ventricle at the end of systole. Left ventricular end *diastolic* volume (LVEDV) is the amount of blood that is in the ventricle just before ejection occurs. The left ventricle never ejects the entire volume it receives during diastole. The portion of the volume it does eject is referred to as **ejection fraction** (EF), which is approximately 70% of the total volume at the end of diastole.

Do You UNDERSTAND?

DIRECTIONS: **Fill in the blanks to complete the following statements.**

1. The cardiac conduction system provides electrical activation to cause the heart to ________________________________

   ________________________.

2. During systole, the ____________________ valves are open and the ____________________ ____________________ are closed.
3. During diastole, the ____________________ valves are open and the ____________________ ____________________ are closed.
4. Atrial contraction is referred to as atrial ____________________ ____________________ and is responsible for as much as ____________________ ____________________ % contribution to CO.
5. The left ventricle never ejects the entire volume it receives during systole. The portion of blood that the left ventricle ejects during systole is referred to as ____________________.
6. The volume of blood that is in the ventricle just before ejection occurs is called ____________________ ____________________ ____________________.

What IS Blood Pressure?

If flow or resistance is altered, then pressure is affected. This principle of physics can be applied to BP. Narrowed vessels increase resistance and increase pressure. Conversely, dilated vessels decrease resistance and decrease pressure.

$$BP = CO \times SVR$$

Normal values:
Systolic: 100 to 139 mm Hg
Diastolic: 60 to 90 mm Hg

BP is defined as the tension exerted by blood on the arterial walls. Monitoring BP is based on the following equation:

$$\text{Pressure} = \text{Flow} \times \text{Resistance}$$

SVR is a reflection of peripheral vascular resistance and is the opposition to blood flow from the blood vessels. It is affected by the tone of the blood vessels, blood viscosity, and resistance from the inner lining of the

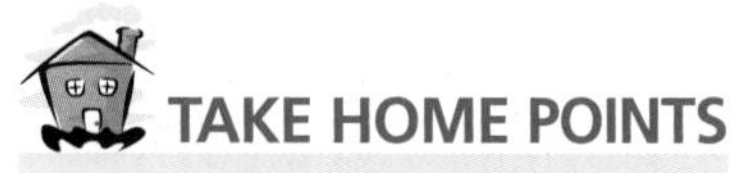

CO and peripheral vascular resistance directly affect BP. If a patient's BP decreases, then either the flow (CO) or the resistance (SVR) will change.

Answers: **1. contract; 2. semilunar, AV valves; 3. AV, semilunar valves; 4. kick, 30; 5. ejection fraction; 6. left ventricular end diastolic volume.**

Factors Influencing Arterial Blood Pressure

- Mean arterial blood pressure
  - Peripheral resistance
    - Blood viscosity (influenced by hematocrit)
    - Arteriolar lumen size (influenced by sympathetic nervous system)
  - Autonomic control
  - Cardiac output
    - Heart rate
      - Sympathetic and parasympathetic nervous system
    - Stroke volume
      - Left ventricular end–diastolic volume (preload)
        - Intraventricular pressure
          - Autonomic control
          - Atrial pressure
          - Venous pressure
            - Blood volume
            - Renin-angiotensin system
          - Venous return

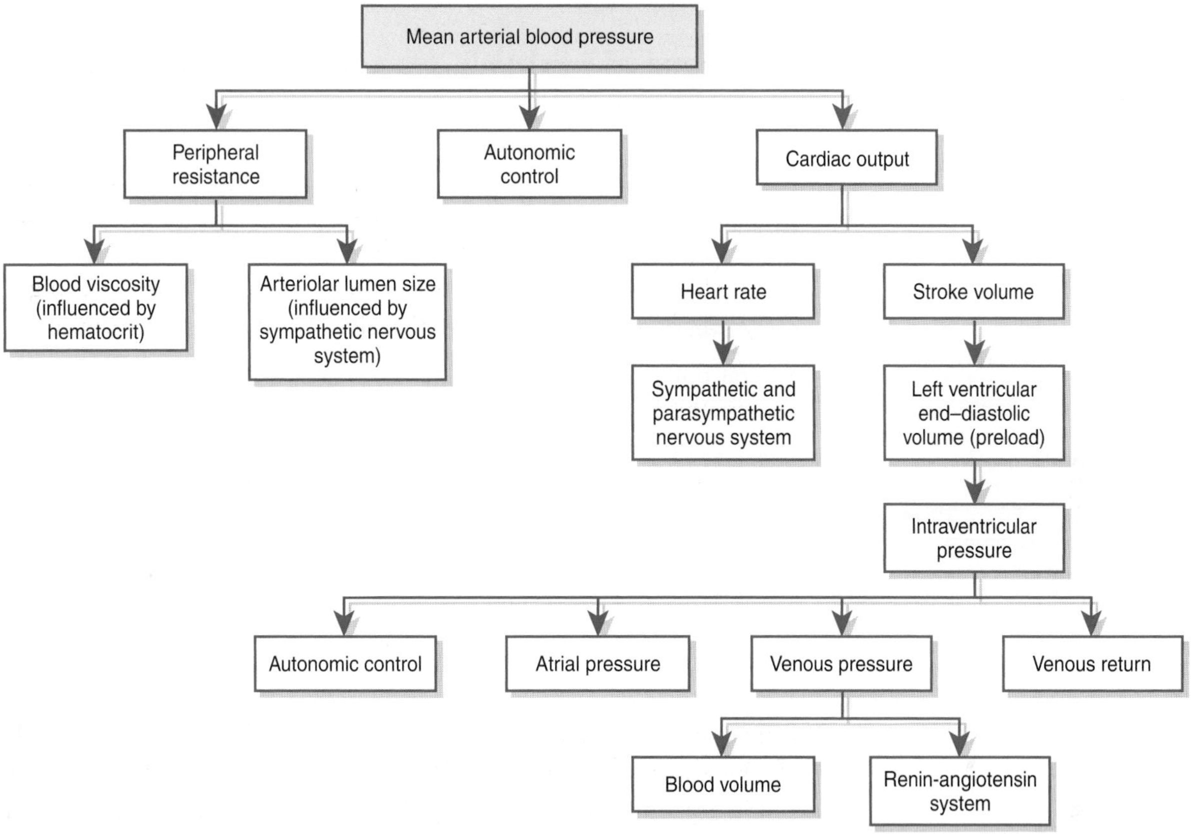

(From Sole ML, Lamborn ML, Hartshorn JC: Introduction to critical care nursing, *ed 3, Philadelphia, 2001, WB Saunders.)*

blood vessels. SVR is also the resistance against which the left ventricle pumps; it usually has an inverse relationship with CO.

$$\text{SVR} = \frac{\text{Mean Arterial Pressure (MAP)} - \text{CVP} \times 80}{\text{CO}}$$

The diameter of the blood vessel is one of the major factors that influence SVR. SVR decreases when the blood vessels relax, and it increases with the narrowing of the blood vessels. Vasoactive drugs are often used in the critical care setting to change the size of the arterioles to decrease or increase BP.

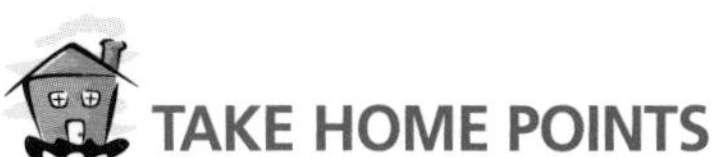

TAKE HOME POINTS

If the SVR decreases, then the CO increases. SVR increases to maintain BP when the CO decreases.

Normal value:
800 to 1200 dynes/sec/cm^{-5}

What You NEED TO KNOW

Elevations of Systemic Vascular Resistance

The two primary reasons for elevations in SVR are vascular disturbances, such as vasoconstriction caused by hypertension, or excessive catecholamine release and compensatory responses to maintain BP in decreased CO. In addition, elevations of SVR increase the workload of the heart and myocardial oxygen consumption.

Decreases in Systemic Vascular Resistance

Several potential causes for decreased SVR exist, including sepsis and neurologically mediated vasomotor tone loss. When SVR decreases, CO increases in an attempt to maintain BP.

TAKE HOME POINTS

- Common medications and habits can often change SVR. For example, smoking and stress can cause vasoconstriction.
- Vasodilators enlarge **(dilate)** the size of the arterioles in an attempt to decrease BP.
- Vasoconstrictors shrink **(constrict)** the size of the arterioles in an attempt to increase BP.

What IS Cardiac Output?

CO is the amount of blood ejected from the heart in 1 minute. CO has two components: SV and HR. A major goal in assessing CO is ensuring adequate oxygenation.

$$CO = SV \times HR$$

Normal values: 4 to 8 L/min

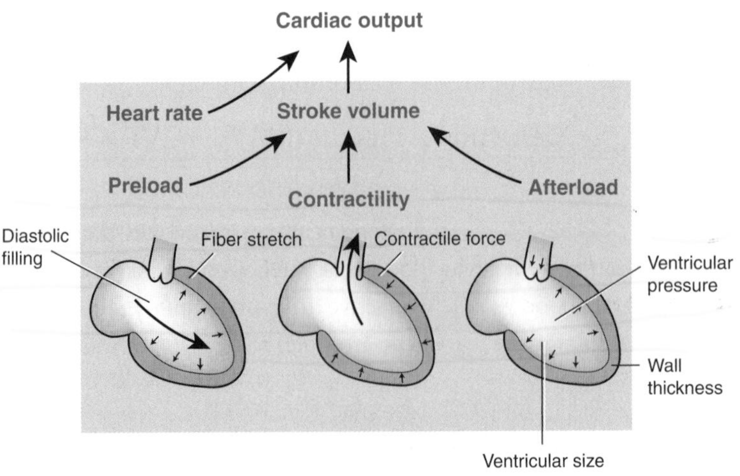

CO = SV × HR

What IS Stroke Volume?

SV is the amount of blood ejected from the heart with each beat. The three factors that influence SV are preload, afterload, and contractility.

What You NEED TO KNOW

Preload

Preload is the filling volume of the ventricle at the end of diastole. It reflects the amount of cardiac muscle stretch at end diastole just before contraction. Preload is dependent on the volume of blood returning to the heart. Venous tone and the actual amount of blood in the venous system influence this volume. Preload is measured by obtaining a pressure measurement with a pulmonary artery (PA) catheter. This pressure is referred to as a *pulmonary artery occlusion pressure/pulmonary artery wedge pressure* (PAOP/PAWP).

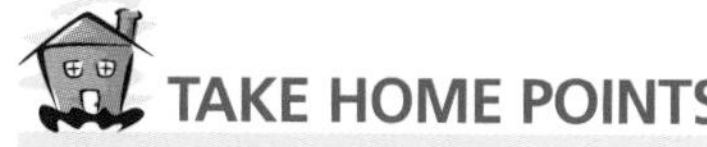

- Preload is directly related to the force of myocardial contraction.
- An enlarged heart will increase preload because the volume in the ventricle is larger, and is measured by an elevated PAWP.

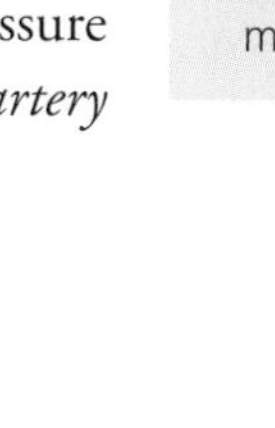

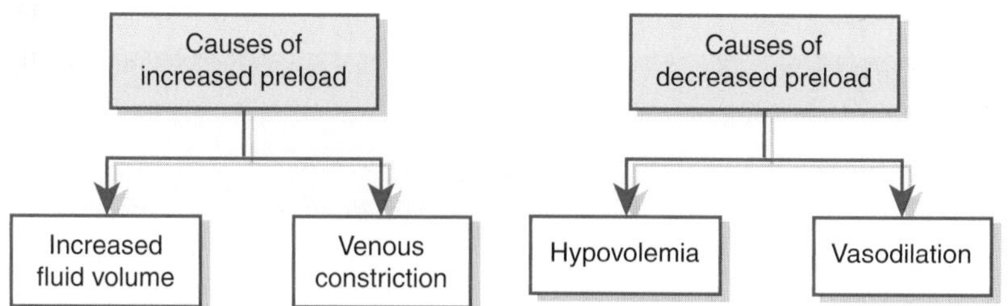

(From Sole ML, Lamborn ML, Hartshorn JC: Introduction to critical care nursing, *ed 3, Philadelphia, 2001, WB Saunders.)*

Afterload

Afterload is the amount of resistance against which the left ventricle pumps. It is primarily influenced by the blood vessels, but blood viscosity, flow patterns, and valves can also have an effect. The greater the resistance, the more the myocardium has to work to overcome the resistance. Afterload is determined by BP and arterial tone.

Left ventricular afterload is measured by the assessment of the SVR. Pulmonary vascular resistance (PVR) measures the resistance against which the right ventricle works.

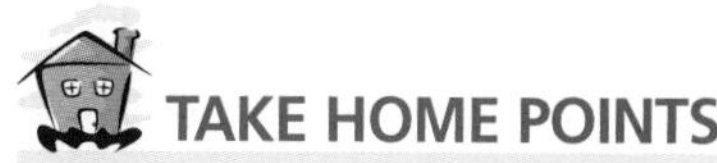

Vasoconstriction results from an increase in systemic arterial tone, which increases BP and causes an increase in afterload.

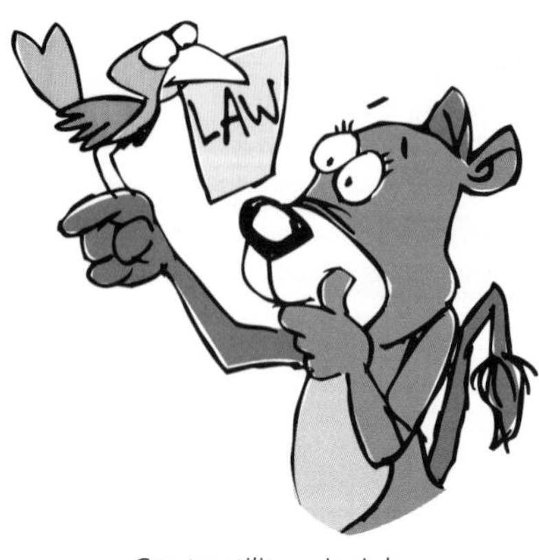

Contractility principle.

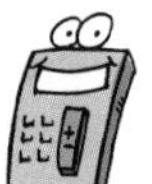
Left VSWI = MAP − PCWP × SV Index (SVI) × 0.0136
Normal value: 40 to 70 gm/m^2/beat
SVI = CO ÷ Body Surface Area (BSA)
Normal value: 33 to 47 ml/beat/m^2

Contractility

Contractility is defined as the strength of myocardial fiber shortening during systole. It allows the heart to work independently, regardless of changes in preload, afterload, or fiber length. Because contractility is a determinant of SV, it affects ventricular function. Preload is one factor that directly influences contractility because of the physiologic principle referred to as the **Frank-Starling law**, which states, "The greater the stretch, the greater the force of the next contraction."

Increases in preload (end-diastolic volume) maximally increase SV. However, in cases of compromised cardiac or pulmonary function, volume and pressure relationships are not directly linear. Ventricular stroke work index (VSWI) is a useful measurement of myocardial contractility.

Heart Rate

The number of heartbeats per minute is important in maintaining CO and is included in the CO formula. When contractility is depressed or if CO is decreased, then the HR will increase to maintain sufficient blood flow for metabolic demand.

Manipulation of Cardiac Output

Stroke Volume					Heart Rate	
Preload		Afterload (Systemic Vascular Resistance)		Contractility		
Increased	Decreased	Increased	Decreased	Decreased Contractility	Increased	Decreased
Diuretics Venodilators	Fluids Vasoconstrictors	Arterial vasodilators	Vasoconstrictors	Positive inotropes	Beta-blockers and calcium channel blockers to decrease heart rate	Sympathometics Cardiac pacing

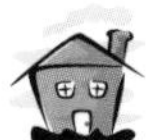
TAKE HOME POINTS

As resistance to left ventricular ejection (afterload) increases, left ventricular work increases and SV may decrease.

Physiologic Principles that Affect Cardiac Performance

Factors that influence cardiac performance include the Frank-Starling law of the heart, the ability to influence contractility of the muscle fibers of the heart (**inotropism**), any changes in HR or regularity of rhythm

(force-frequency ratio), and miscellaneous influences such as the sympathetic or parasympathetic nervous system responses.

Frank-Starling law of the heart. Augmenting ventricular filling during diastole before the onset of a contraction will increase the force of that next contraction during systole.

Inotropism. Inotropism is the ability to influence contractility of muscle fibers. A positive inotrope enhances contractility. A negative inotrope depresses contractility.

Force-frequency ratio. Any changes in HR or rhythm can change diastolic filling time of the ventricles, therefore altering fiber stretch and the force of the next contraction. This ratio influences SV and CO. In addition, the majority of coronary artery filling occurs during diastole. When HRs increase, myocardial oxygen demand increases; however, when diastolic filling time is shortened, coronary artery filling decreases. This ratio results in an imbalance between the supply and demand of myocardial oxygen.

Miscellaneous influences. Factors such as hypoxia, hyperkalemia, hypercarbia, hyponatremia, and myocardial scar tissue also can decrease myocardial contractility. Sympathetic stimulation increases myocardial contractility, and parasympathetic stimulation (via the vagus nerve) depresses the SA node, atrial myocardium, and AV junctional tissue.

Normal Adult HR: 60 to 100 beats/min
Bradycardia: <60 beats/min (lengthens diastolic filling time)
Tachycardia: >100 beats/minute (shortens diastolic filling time)

Do You UNDERSTAND?

DIRECTIONS: **Fill in the blanks to complete the following statements.**

1. CO = ________________ ________________ × ________________ ________________.
2. Preload, afterload, and contractility are determinants of ________________.
3. Preload is defined as ________________.
4. Afterload is defined as ________________.
5. PAWP measures ________________.
6. SVR measures ________________.

DIRECTIONS: Match the descriptions in Column A with the terms in Column B.

Column A	Column B
_____ 7. Decreases myocardial contractility	a. Sympathetic stimulation
_____ 8. Increases myocardial contractility	b. Influencing contraction
_____ 9. Inotropism	c. Frank-Starling law
_____ 10. "The greater the stretch, the greater the next force of contraction"	d. Hyperkalemia, hypoxia, hypercarbia, hyponatremia

What IS Hemodynamic Monitoring?

Hemodynamics or pressures of the cardiovascular and circulatory system can be measured by invasive methods such as direct arterial BP monitoring, CVP monitoring, and indirect measurements of left ventricular pressures via a flow-directed, balloon-tipped catheter (e.g., PA catheters, Swan-Ganz catheters).

The goals of hemodynamic monitoring include ensuring adequate perfusion, detecting inadequate perfusion, titrating therapy to specific end points, qualifying the severity of illness, and differentiating system dysfunction (e.g., differentiating between cardiogenic and noncardiogenic pulmonary edema).

Direct Arterial Blood Pressure Monitoring

Direct intraarterial monitoring allows for accurate, continuous monitoring of arterial BPs. It also provides a system for continuous sampling of blood for arterial blood gases without repeated arterial punctures. Clinical considerations include the potential complications of thrombosis, embolism, blood loss, and infection. Invasive intraarterial monitoring is considered to be more accurate and reliable than noninvasive types of BP monitoring.

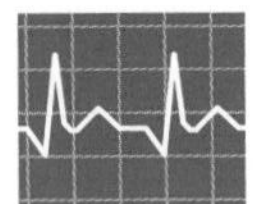

Monitoring: Normal CVP or RAP values are 0 to 6 mm Hg.

Answers: 1. stroke volume, heart rate; 2. stroke volume; 3. left ventricular end diastolic volume; 4. resistance against which the left ventricle has to pump; 5. preload; 6. afterload; 7. d; 8. a; 9. b; 10. c.

Hemodynamic monitoring. *(From Sole ML, Lamborn ML, Hartshorn JC:* Introduction to critical care nursing, *ed 3, Philadelphia, 2001, WB Saunders.)*

Right Atrial Pressure Monitoring

Measuring pressures from the right atrium can be referred to as right atrial pressures (RAP) or CVPs. Measuring pressure from the superior or inferior vena cava (CVP) or from the right atrium (RAP) is a direct method. The pressures between these two areas are essentially equal. Because the tricuspid valve (i.e., AV valve between the right atria and right ventricle) is open during diastole, a RAP measurement can reliably reflect right ventricular end diastolic pressure (RVEDP). Any condition that changes venous tone, blood volume, or contractility of the right ventricle can cause an abnormality in RAP values.

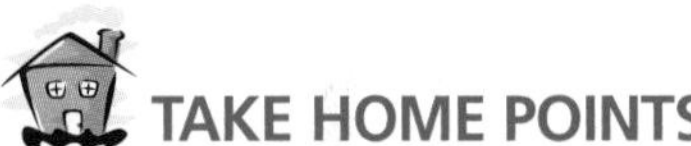

TAKE HOME POINTS

Low RAP or CVP measurements can reflect hypovolemia or extreme vasodilation. High RAP measurements can reflect hypervolemia, or severe vasoconstriction, or conditions that reduce the ability of the right ventricle to contract (i.e., pulmonary hypertension and right ventricular failure).

Left Atrial Pressure Monitoring

Direct left atrial pressure (LAP) monitoring is not routinely used except in cardiac surgical procedures, cardiac catheterization laboratories, and after open-heart procedures. Most often, a catheter is inserted during cardiac surgery with the distal end tunneled through an incision in the

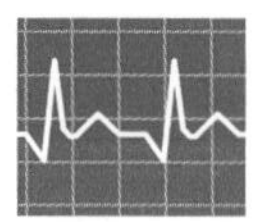

Monitoring: Normal PA catheter values:
Right ventricular pressures: Systolic 15 to 25 mm Hg
Diastolic 0 to 6 mm Hg
PA pressures: Systolic 15 to 25 mm Hg
Diastolic 8 to 15 mm Hg
PA occlusion pressure: 6 to 12 mm Hg

chest wall. LAP monitoring provides the ability to observe the pressures in the left atrium; however, air embolism and system debris are major complications that can obstruct a coronary or cerebral artery. To prevent the possibility of complications, connections must be tight and caps should be on stopcocks to avoid air entering or administering medications and fluids through this line.

Pulmonary Artery Monitoring

The PA catheter is a multilumen, balloon-tipped catheter that is inserted through the venous system into the right side of the heart and into the PA. The catheter may be inserted at the bedside from an antecubital vein, external jugular vein, subclavian artery, or any other peripheral vein into the PA through a percutaneous introducer. Fluoroscopy is not required because the pressure tracing can identify the positioning on the monitor. The catheter is inserted with the balloon deflated; however, when the catheter enters the right atrium, the balloon is inflated, allowing it to float with the flow of blood into the PA. When the balloon is deflated, the catheter directly measures PA pressures. With balloon inflation, the catheter floats into a pulmonary arteriole and wedges itself in a smaller lumen. The opening of the catheter beyond the inflated balloon reflects pressures distal to the PA (i.e., passive runoff of pulmonary venous blood in the left atrium). This PCWP, also referred to as the PAOP, indirectly measures left ventricular function because the mean PCWP or PAOP and left atrial pressures closely approximate LVEDP in patients with normal mitral valve function.

The other lumen of the catheter allows for monitoring of right atrial pressures (CVP). An additional port, referred to as the *thermistor*, allows for the measurement of CO. PA catheters may also have additional lumens, which allow for intravenous administration of solutions or insertion of pacemaker electrodes for the purpose of transvenous pacing. Other catheters also have the ability to monitor CO or mixed venous oxygen saturation continuously. The PA catheter is used to monitor high-risk, critically ill patients with goals that include the detection of adequate perfusion and the diagnosis and evaluation of the effects of therapy. This at-risk patient group also includes those with a variety of cardiopulmonary problems, including acute myocardial infarction, severe angina, cardiomyopathy, right and left ventricular failure, and pulmonary diseases. In addition, PA monitoring is a valuable tool for observing fluid balance in the critically ill patient at risk for other cardiopulmonary problems.

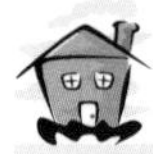

TAKE HOME POINTS

It is important to remember that changes in PCWP are not always equal to volume changes because the PCWP is not the only parameter involved in muscle stretch. Patients who have compliant left ventricles can have large volume changes without large changes in pressure; conversely patients with noncompliant ventricles may have extreme volume changes without PCWP increases.

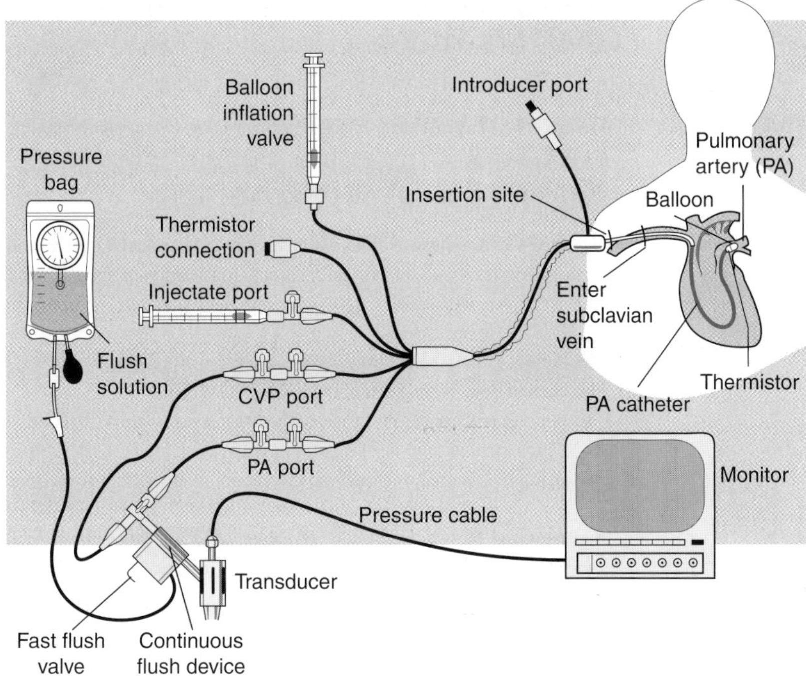

Pulmonary artery monitoring. *(From Bucher L, Melander S:* Critical care nursing, *Philadelphia, 1999, WB Saunders.)*

What You DO

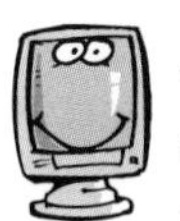

www.pacep.org
www.edwards.com/Products/PACatheters/placementvideo.hym?WT.ac=SGPAC

To monitor hemodynamics, the equipment must include a transducer, amplifier, display monitor, catheter system, and tubing filled with fluid. This system provides the ability to monitor a pressure waveform that is displayed as a digital readout on the oscilloscope.

Nursing interventions for hemodynamic monitoring include (1) providing patient education about the procedure, (2) ensuring that the appropriate procedure consent forms are signed, (3) setting up the equipment, (4) preparing the line, (5) assisting the physician with catheter insertion, (6) monitoring the pressures, and (7) making clinical decisions per institutional policy. The nurse should also be alert to potential complications.

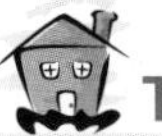

TAKE HOME POINTS

Even though hemodynamic monitoring is an important assessment tool for the critical care nurse, it is still essential to assess your patient and put everything together to make sure everything makes clinical sense. Sometimes, numbers are just numbers and the patient does not look like what the numbers suggest.

References

Ahrens T, Taylor L: *Hemodynamic waveform analysis,* Philadelphia, 1992, WB Saunders.

Alspach J, et al: *AACN core curriculum for critical care nursing,* ed 6, Philadelphia, 2006, WB Saunders.

Brown CV, Showmaker WC, Woo CC, et al: Is noninvasive hemodynamic monitoring appropriate for elder critically injured patient? *Journal of Trauma,* 2005;58:102-107.

Chernecky C, Berger B: *Laboratory tests and diagnostic procedures,* ed 5, Philadelphia, 2008, WB Saunders.

Chulay M, Burns SM: *American Association of Critical Care Nurses essentials of critical care nursing,* New York, 2006, McGraw Hill.

Darovic GO: *Handbook of hemodynamic monitoring,* 2nd ed., Philadelphia, 2004, WB Saunders.

Dickens JJ: Central venous oxygenation saturation monitoring: a role for critical care. *Current Anaesthesia* & *Critical Care* 2004;15:378-382.

George-Gay B, Chernecky C: *Clinical medical-surgical nursing: a decision making reference,* Philadelphia, 2002, WB Saunders.

Hodges RK, Garrett K, et al: *Hemodynamic monitoring,* St. Louis, 2005, Elsevier Saunders.

Miller LR: Case studies in hemodynamics, *AACN 2008 NTI & critical care exposition proceedings manual,* Chicago, 2008, AACN.

Morton PG, Fontaine DK, Hudak CM, Gallo BM: *Critical care nursing: a holistic approach,* 8th ed, Philadelphia, 2005, Lippincott Williams & Wilkins.

Sole ML, Klein DG, Moseley MJ: *Introduction to critical care nursing,* 4th ed, St. Louis, 2005, Elsevier Saunders.

Urden LD, Stacy KM, Lough ME: *Thelan's critical care nursing diagnosis and management,* 5th ed, St. Louis, 2005, Elsevier.

NCLEX® Review

1. At the end of diastole, the degree of ventricular stretch is referred to as:
   1 Preload.
   2 Afterload.
   3 Contractility.
   4 Cardiac output (CO).

2. The cardiac conduction system is the stimulus for:
   1 Atrial filling.
   2 Ventricular contraction.
   3 Systemic vascular resistance (SVR).
   4 Afterload.

3. The formula for CO equals:
   1 Stroke volume × heart rate (HR).
   2 Patient weight × HR.
   3 Contractility × HR.
   4 Stroke volume × contractility.

4. Which of the following is not a determinant of stroke volume?
   1 Contractility.
   2 Preload.
   3 HR.
   4 Afterload.

5. Preload is:
   1 A measurement of SVR.
   2 A measurement reflecting contractility.
   3 Reflective of left ventricular end-diastolic volume.
   4 Reflective of CO.

6. Afterload is reflective of:
   1 Pulmonary capillary wedge pressure (PCWP).
   2 CO.
   3 Contractility.
   4 SVR.

7. A substance that affects contractility is referred to as:
   1 Chronotropic.
   2 Inotropic.
   3 Vasoactive.
   4 Vasodilatory.

8. Preload can be measured with a pulmonary artery catheter by obtaining:
   1 SVR.
   2 PCWP.
   3 Left ventricular stroke work index (LVSWI).
   4 Pulmonary artery systolic pressure.

9. The sum of resistance in peripheral arterioles reflected in mean aortic pressure is:
   1 Pulmonary vascular resistance (PVR).
   2 SVR.
   3 Mean arterial pressure (MAP).
   4 PCWP.

10. Miscellaneous influences that *decrease* contractility include:
    1 Hypoxia, hyperkalemia, sympathetic stimulation.
    2 Hypercarbia, hyponatremia, sympathetic stimulation.
    3 Hypoxia, myocardial scar tissue, parasympathetic stimulation.
    4 Hypokalemia, hypernatremia, parasympathetic stimulation.

NCLEX® Review Answers

1.3 Contractility is the degree of ventricular stretch. Preload is the volume in the left ventricle at the end of diastole. Afterload is the resistance against which the left ventricle has to work. CO is the amount of blood ejected from the ventricles in 1 minute.

2.2 The electrical conduction system provides the stimulation for depolarization of cardiac cells, resulting in contraction. Right atrial filling results from venous return to the heart. Left atrial filling results from return from the pulmonary capillary bed via the pulmonary veins. SVR is reflective of afterload. Afterload is the resistance against which the left ventricle works.

3.1 The formula for CO is CO = stroke volume × HR. The CO formula does not include patient weight. Contractility is one of the parameters that influence stroke volume, and preload and afterload should also be considered. Stroke volume is included in the formula for CO, but contractility is one of the parameters for stroke volume.

4.3 HR is *not* a parameter of stroke volume; however, it is part of the formula for CO. Preload, afterload, and contractility *are* parameters of stroke volume.

5.3 Preload is a measurement of left ventricular end diastolic pressure, which is reflective of left ventricular end diastolic volume. Preload is a measurement of left ventricular end diastolic pressure and is not the only parameter considered in CO.

6.4 Afterload is the resistance against which the left ventricle works and is measured by obtaining SVR. PCWP is reflective of preload. CO considers stroke volume and HR. Afterload is the resistance against which the left ventricle works and is measured by obtaining SVR.

7.2 Inotropic means affecting contractility. Chronotropic refers to affecting rate; vasoactive means affecting the blood vessels; vasodilatory means causing dilation of the vessels.

8.2 A PCWP is reflective of left ventricular end diastolic volume or pressure (or preload). SVR is reflective of afterload. LVSWI is reflective of contractility. Pulmonary artery systolic pressure reflects pressure in the pulmonary artery during systole when the mitral valve is closed, thus only reflecting left atrial pressure.

9.2 SVR is a reflection of the peripheral resistance during mean aortic pressure. PVR reflects the resistance against which the *right* ventricle works (the resistance from the lungs). MAP is a reflection of the perfusion pressure to vital organs. PCWP reflects left ventricular end diastolic pressure.

10.3 Hypoxia, myocardial scar tissue, and parasympathetic stimulation *decrease* contractility. Miscellaneous influences that decrease myocardial contractility include hypoxia, hyperkalemia, hypercarbia, hyponatremia, and myocardial scar tissue. Sympathetic stimulation increases contractility.

Shock Trauma

Chapter 2

What You WILL LEARN

After reading this chapter, you will know how to do the following:

- ✔ Differentiate between the various shock states.
- ✔ Describe the physical manifestations most commonly associated with the various shock states.
- ✔ Compare and contrast various shock states.
- ✔ Identify appropriate nursing interventions for the treatment of shock states.
- ✔ Discuss the complications of the various shock states.
- ✔ Describe prevention approaches that can be instituted in the critical care environment.

evolve
See http://evolve.elsevier.com/Schumacher/criticalcare for additional NCLEX® review questions.

What IS Anaphylaxis and Anaphylactic Shock?

Anaphylaxis is a life-threatening hypersensitivity or pseudoallergic reaction to an exogenous agent. These severe reactions can be either immune mediated (**anaphylactic**) or chemically mediated (**anaphylactoid**).

Anaphylaxis is the result of an antigen-antibody reaction and is usually observed in individuals with allergies. The immune response is directed against substances that are not inherently harmful to the body and that enter through either the skin or the respiratory tract. Substances such as foods, food additives, environmental agents (e.g., pollens, molds, animal dander), diagnostic agents, medications, blood or blood products, or venoms (e.g., bee stings, snakebites) can trigger an immune-mediated reaction.

Typically, the initial exposure to the allergy-inducing agent (**allergen**) results in the formation of an antibody called *immunoglobulin E* (IgE) specific for that allergen. This first exposure to the antigen is known as the *primary immune response.* No clinical evidence of the exposure is usually observed at this time. The antibodies accumulate and attach themselves to the membrane of mast cells, which contain large amounts of histamine, and to the basophils in the plasma. The mast cells and basophils are both dispersed throughout the body, where they wait for the next allergen exposure. Subsequent exposures to the allergen produce a *secondary immune response.* The antigen and the IgE antibody interact to trigger the rupture of the mast cells, which is called *degranulation.* The mast cells then release chemical mediators such as histamine, eosinophilic chemotactic factor of anaphylaxis (ECF-A), leukotrienes (formerly known as slow-reacting substance of anaphylaxis [SRS-A]), platelet-activating factors (PAF), kinins, and prostaglandins. Histamine is believed to be the most important cause of the symptoms associated with allergic reactions. The substances released cause vasodilation, increased capillary permeability, and smooth muscle contraction. This reaction is followed by evidence of symptomatic clinical changes, which precipitates **anaphylactic shock.**

Anaphylactoid reactions reflect the release of histamine from mast cells and basophils in response to the administration of a drug (chemical mediator). The histamine released is independent of an antigen-antibody interaction, but the signs and symptoms are exactly the same. In contrast to anaphylactic reactions that need prior exposure, anaphylactoid reactions may occur without prior exposure to a drug. Although anaphylactoid reactions can be as life threatening as anaphylactic reactions, they tend to be self-limiting (5 to 10 minutes) because of the short half-life of histamine in the plasma (see Color Plate 1 of the insert for mediator response and clinical manifestations).

TAKE HOME POINTS

- Anaphylactic reactions need prior exposure; anaphylactoid reactions may occur without prior exposure.
- Anaphylactic reactions have the possibility of increasing with each exposure.
- Anaphylactic reactions may manifest immediately or be delayed.

What You NEED TO KNOW

Anaphylactic and anaphylactoid reactions, which are clinically indistinguishable, may become rapidly fatal if appropriate therapy is not promptly initiated.

Symptoms of anaphylaxis usually occur within seconds to minutes of injection of the causative agent, although symptoms may be delayed up to 1 hour after exposure. Histamine triggers physiologic changes by promoting vasodilation and increasing capillary-venous permeability, which is clinically evidenced by redness, warmth, and swelling.

Anaphylactic and anaphylactoid reactions are associated with acute medical emergencies that ultimately involve compromised cardiovascular and respiratory systems.

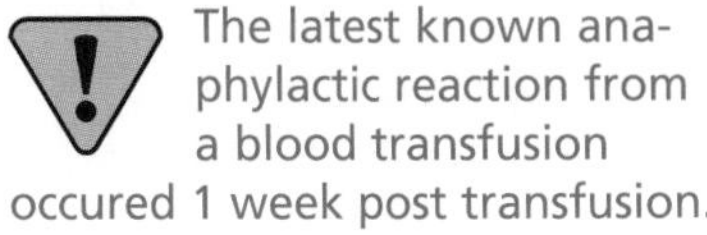

The latest known anaphylactic reaction from a blood transfusion occured 1 week post transfusion.

The first dermatologic symptoms include pruritus, generalized erythema, urticaria (usually on the chest and then on the face), and angioedema. Angioedema is a result of fluid leaking into the interstitial space, which causes a swelling of the face, oral cavity, and lower pharynx. The patient may become restless, anxious, and apprehensive with the complaint of a sense of impending doom—an ominous sign that should never be taken lightly by a critical care nurse. Smooth muscle constriction gives rise to signs of gastrointestinal (GI) and genitourinary distress including vomiting, diarrhea, cramping, abdominal pain, urinary incontinence, or vaginal bleeding.

Pulmonary manifestations include laryngeal edema, bronchoconstriction, bronchorrhea, or pulmonary edema. Clinical signs and symptoms of laryngeal edema include inspiratory stridor, hoarseness, dysphonia, and difficulty swallowing. The patient may complain of the feeling of a lump in his or her throat, which is caused by soft tissue swelling. Bronchoconstriction can cause chest tightness, dyspnea, and wheezing, which can be frightening for the patient.

With cardiovascular involvement, the patient may complain of dizziness or changes in his or her level of consciousness (LOC). The patient may feel faint or weak, or may complain of palpitations. Typically, the electrocardiogram (ECG) shows tachycardia, supraventricular arrhythmias, myocardial ischemia, and possibly infarction. Tachycardia and syncope may lead to the development of hypotension and severe cardiovascular compromise.

The net effect of this downward spiral is significant hypotension and a decreased systemic vascular resistance (SVR) because of the leaky capillaries and postcapillary venules. Anaphylactic shock occurs as a result of an extreme decrease in venous return from the vasodilation and lowered intravascular volume. Assessment of the patient in anaphylactic shock shows hemodynamic compromise of cardiac function, including decreased SVR, decreased stroke volume, decreased afterload, decreased end-diastolic volume, and decreased mixed venous oxygenation saturation. These hemodynamic responses lead to an overall decrease in cardiac output (CO) with ineffective

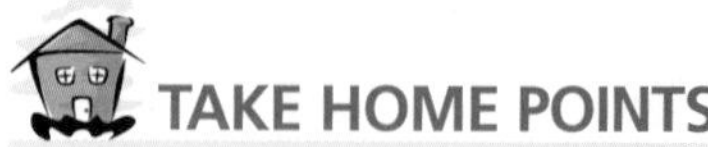

- Anaphylactic shock occurs as a result of an extreme decrease in venous return from vasodilation and lowered intravascular volume, which results in severe cardiovascular and respiratory compromise.
- Anxiety and restlessness may be exhibited due to a sense of impending doom.

tissue perfusion. Once the patient has reached the level of shock, any number of organ systems can be affected. During the time of decreased CO with a drop in blood volume, the body protects itself by diverting oxygenated blood to organs of highest priority. These organs include the heart, brain, and kidneys. Although the major organs are receiving most of the blood volume at this time, ineffective tissue perfusion is still taking place, which leads to cell death and lactic acidosis. Depending on the extent of hypoperfusion, the body's organs may or may not recover with appropriate therapy. Rapid recognition and treatment is the mainstay of preventing morbidity and mortality.

What You DO

Medical Management and Treatment

The key to successful treatment of anaphylactic and anaphylactoid reactions is an astute clinician who recognizes the problem early and takes immediate life-saving actions. The steps taken in treatment may need to be done simultaneously to ensure patient safety. The first step in treating an anaphylactic reaction is to immediately discontinue use of the causative agent, even when the product is only under suspicion. This prevents further recruitment of mast cells and the release of their mediators. The second step, the hallmark of treatment, is to administer epinephrine (Adrenaline). If the adult patient does not have an existing intravenous (IV) or vascular access device in place, epinephrine (Adrenaline) should be subcutaneously administered at a dose of 0.2 to 0.5 mL of a 1:1000 solution. This dose may be repeated every 10 to 15 minutes as needed. If the patient does have an IV in place, the dose should be 1 to 2.5 mL of a 1:10,000 solution (0.1 to 0.25 mg) in an adult. The dose may be increased to 0.3 to 0.5 mg and repeated every 5 to 15 minutes as needed. Epinephrine (Adrenaline) promotes vasoconstriction, inhibits bronchoconstriction, and inhibits the release of mediators from stimulated mast cells or basophils by stimulating the production of cyclic adenosine monophosphate (cAMP).

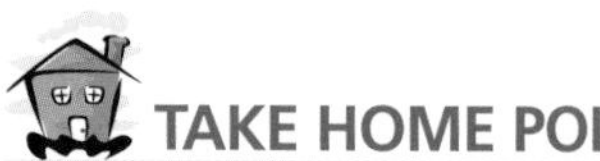

Epinephrine can also be administered via the endotracheal tube in smaller doses, 1 to 2.5 mL of a 1:10,000 solution for an adult (1 mg Epinephrine in a 10-mL solution).

FIRST-LINE AND INITIAL TREATMENT FOR ANAPHYLACTIC AND ANAPHYLACTOID REACTIONS

- Find the cause and discontinue it.
- Administer epinephrine (Adrenaline).
- Provide oxygen.
- Administer antihistamines or beta-2 agonists.
- Administer corticosteroids.

The third step involves the ABCs of patient care: *airway, breathing,* and *circulation*. The nurse must support the patient's airway while administering supplemental oxygen up to 100%. The most appropriate oxygen-delivery device available should be used, either a nasal canula or facemask. Changes in pulmonary capillary leakage with mismatching ventilation and perfusion can take place for several days after an allergic reaction; therefore, the nurse should consider endotracheal intubation with mechanical ventilation until the patient's situation stabilizes. Oral tracheal intubation can be unsuccessful—even in the most experienced hands—in the patient with severe laryngeal edema. If the patient cannot be orally intubated, immediate action should be taken to provide oxygen to the patient. An experienced professional can perform emergency measures (e.g., cricothyrotomy, surgical tracheotomy) to establish an airway. If cardiac arrest or a total loss of blood pressure (BP) or pulse occurs, resuscitative doses of epinephrine are administered at a dose of 0.01 mg/kg along with rapid volume expansion and cardiopulmonary resuscitation (CPR). A patient experiencing airway, respiratory, or cardiovascular compromise should be admitted to an intensive care unit (ICU) for treatment and monitoring. Vital signs including BP, heart rate and rhythm, oxygen saturation, and neurologic status must be frequently assessed. Often, the patient needs a pulmonary artery catheter to monitor cardiac function, an arterial line for continuous monitoring of BP, and frequent blood sampling to evaluate arterial blood gases.

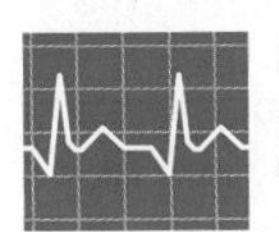

Monitoring the patient's ABCs is crucial.

Secondary treatment for anaphylaxis takes place once the patient's condition improves and measures to prevent further compromise can be initiated. Secondary therapy includes administering antihistamines or beta-2 agonists. If the patient experiences bronchospasms, albuterol inhalation treatments should be initiated to keep the airways open. Diphenhydramine (Benadryl) is used to inhibit the histamine response, and corticosteroids are used to prevent a delayed allergic reaction and to stabilize the capillary membranes. Fluid replacement and positive inotropic agents may need to be ongoing if hypotension persists as a result of increased capillary permeability. The vasoactive agents may help reverse the effects of the myocardial depression and vasodilation from the chemical mediators.

The management of a patient with an anaphylactic reaction should always include an investigation to find the causative agent, to prevent future reactions. Because the allergic reaction may return, the patient should be observed in the ICU even after he or she has recovered from an anaphylactic reaction.

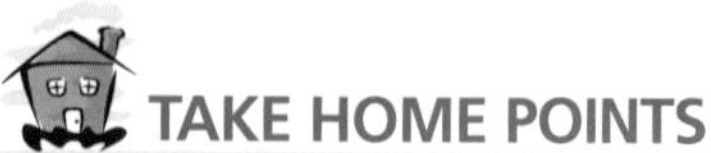

Life-threatening situations may occur up to 8 hours without symptoms.

Nursing Management and Prevention

Because it is not possible to predict which patient may experience an anaphylactic reaction, the critical care nurse should become suspicious of any change in behavior or patient presentation when administering medications, blood products, or diagnostic products. The critical care nurse should take a thorough admission assessment of all patients, including any history of allergies to foods, environmental agents, or medications. It is possible that patients may not have an anaphylactic reaction to the antigen with the second exposure but will to a third. Many times the repeating exposures are less severe than the initial event; however, this outcome is not predictable. Unfortunately, most severe allergic reactions leading to anaphylactic shock occur unexpectedly.

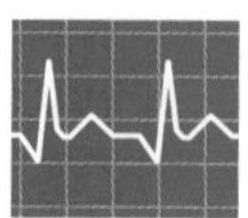

By maintaining continued vigilance, the critical care nurse can provide the patient with needed attention in case signs of allergic reaction return. These signs may include only mild dermatologic changes or more severe respiratory or cardiovascular compromise.

Prevention is the ideal way for the nurse to manage severe anaphylactic and anaphylactoid reactions. Nurses in the critical care areas are responsible for identifying patients with allergies along with the type of reaction the patient experiences with exposure. Factors that improve a patient's survival during an anaphylactic episode include (1) decreasing the length of time between exposure and onset of symptoms, (2) determining route and dose of the agent, (3) identifying length of time between onset of symptoms and initiation of therapy, and (4) determining overall sensitivity of the patient.

TAKE HOME POINTS

A thorough admission history can be helpful, but the astute nurse must also keep in mind that exposure without symptoms does not eliminate the possibility of an anaphylactic reaction.

Depending on the patient's symptoms, the critical care nurse should prioritize interventions. Nursing interventions should first include recognizing the problem and instituting measures to prevent further compromise such as anaphylactic shock. With knowledge that the hallmark of management for anaphylaxis is the administration of epinephrine (Adrenaline), maintaining the patient's ABCs, positioning the patient to optimize breathing, and administering oxygen. The astute critical care nurse also knows that an anaphylactic reaction ultimately produces leaky

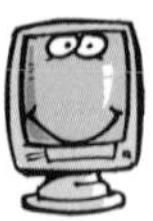

www.anaphylaxis.com

capillaries and that the patient will require fluid volume replacement. Therefore, establish two large-bore peripheral IV lines in the patient. Overall, the critical care nurse should provide the patient comforting measures, including emotional support during the crisis until subsequent treatment is determined. Finally, thorough documentation and a patient alert bracelet for allergies are essential.

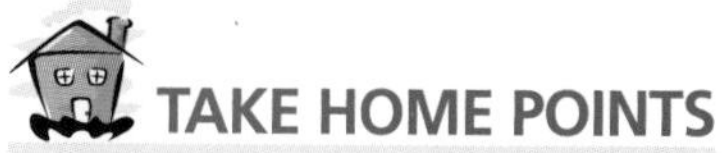

TAKE HOME POINTS

Utilize current implanted ports and central lines if available.

Do You UNDERSTAND?

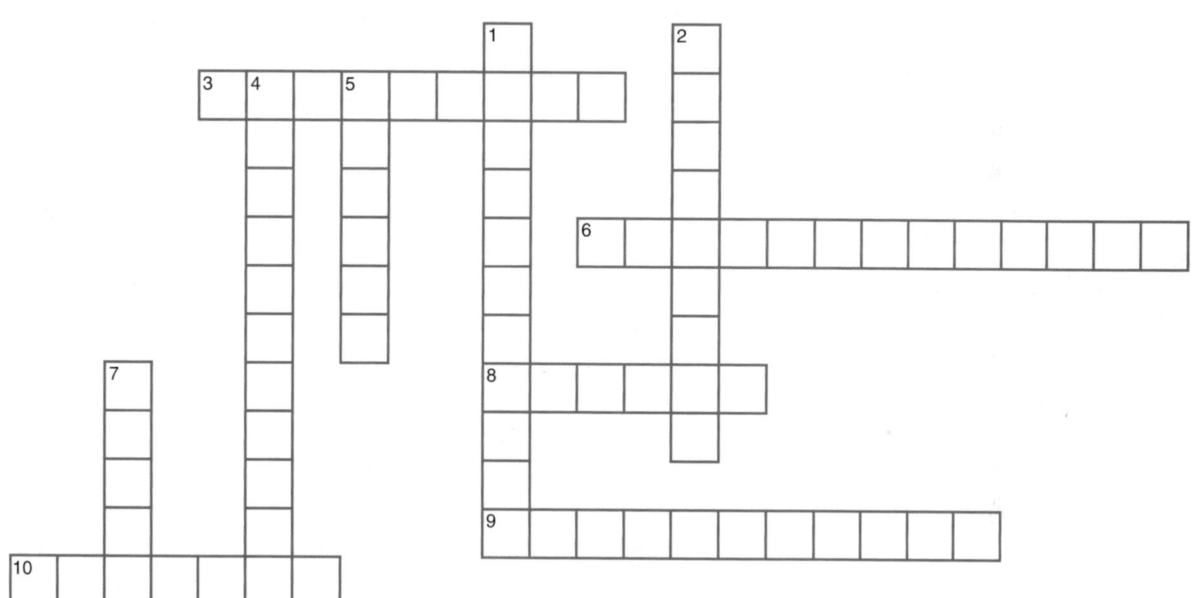

DIRECTIONS: Complete the following crossword puzzle.

Across

3. Anaphylactic reactions are immune-mediated responses by IgE bound to mast cell membranes and _______.

Down

1. The first step in treating a possible anaphylactic reaction is to _______ the causative agent.

Across

6. Anaphylactic reactions need prior exposure; _____ reactions may occur without prior exposure.
8. Anaphylactic reactions are _____ mediated responses.
9. _____ is the hallmark of management for anaphylaxis.
10. Classic signs of a histamine-triggered reaction include _____, warmth, and swelling.

Down

2. _____ triggers physiologic changes in the body by promoting vasodilation and increasing capillary-venous permeability.
4. _____ is a life-threatening hypersensitivity or pseudoallergic reaction to an exogenous agent.
5. When treating anaphylaxis, the nurse should maintain the patient's airway while administering _____.
7. Common causes of an anaphylactic reaction include foods, environmental agents, medications, _____ or blood products, or venoms.

What IS Cardiogenic Shock?

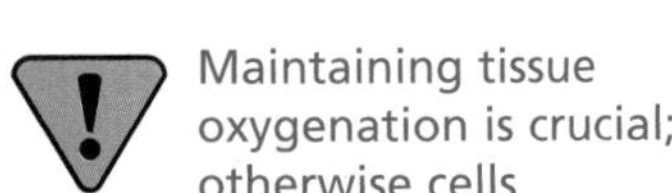

Maintaining tissue oxygenation is crucial; otherwise cells begin to die.

Cardiogenic shock is a special kind of shock during which the heart does not adequately pump enough blood to the body's tissues. When the heart does not contract adequately, blood flow to tissues decreases and oxygen delivery falls. When oxygen delivery falls below critical levels, tissues fail to function and eventually break down **(cellular destruction)** and die. When enough tissues die, the entire body dies.

Pathophysiology

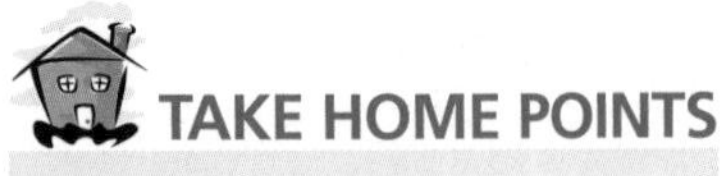

TAKE HOME POINTS

Acute myocardial infarction is the main cause for cardiogenic shock.

Cardiogenic shock is due to decreased functioning of the heart, which leads to decreased forward flow of oxygenated blood to the tissues. The most common cause of cardiogenic shock is a heart attack **(myocardial infarction)** that can damage 40% or more of the ventricle.

Answers: *Across:* **3. basophils; 6. anaphylactoid; 8. immune; 9. epinephrine; 10. redness.**
Down: **1. discontinue; 2. histamine; 4. anaphylaxis; 5. oxygen; 7. blood.**

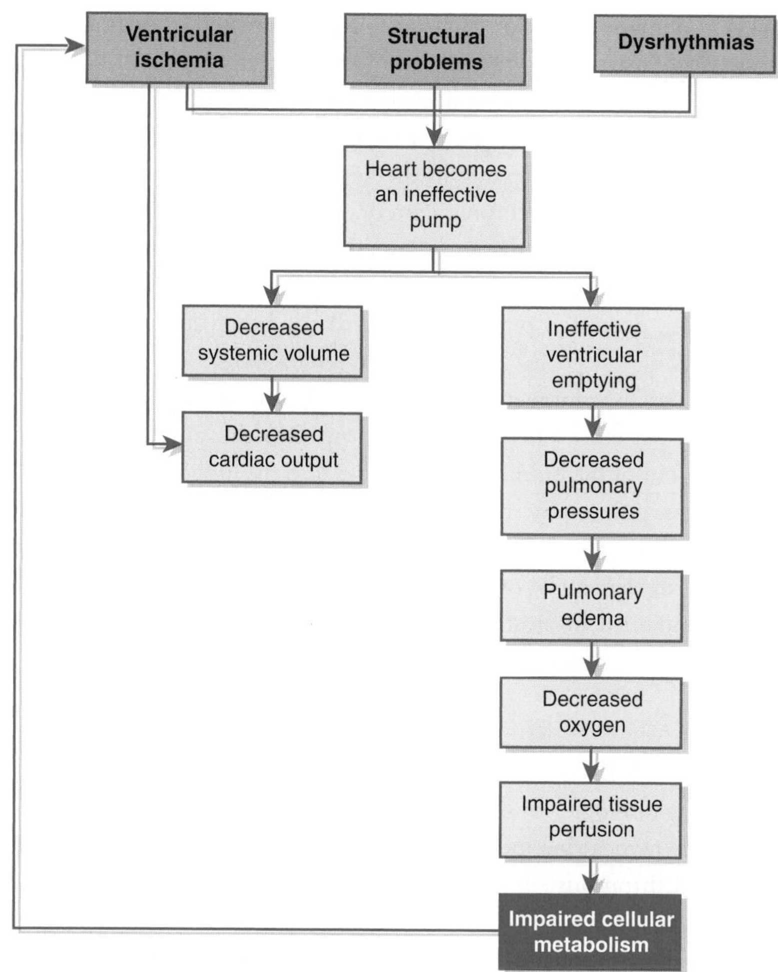

Causes and physiology of cardiogenic shock. *(From Phipps W et al:* Medical-surgical nursing: health and illness perspectives, *ed 7, St Louis, 2003, Mosby.)*

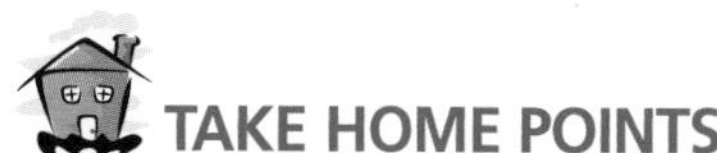

The left ventricle is more likely damaged during a heart attack.

Ventricular function is very important to cardiac function because this chamber of the heart performs most of the work in moving the blood forward in the body. When the ventricle is damaged, it does not empty completely, which causes a decreased stroke volume. Stroke volume is the amount of blood pumped out of the heart during each contraction or heart beat. The CO, or the amount of blood pumped out of the heart every minute, also decreases. As stroke volume and CO decrease, blood builds up in the heart. When blood builds up in the heart, the left ventricular end diastolic volume (LVEDV) increases. An increased LVEDV increases the amount of oxygen the heart needs (oxygen demand) to do its work. This increased demand occurs because the heart has to try to pump out a larger volume of blood.

An increased LVEDV also decreases the amount of blood that flows through the coronary arteries. This happens because the blood in the ventricle increases the pressure in the heart muscle. As pressure increases in the heart muscle, the coronary artery decreases in size, which results in decreased blood flow in the coronary arteries. This decreased blood flow decreases the amount of oxygen that is delivered to the heart muscle. Once again, decreased oxygen delivery to the heart can lead to cardiac hypoxia.

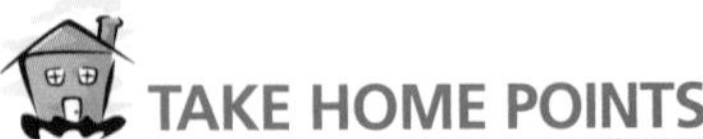

Hypoxia in cardiac tissues leads to a further decrease in cardiac functioning and continues to compromise cardiovascular function.

As the cardiovascular system becomes more damaged, a vicious cycle develops, which may lead to patient deterioration and death if left untreated.

As the stroke volume and CO decrease, blood also backs up into the pulmonary system. When blood backs up into the pulmonary system, fluid leaks out of the pulmonary capillaries into the lung tissue and alveoli, which causes pulmonary edema. Pulmonary edema hinders the movement of oxygen from the alveoli to the blood in the pulmonary capillaries. Decreased movement of oxygen from the alveoli to the blood reduces the oxygen contained in arterial blood (oxygen content). Decreased oxygen content in arterial blood can lead to tissue hypoxia.

At-Risk Populations

Patients at risk for developing cardiogenic shock often have one of the following pathologic conditions:

- Acute myocardial infarction (ST segment elevation MIs- STEMIs)
- Atrial thrombus
- Cardiac contusion
- Cardiac tamponade
- Cardiac tumor
- Cardiomyopathic conditions
- Cardiopulmonary arrest
- Dysrhythmias
- Endocarditis
- Myocarditis
- Open heart surgery
- Pheochromocytoma
- Pneumothorax
- Pulmonary embolus
- Septic shock
- Valvular dysfunction (mitral or aortic regurgitation, mitral stenosis)
- Ventricular aneurysm

What You NEED TO KNOW

Clinical Manifestations

Many clinical manifestations can appear in the patient with cardiogenic shock; these manifestations depend on the severity of the shock, other underlying conditions in the patient, and the cause of the pump failure. Some clinical manifestations are a result of the pump's failure, whereas others are the result of the body's response to the shock.

Cardiovascular signs of cardiogenic shock include a low systolic BP of less than 90 mm Hg. Tachycardia develops in response to the low BP and decreased CO (less than 2.2 L/min). As the heart continues to fail, the pulse becomes "weak and thready." Catecholamines are released in response to the low BP. The catecholamines cause the BP to rise as a result of an increase in the heart rate and peripheral vascular constriction. Severe vasoconstriction causes the pulses to feel weak and thready. Capillary refill is sluggish, and peripheral tissues begin to show signs of hypoxia as a result of decreased blood flow and oxygen delivery. The heart cannot continue to respond to the catecholamines because of a lack of oxygen, which is needed for heart contraction. Oxygen is also needed to maintain vessel constriction. If oxygen delivery is not restored, the heart becomes more hypoxic, experiences more damage, and becomes even less able to pump blood. The CO continually falls and leads to a continual increase of tissue hypoxia.

As the heart becomes more hypoxic, ischemic changes may be observed on an ECG. These changes are often seen as ST segment changes

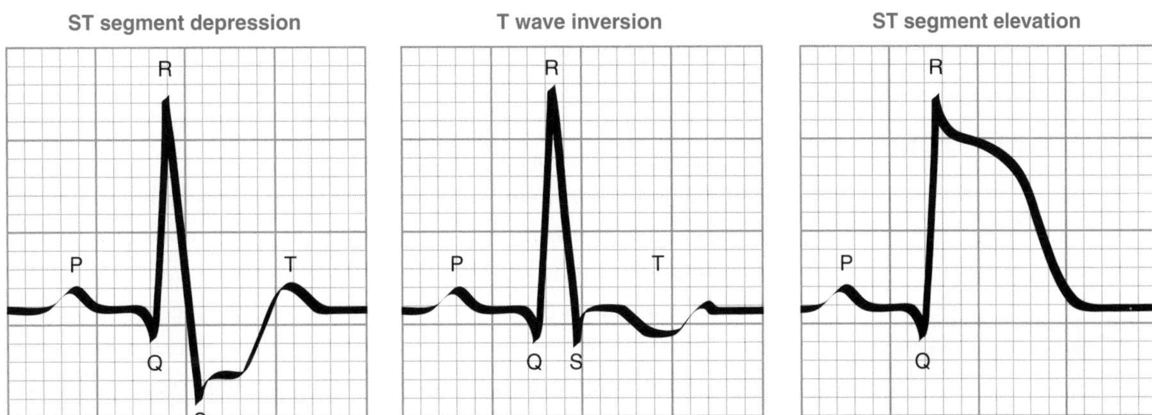

(From Phipps W et al: Medical-surgical nursing: health and illness perspectives, *ed 7, St Louis, 2003, Mosby.)*

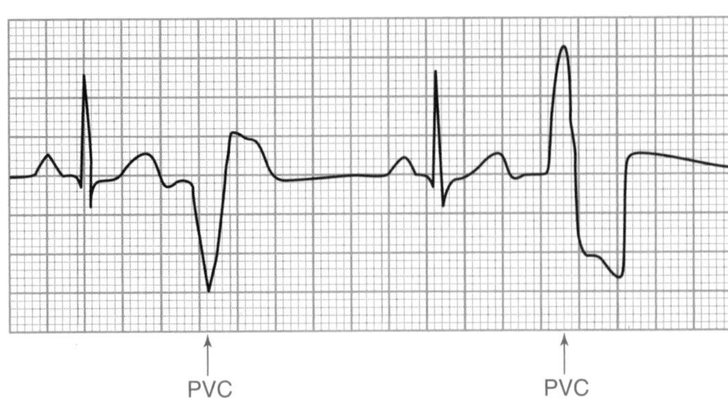

Premature ventricular contractions on ECG. *(From Chernecky C et al:* Real-world nursing series: ECGs & the heart, *Philadelphia, 2002, WB Saunders.)*

or premature ventricular contractions (PVCs). The patient may also complain of chest pain or tightness.

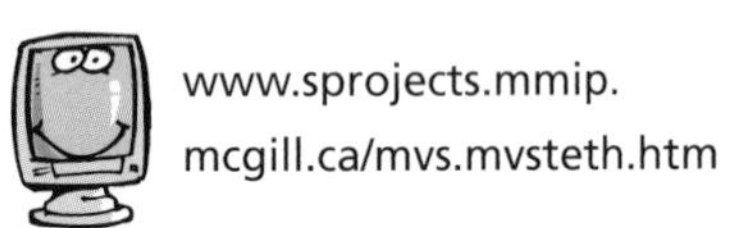
www.sprojects.mmip.mcgill.ca/mvs.mvsteth.htm

As CO decreases, blood backs up into the heart and lungs. Fluid leaks out from the pulmonary capillaries into the lungs. Fluid in the lungs causes crackles and diffuse pulmonary edema when the patient breathes. Oxygen does not cross as easily from the alveoli into the blood because of the fluid in the alveoli and capillary membrane. As a result, arterial blood is less oxygenated and oxygen saturation falls. Oxygen saturation may be measured by direct arterial blood sampling or estimated through pulse oximetry measurements. In instances of severe hypoxia, the patient may have dark-colored nail beds and mucous membranes.

The central nervous system (CNS) depends on blood flow and oxygen for proper functioning. Decreased blood flow and hypoxia can lead to anxiety, confusion, lethargy, and coma; however, the first sign is often a change in mental status.

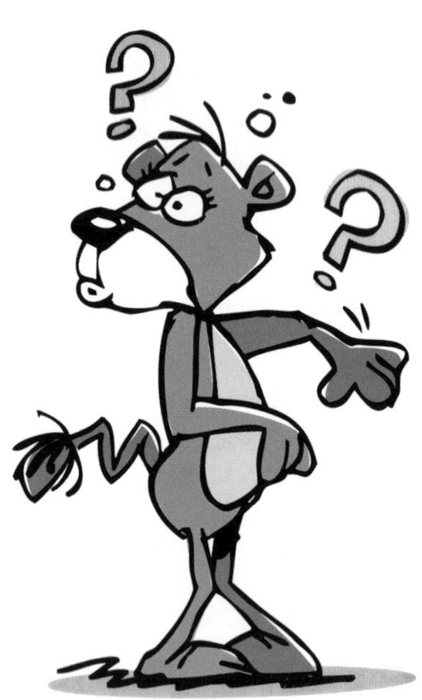
Confusion from decreased blood flow and hypoxia.

Cardiogenic shock also affects the GI system. Patients are often nauseated and experience decreased bowel sounds because of a lowered BP. As the shock becomes severe, blood flow can fall so low as to cause bowel ischemia and infarction (death).

The renal system is also very sensitive to decreases in blood flow and oxygen supply. The kidneys require a constant supply of oxygen from the blood to do their job. The kidneys have the ability to regulate a constant blood flow despite a range of BP levels. This ability is termed *autoregulation.* Autoregulation allows the kidneys to have a constant blood flow, although the mean arterial BP may range from 50 to 150 mm Hg. If the mean arterial BP falls below 50 mm Hg, blood flow to the kidneys also falls and the kidneys become hypoxic. During times of hypoxia, the kidneys are less able to regulate the body's fluids and electrolytes, as well as excrete waste products and metabolize medications. Decreased blood flow in the kidneys causes urine output to fall, and peripheral edema ensues. The kidneys can be damaged by the decrease in blood flow and lack of oxygen. Vasoconstriction in the kidneys from catecholamines often worsens kidney damage. Severe or prolonged decreases in blood flow and oxygenation can lead to renal insufficiency and failure.

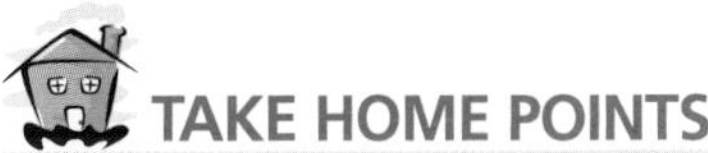

TAKE HOME POINTS

The prognosis is poor for patients who develop cardiogenic shock. The risk of dying is between 70% and 80%.

What You DO

To prevent cardiogenic shock, all treatments must be aimed at restoring blood flow and oxygenation and administered early and quickly to limit organ damage. Emergent cardiac revascularization through thrombolytic therapy, angioplasty, or bypass surgery is often needed to decrease mortality in patients experiencing myocardial ischemia. To prepare the patient for thrombolytic therapy, the nurse should review the patient history to determine patient age, onset of symptoms, medications, allergies, presence of hypertension, and recent history of surgery, trauma, bleeding, or stroke. Preparing for angioplasty or bypass surgery requires the standard preoperative assessment and work-up unless emergency circumstances preclude an in-depth surgical preoperative work-up.

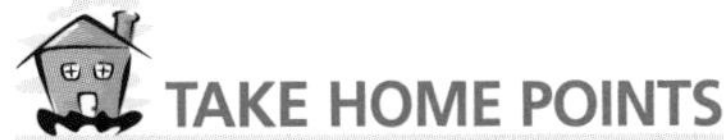

TAKE HOME POINTS

Treatment goal is to restore blood flow and oxygenation to the tissues to limit tissue and organ damage.

Patients at risk for or experiencing cardiogenic shock may require total circulatory support from mechanical devices such as an intraaortic balloon pump (IABP), a left ventricular assist device (LVAD), extracorporeal life support (ECLS), or pharmacologic interventions. Additionally, oxygen therapy and respiratory support may assist in increasing oxygen supply to a failing heart.

Mechanical Circulatory Support Devices

The IABP works by inflating during diastole and deflating during systole. Systolic deflation helps move blood out of the heart by reducing the afterload or the resistance against which the heart has to pump. When the balloon deflates, a space is created that has less resistance, enabling the heart to send blood. By decreasing afterload, the workload of the heart is decreased and the amount of oxygen needed to do the work is decreased (see Color Plate 2 for IABP placement and balloon effects).

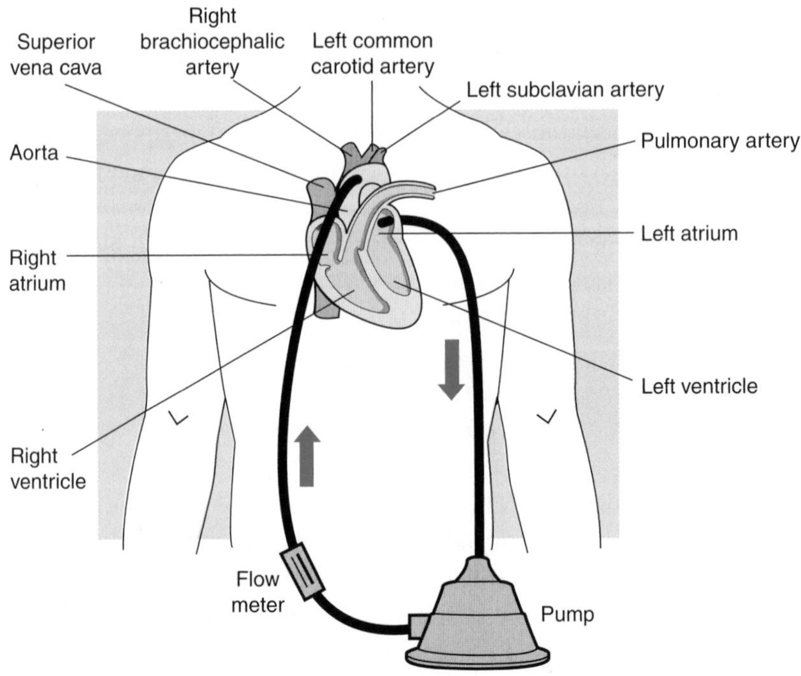

Circulatory support for cardiogenic shock. *(From Chernecky C et al:* Real-world nursing series: ECGs & the heart, *Philadelphia, 2002, WB Saunders.)*

When the balloon inflates during diastole, blood is "pushed" into the coronary arteries on either side of the aorta. This action increases the blood flow through the coronary arteries to the heart muscle. By increasing blood flow to the heart muscle, oxygen delivery is also increased. Increasing oxygen delivery to the heart muscle increases the oxygen supply to the heart, and helps reduce cardiac hypoxia. Thus, by decreasing afterload and increasing coronary artery perfusion, the IABP decreases cardiac workload, decreases myocardial oxygen demand (MVO_2), and increases myocardial oxygen supply, which allows the heart to function more efficiently.

An LVAD increases CO by helping the left ventricle pump blood to the periphery. By helping the heart work, the LVAD allows the heart to rest and not work so hard while the body tries to repair the damage. An LVAD is often used as a last resort in patients with severe cardiogenic shock.

ECLS relieves both the heart and lungs of part of their workload by circulating blood outside of the body through an external membrane for oxygenation to occur and then return the blood to the body to be circulated. ECLS is often used as a bridge to heart transplantation.

LVADs, ECLS, and IABP catheters are inserted surgically. The use of these devices requires that the patient be anticoagulated to prevent blood clot formation that could cause an embolus around the device. Nursing care involves monitoring the coagulation status of the patients, so clotting is adequately reduced. The patient, surgical site, and equipment connections should also be monitored for bleeding and exsanguination. The IABP, LVAD, and ECLS therapies are not permanent solutions but are used to help the heart recover from the shock phase.

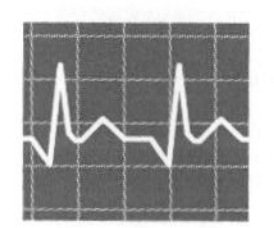

The patient's coagulation status must be closely monitored to prevent the ECLS, LVAD, or IABP devices from becoming clotted.

Pharmacologic Intervention

The cause of cardiogenic shock may be left heart failure (most common), right heart failure, or cardiac tamponade. A number of available pharmacologic agents for treatment are available, and the best combination is determined by the cause of the pump's failure and the patient's response. Some of the more common agents include the following:

- Dopamine (Intropin): Increases renal perfusion at lower doses and causes an increase in CO, heart rate, and systemic arterial pressure at higher doses, which increases the pumping action of the heart (positive inotropic).
- Dobutamine (Dobutrex): Increases the pumping action of the heart (positive inotropic) and CO and decreases ventricular filling pressure.
- Norepinephrine (Levophed): A profound peripheral vasoconstrictor that is used in patients with extremely low systolic pressure (<70 mm Hg) to prevent total circulatory collapse.
- Milrinone (Primacor): Promotes arterial vasodilation and reduces preload and afterload while increasing the pumping action of the heart (positive inotropic).
- Sodium nitroprusside (Nipride): Decreases arterial resistance and is often used to decrease SVR, afterload, and systolic BP.
- Nitroglycerin (Nitrol, Tridil): Decreases venous resistance and increases coronary artery dilation to assist with decreasing anginal pain.
- Diuretics: Decrease body water, pulmonary edema, and systemic fluid overload.

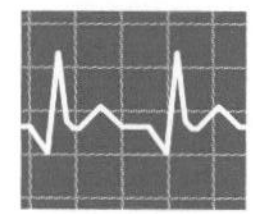

The patient needs to be monitored carefully while medications are being adjusted and titrated. Attention must be paid to the effects on the patient's heart rate, BP, and hemodynamic readings to optimize cardiac function.

Oxygen Therapy

The goal of oxygen therapy is to improve arterial blood oxygenation to increase oxygen supply to the tissues. A measurement of oxygen tension in the arterial blood (PaO_2) of greater than 80 mm Hg on blood gas analysis and an oxygen saturation of greater than 90% is considered normal. Patients experiencing myocardial ischemia or who are at risk for cardiogenic shock should receive supplemental oxygen. The patient's condition may require use of mechanical ventilation with the addition of positive end-expiratory pressure to help meet the goals of adequate oxygenation.

Medication, Doses, and Sites of Action

Medication	Action	Receptor	Dose Range
Dopamine (Intropin)	Increases blood pressure, cardiac output, urine output	**Small doses:** <2 µg/kg/min—stimulates dopaminergic sites **Medium doses:** 3 to 10 µg/kg/min—stimulates dopamine and β-adrenergic sites **Large doses:** >10 µg/kg/min—stimulates α-adrenergic sites	0.5 to 20 µg/kg/min, titrated based on hemodynamic response
Dobutamine (Dobutrex)	Positive inotrope with minimal heart rate increase	β-1 agonist	Starting with 2.0 µg/kg/min, titrated to 40 µg/kg/min
Milrinone (Primacor)	Positive inotrope	Vascular smooth muscle dilator	Loading dose: 50 µg/kg over 10 min Infusion: 0.375 to 0.750 µg/kg/min
Nitroglycerin (Nitrol, Tridil)	Decreases blood pressure, decreases angina	Dilates coronary arteries, dilates peripheral veins	IV: Start 5 µg/min, titrated upward, based on hemodynamic response
Norepinephrine (Levophed)	↑ BP through vasoconstriction and there is also some positive inotropic effects	β-1, β-2, and α-adrenergic agonist	Starting with 2.0 µg/min, titrated to 12 µg/min, based on hemodynamic response
Sodium nitroprusside (Nipride)	Lowers blood pressure, decreases cardiac preload and afterload	Peripheral arteriole and venous smooth muscle dilator	0.3 to 10.0 µg/kg/min

Do You UNDERSTAND?

DIRECTIONS: Complete the following crossword puzzle.

Across

2. Embolus
4. Type of shock
8. He has had three _____ bats
9. What the heart does
10. James Bond
11. Contracting ability
13. Has four chambers
15. Not enough oxygen in the tissues causes this

Down

1. Candy _____
3. Diplomacy
5. Chest pain
6. Increases pumping action of the heart
7. Decreases afterload (*abbreviation*)
10. Cardiogenic _____
12. Dynamite (*abbreviation*)
14. Hazard

Answers: *Across:* **2. clot; 4. cardiogenic; 8. at; 9. pump; 10. spy; 11. inotropic; 13. heart; 15. ischemia.**
Down: **1. bar; 3. tact; 5. angina; 6. dopamine; 7. IABP; 10. shock; 12. TNT; 14. risk.**

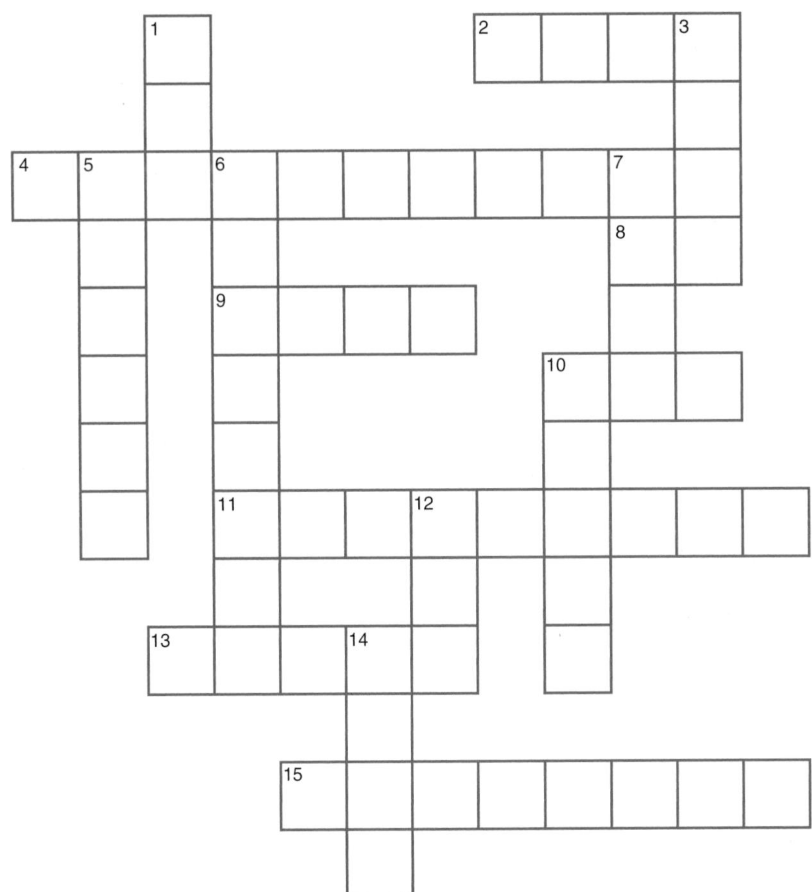

What IS Hypovolemic Shock?

Hypovolemic shock, the most common form of shock, is caused from an inadequate circulating blood volume in the intravascular bed. As with all forms of shock, circulating oxygenated blood flow to the body organs decreases. This lack of oxygenated blood leads to inadequate tissue perfusion, causing cellular hypoxia, organ failure, and death.

TAKE HOME POINTS

- The hallmark of all forms of shock is impaired tissue perfusion.
- The most common cause of hypovolemic shock is hemorrhage.

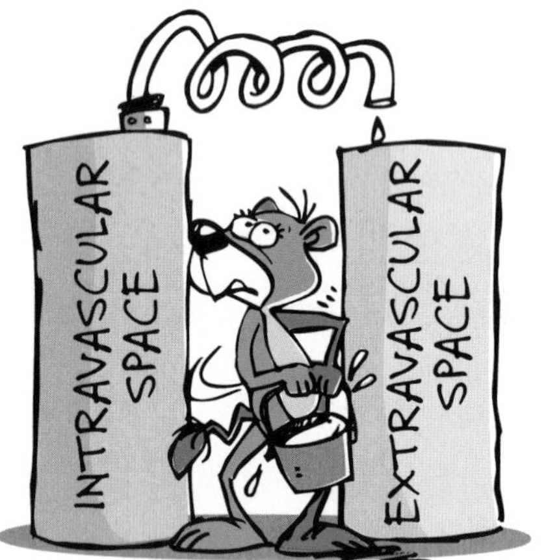

Third spacing causes edema and absolute hypovolemia.

What You NEED TO KNOW

The causes of hypovolemic shock can be divided into two categories: *absolute hypovolemia* and *relative hypovolemia.* Absolute hypovolemia occurs as a result of fluid loss from the intravascular space (external fluid loss, internal fluid shifting, called *third spacing*). Relative hypovolemia occurs as a result of vasodilation and an increase in vascular capacitance in comparison to the amount of circulating volume.

Causes of Hypovolemic Shock

Absolute Losses	Relative Losses
GI status (diarrhea, vomiting, GI suction, ostomies, fistulas)	Increase capillary membrane permeability (sepsis, anaphylaxis, thermal injuries, spinal shock)
Hemorrhage (trauma, surgery, GI bleeding, DIC, thrombocytopenia, hemophilia, ruptured spleen, arterial dissection/rupture, hemorrhagic pancreatitis, hemothorax, long bone fractures, pelvic fractures)	Vasodilation (sepsis, anaphylaxis, loss of sympathetic stimulation)
Plasma losses (thermal injuries, exudative lesions, decreased oral fluid intake)	Sequestration of fluid as a result of decrease colloidal osmotic pressure (cirrhosis, intestinal obstruction, ileus, peritonitis, severe sodium depletion, hypopituitarism)
Renal losses (massive diuresis; hyperglycemic osmotic diuresis, diabetes insipidus, Addison's disease)	

GI, Gastrointestinal; *DIC,* disseminated intravascular coagulation.

Pathophysiology of Hypovolemic Shock

As the circulating blood volume decreases, the venous return to the right side of the heart decreases. This leads to a decrease in cardiac filling pressure and volume, which is known as the *preload* or the *end-diastolic volume.* A decrease in preload results in a decrease in stroke volume and CO. The decrease in CO leads to hypotension and a subsequent decrease in oxygenated blood flow to the organs and inadequate tissue perfusion. The baroreceptors in the aortic notch and carotid sinuses sense a decrease in circulating blood volume, which stimulates the sympathetic branch of the autonomic nervous system. The fibers of the sympathetic nervous system (SNS), as well as the medullary portion of the adrenal glands, release two neurotransmitter substances—epinephrine and norepinephrine.

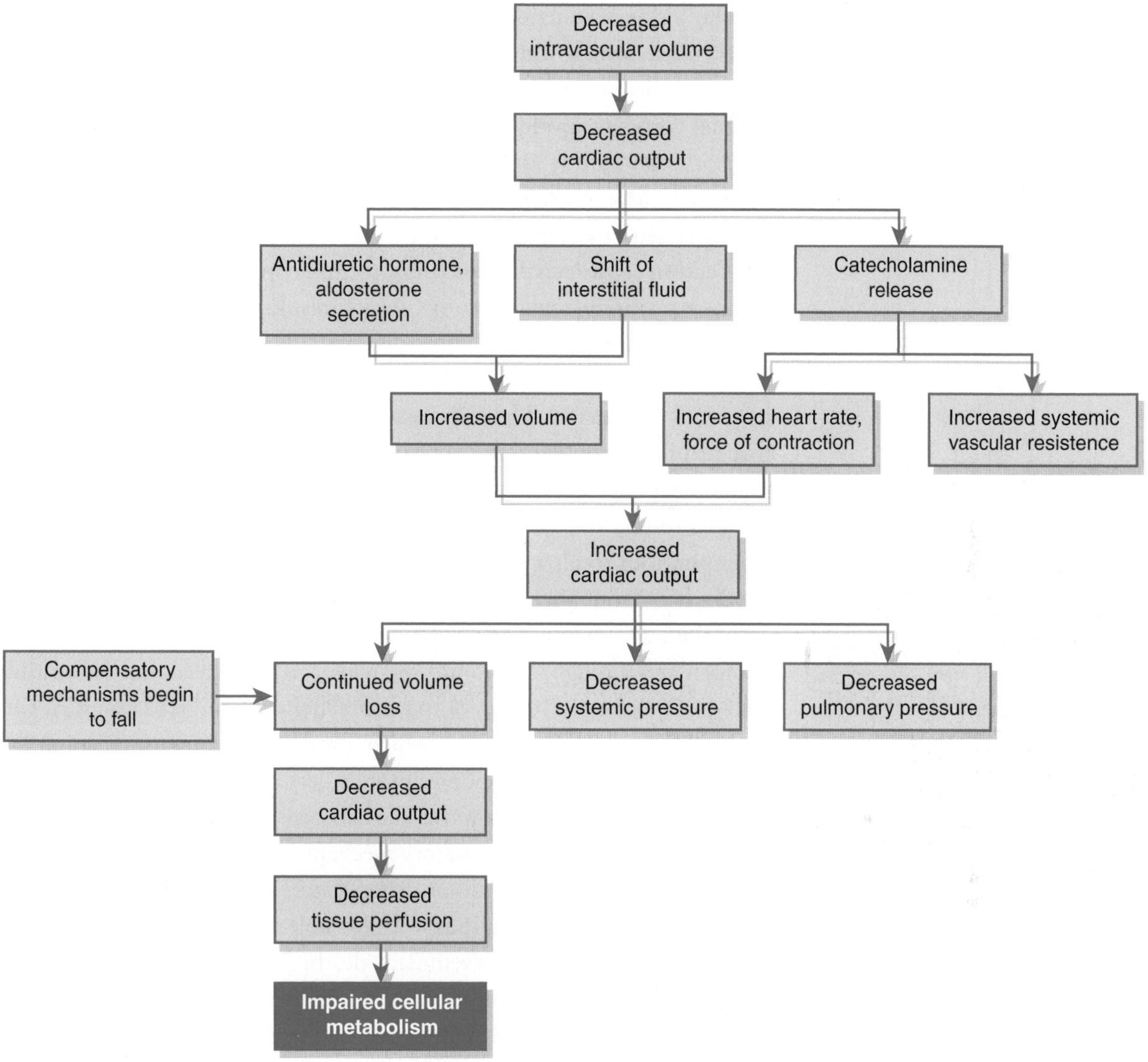

Decreased intravascular volume
Decreased cardiac output
Antidiuretic hormone, aldosterone secretion
Shift of interstitial fluid
Catecholamine release
Increased volume
Increased heart rate, force of contraction
Increased systemic vascular resistence
Increased cardiac output
Compensatory mechanisms begin to fall
Continued volume loss
Decreased systemic pressure
Decreased pulmonary pressure
Decreased cardiac output
Decreased tissue perfusion
Impaired cellular metabolism

Pathophysiology of hypovolemic shock. *(From Phipps et al:* Medical-surgical nursing: health and illness perspectives, *ed 7, St Louis, 2003, Mosby.)*

Epinephrine and norepinephrine increase heart rate and strengthen the contractile force of the heart in an attempt to increase CO. These neurotransmitter substances also cause systemic vasoconstriction to maintain arterial BP. The vasoconstriction shunts much needed blood flow away from nonvital organs such as the skin, GI tract, kidneys, and musculoskeletal system. This vasoconstriction is part of the body compensatory mechanism, which maintains oxygenated blood flow and tissue perfusion to the vital organs, specifically to the brain and heart.

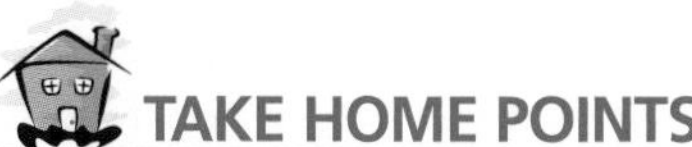

TAKE HOME POINTS

The body attempts to compensate for the decrease in blood volume and decline in tissue oxygenation through the release of epinephrine and norepinephrine, which results in vasoconstriction and an increased heart rate.

The kidneys contribute to vasoconstriction by releasing a substance called *renin,* which stimulates the lungs to produce a powerful vasoconstrictor substance called *angiotensin II.* Angiotensin II stimulates the adrenal cortex to produce *aldosterone,* which acts on the renal tubules by reabsorbing sodium and, consequently, water. The posterior pituitary releases a vasoconstrictor substance called *antidiuretic hormone* (ADH) (**vasopressin**) in response to the decreased circulating blood volume. This action causes renal water reabsorption, conservation of fluid, and an increase in intravascular volume, which results in a decrease in urinary output.

As blood flow decreases and tissue perfusion becomes inadequate, cellular hypoxia occurs. The cells resort to anaerobic metabolism in an effort to produce adenosine triphosphate (ATP) for energy. This type of metabolism produces an accumulation of lactic acid, which causes acidosis. The respiratory system compensates by increasing the rate and depth of respirations to blow off carbon dioxide and raise the blood pH, which produces a compensatory respiratory alkalosis.

In the early, reversible stage of hypovolemic shock, the body attempts to compensate through SNS outflow, which is evidenced by tachycardia, tachypnea, decreased urinary output, apprehension, and restlessness, as well as cutaneous vasoconstriction, which produces pallor and diaphoresis. These pathophysiologic responses protect perfusion to the brain and heart and restore homeostasis. However, the compensatory mechanisms are short lived. As the patient's compensatory mechanisms fail, shock progresses and, as the patient's clinical condition deteriorates, metabolic acidosis and hypoxia are produced, which leads to irreversible shock and cell death, organ ischemia and failure, and eventually death. The hypoxia and decreased perfusion to organs such as the brain cause the patient to be confused, restless, uncooperative, possibly combative, and perhaps comatose.

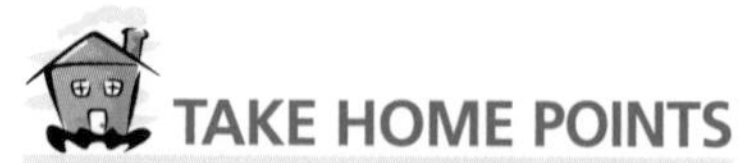

TAKE HOME POINTS

The refractory or irreversible stage of shock means that all attempts to restore homeostasis have failed and cells begin to die.

Clinical Manifestations of Hypovolemic Shock

The clinical manifestations of hypovolemic shock depend on the severity and rate of volume loss, the patient's ability to compensate, the patient's age, and the presence of preexisting illnesses. The clinical manifestations of shock continue to progress in stages, regardless of the type of shock. The signs and symptoms of each stage are a reflection of the volume of loss and the body's response.

The reversible, compensatory stage occurs with a fluid loss of 15% to 30% or up to 1500 mL. The goal of this stage is to restore oxygenation and perfusion to the cells. The patient may exhibit normal BP readings and narrowed pulse pressure (the difference between the systolic and diastolic BP, which is normally 40 mm Hg). In addition, the patient may also develop tachycardia, tachypnea (creating a respiratory alkalosis), hypoxia, decreased urinary output, thirst, pale and cool skin, delayed capillary refill (less than 2 seconds), and changes in the LOC (e.g., confusion, restless, anxiousness).

During the reversible or compensatory stage, it is easy to overlook the occurring manifestations as hypovolemic shock.

If the underlying problem is not corrected, the patient then enters the progressive stage of shock. This stage begins with a fluid loss of 30% to 40% or up to 2000 mL. In this stage, the compensatory mechanisms begin to fail, tissue perfusion becomes ineffective for the body organs to function, heart rate increases, cardiac dysrhythmias develop, and the CO, cardiac index, right atrial pressure, and pulmonary artery wedge pressures decrease. The SVR increases as a result of the continued vasoconstriction of the arterial system. The prolonged vasoconstriction decreases capillary blood flow to the tissues, which contributes to cellular hypoxia, anaerobic metabolism, and acidosis. Prolonged capillary vasoconstriction causes the vessels to become clogged, which impedes blood flow. Eventually, the capillary hydrostatic pressure increases, leading to third spacing of fluid and edema. The fluid shift is further aggravated as capillary permeability is increased and the colloidal osmotic pressure is decreased from loss of proteins. As fluid shifts out of the intravascular space into the extravascular space, hypovolemia increases. The patient becomes hypotensive with a narrowed pulse pressure.

Hypotension is a late sign. Patients can lose 30% or more of their intravascular volume before signs and symptoms appear.

As the respiratory system fails, the patient can develop pulmonary edema and the arterial blood gases can deteriorate to reflect a respiratory and metabolic acidosis with continued hypoxemia. The oliguria progressively worsens and becomes unresponsive to treatment. As the kidneys lose function, the blood urea nitrogen (BUN) and creatinine levels increase. The patient's LOC continues to deteriorate as cerebral perfusion decreases. The patient becomes increasingly lethargic, confused, and eventually comatose. During this stage, organs become dysfunctional and all body systems are affected. As one organ system fails, the others eventually become dysfunctional, leading to multiorgan dysfunction syndrome (MODS). (Refer to the discussion on MODS later in Chapter 12.)

Once the body systems are no longer responsive to treatment and multiple organ failure ensues, the patient is in the refractory or irreversible stage of shock. This final stage of shock occurs with a fluid volume loss of greater than 40% or more than 2000 mL. In this stage, the compensatory mechanisms have been completely exhausted and organ failure has occurred. Death is imminent in this stage. Once brain damage

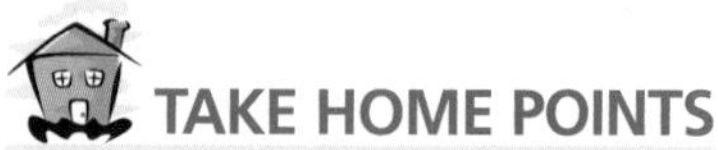

The outcome of the irreversible stage of shock is patient death.

occurs, sympathetic tone is lost. The severe tachycardia becomes bradycardia with continued hypotension until cardiopulmonary arrest. The patient becomes unresponsive. The acidosis, fluid shifts, edema, oliguria, and anuria also become severe. A variety of clinical manifestations may occur in response to the failure of other body systems. All systems do not have to fail for death to ensue. The patient has a 90% to 100% mortality rate when only three body systems fail.

What You DO

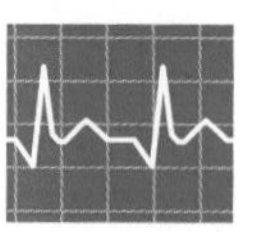

The patient's BP, heart rate, urine output, and laboratory and hemodynamic readings must be monitored to evaluate the effectiveness of treatments and to adjust treatments as necessary.

Treatment of the patient in hypovolemic shock is focused on identifying and treating the underlying cause. The care of these patients involves maintaining oxygenation and perfusion by keeping the mean arterial pressure (MAP) equal to or greater than 60 mm Hg. These patients are treated according to their BP, urine output, hemodynamic parameters, laboratory results, and clinical status. The patient in hypovolemic shock may require massive fluid resuscitation and diligent monitoring of the patient's intake and output to stay ahead of the patient's fluid needs. The goal of fluid resuscitation is to restore intravascular volume, maintain oxygen-carrying capacity, and restore venous return and CO necessary for adequate tissue perfusion.

Equation for calculating MAP:

$$\text{MAP} = \frac{\text{Systolic BP} + 2(\text{Diastolic BP})}{3}$$

FIRST-LINE AND INITIAL TREATMENT FOR HYPOVOLEMIC SHOCK

Goal: Restore homeostasis and intravascular volume.
Intervention: Infuse IV fluids and/or blood products.

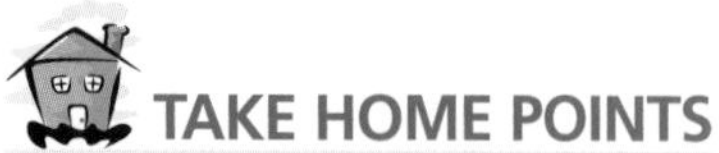

Utilize existing central lines such as ports or PICCs for fluid administration.

The patient requires at least two large-bore (14- or 16-gauge) IV catheters, preferably in the antecubital veins for rapid administration of fluid. These fluids may need pressure-bagged or rapid-infusion devices. The patient may also need a central line for administering fluids and vasoactive drugs, as well as for monitoring the central venous pressure (CVP).

Because renal blood flow is sensitive to the CO, an increase or decrease in CO affects the urinary output. It is imperative to monitor the urinary output of the patient with hypovolemic shock: It is a valuable indicator of the patient's fluid status. Adequate fluid replacement should yield a urinary output of at least 0.5 mL/kg/hr.

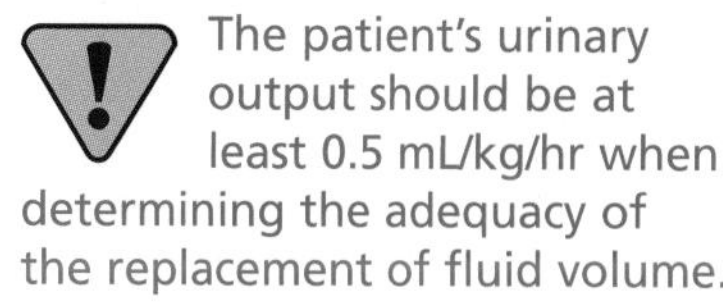

The patient's urinary output should be at least 0.5 mL/kg/hr when determining the adequacy of the replacement of fluid volume.

Crystalloids, colloids, and blood and blood products are used to treat hypovolemic shock. Crystalloids, the first-line choice of treatment, are inexpensive and move rapidly and freely within the intravascular and extravascular spaces. The recommended initial treatment is 1 to 2 L bolus rapidly infused for adults. When given in sufficient amounts according to the patient's underlying condition and needs, crystalloids can be just as effective as colloids in restoring intravascular volume. Crystalloids may be given in large volumes, but evaluation is needed because greater than 4 to 5 L can cause internal and external edema. The crystalloid of choice is Ringer's lactate. Normal saline can be used as a second choice, but it can potentially cause hyperchloremic acidosis, which is made worse in the presence of renal impairment.

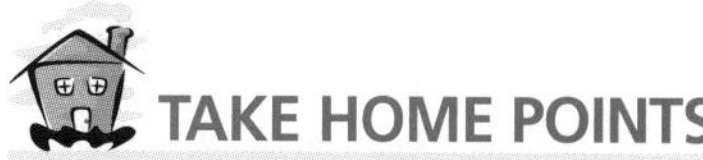

TAKE HOME POINTS

The intravascular half-life of crystalloids is 20 to 30 minutes.

Colloids, a more expensive choice than crystalloids, contain proteins that increase the intravascular osmotic pressure and pull fluid out of the extravascular space into the intravascular space to expand the plasma volume. Colloids stay in the intravascular space longer than crystalloids; they have a half-life between 3 to 6 hours. General indications for colloid administration include patients with severe intravascular fluid deficits and severe hypoalbuminemia or conditions associated with large protein losses. Colloids are sometimes used with crystalloids when volume replacement has exceeded 3 to 4 L of crystalloids.

Unlike crystalloids, colloids are given in small volumes. Albumin and Plasmanate are colloid solutions that are administered when volume loss is caused by a loss of plasma proteins and volume rather than by a loss of blood volume. Other synthetic colloids that act as volume expanders include dextran and hetastarch. Dextran is contraindicated in patients with hemorrhagic shock because it decreases platelet adhesiveness and increases bleeding. Additional complications with dextran include allergic reactions and renal damage. Hetastarch has no effect on renal function and is not as likely to cause an allergic reaction; however, it does alter bleeding times. No more than 1 L of either dextran or hetastarch should be administered in a 24-hour period because both produce coagulopathic results.

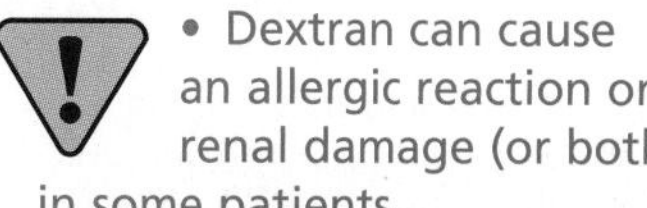

- Dextran can cause an allergic reaction or renal damage (or both) in some patients.
- Dextran and hetastarch infusions alter bleeding times and can produce coagulopathic results.

If bleeding causes hypovolemic shock, the patient can be initially treated with crystalloids. A three-to-one rule is used when replacing blood loss with crystalloids. For every 1 mL of blood loss, 3 mL of crystalloid should be given. Once the blood loss has reached 1500 mL, blood transfusion with packed red blood cells should be administered along with fresh-frozen plasma (FFP) and platelets as needed to restore clotting factors. Clinicians must understand that a loss in total blood volume—not the loss of red blood cells—causes the patient to develop hypovolemic shock (impaired tissue oxygenation and perfusion). A transfusion with packed red blood cells should be initiated when the danger of anemia places the patient at risk for organ ischemia. Transfusions are recommended when the hemoglobin is 7 to 8 g/dl (hematocrit of 21% to 24%); even then the clinician must take into account the rate of blood loss, the presence of cardiovascular or pulmonary disease, and the patient's age. A higher limit of 10 g/dl may be needed if the patient is older or has a co-morbid illness such as cardiac disease. If blood loss is expected to continue at a rapid rate, then higher limits for a transfusion may be indicated or surgical intervention may be needed. Normal saline is the additive fluid of choice for administering blood.

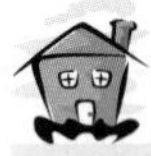

TAKE HOME POINTS

In the treatment of hypovolemia to ensure the effectiveness of vasopressors (i.e., to cause vasoconstriction and to increase BP), the patient must have adequate intravascular volume and not be severely vasoconstricted as a compensatory mechanism.

If volume replacement does not adequately support CO and MAP to ensure and maintain tissue perfusion, then pharmacologic therapy may be used. Vasopressors such as dopamine (Intropin) and norepinephrine (Levophed) can be used to support the BP and increase cardiac contractility. It is imperative that intravascular volume be replaced with fluids to ensure the effectiveness of the vasopressors. The vasoconstriction from the pharmacologic effect can worsen cellular hypoxia and anaerobic metabolism by decreasing capillary blood flow to the tissues if the vascular bed has not been volume loaded and CO sustained with fluids.

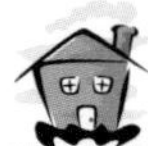

TAKE HOME POINTS

It must be noted that volume loading is the major intervention in the treatment of hypovolemic shock and that drug therapy should be used as a last choice.

Managing the patient's respiratory status is also part of the treatment for hypovolemic shock. All patients should receive 100% oxygen via a non-rebreather mask. Ideally, the patient's oxygen saturation should be 95%, which yields 85% to 100% PaO_2. Arterial blood gases should be frequently monitored for oxygen saturation and acidosis. The patient's respiratory status is affected by the volume loss, and the patient may require mechanical ventilation. If the patient is hemodynamically unstable with a large volume deficit, then early initiation of mechanical ventilation is necessary to influence the best outcome. Mechanical ventilation is the most effective way to improve the patient's oxygenation and acid-base status.

These patients require frequent monitoring of vital signs. Once the patient becomes hypotensive, BP levels should be monitored continuously with an arterial line. Temperature is another important vital sign to monitor. Patients receiving large volumes of fluid or cold blood from the blood bank are at risk for hypothermia. Body temperature should be monitored at least every hour. *Hypothermia* is defined as a body temperature less than 36° C (96° F). When the patient is hypothermic, physiologic changes occur in all body systems. Hypothermia is a cardiac depressant and can predispose the patient to cardiac dysrhythmias. Hypothermia can alter the clotting mechanisms and place the patient at risk for coagulopathic consequences. All fluids should be warmed. The use of external warming devices such as overhead heat lamps, warming blankets, or thermal caps should be used. The clinician must also keep in mind that shivering increases metabolic demands for oxygen up to 400%. This additional demand for oxygen is crucial in the patient who is already suffering from tissue hypoxia.

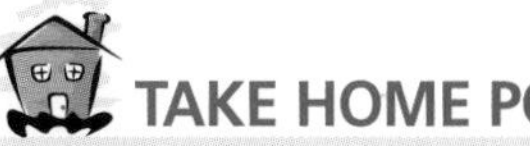

The best treatment for hypothermia is prevention.

Positioning is another important aspect of patient care. If the patient with mild hypovolemia is stable, the best position is supine with the head of the bed elevated 30 to 60 degrees to maintain pulmonary ventilation. Turning the patient every 2 hours has also been shown to improve oxygenation and pulmonary function. However, when the patient is unstable and hypotensive, the best position is supine and flat.

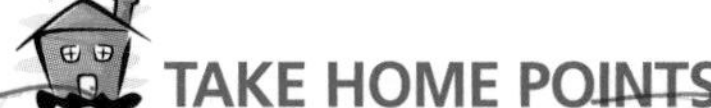

The best position for the unstable patient in hypovolemic shock is supine or flat.

The patient in hypovolemic shock requires vigilance in care with frequent monitoring of vital signs, oxygen saturation, fluid intake, and urine output. These patients need cardiac monitoring, CVP monitoring, and a pulmonary artery catheter for measuring hemodynamic parameters. Monitoring laboratory series (e.g., chemistry profile; hematocrit, hemoglobin, and platelet counts; coagulation studies; arterial blood gases) is necessary.

Do **NOT** attempt to place the patient with hypovolemic shock in the Trendelenburg (head down) position because it stimulates the baroreceptor response and aggravates hypoxia ↓ CO, ↓ heart rate, ↓ BP, ↓ FRC of lungs, and ↑ cerebral venous congestion and ICP.

The hypovolemic patient is a critically ill individual; even patients with mild hypovolemia can rapidly deteriorate. The nurse must remember that hypovolemia affects all organs. The treatment of hypovolemia is volume load and oxygenation.

Do You UNDERSTAND?

DIRECTIONS: **Identify the following statements as *true* (T) or *false* (F).**

______1. Inadequate tissue perfusion, which causes cellular hypoxia, subsequent organ failure, and death from decreased circulating oxygenated blood flow, is the underlying pathophysiologic cause of all forms of shock.

______2. Intestinal obstruction can cause sequestration of fluid as a result of a decrease in colloidal osmotic pressure leading to hypovolemic shock.

______3. The Trendelenburg position is the best position for a patient in hypovolemic shock.

______4. Hypotension is a late sign of shock.

DIRECTIONS: **Fill in the blanks to complete each of the following statements.**

5. Renal blood flow is sensitive to CO. The ____________________ ______________________________________ is the most sensitive indicator of a patient's fluid status and thus the most important for a nurse to monitor when caring for the patient with hypovolemia.
6. The fluid of choice for the initial treatment of hypovolemic shock is ____________________________ ____________________________ ____________________.
7. The initial goal in the resuscitation of a patient in hypovolemic shock is accomplished with fluid volume loading to preserve oxygen perfusion to the tissues by sustaining the ____________________ ____ and the ____________________________ greater than __________ _________ mm Hg.

What IS Septic Shock?

Septic shock is an inflammatory response. The septic process is initiated by the launch of immune mediators that are part of the inflammatory reaction. This process starts a chain of complex interactions that are

Answers: 1. T; 2. T; 3. F; 4. T; 5. urine output; 6. Ringer's lactate; 7. cardiac output, MAP, 60.

controlled by numerous feedback mechanisms. Eventually the immune system is overwhelmed, and the process actually harms the body. *Systemic inflammatory response syndrome* (SIRS) refers to a host's response to a variety of clinical insults, both infectious and noninfectious, and is part of the acute sepsis process.

In the past, it was theorized that the endotoxins released from these microorganisms were the cause of the septic shock state. It is now believed that excessive activation of the host's defense mechanisms cause the clinical syndrome of sepsis rather than the microorganisms themselves. Signs and symptoms of early sepsis can be subtle; therefore, careful monitoring is essential. For this reason, identifying the patients who are at the greatest risk is important. Along with a documented or suspected infection, at least two or more of the following signs and symptoms characterize sepsis:

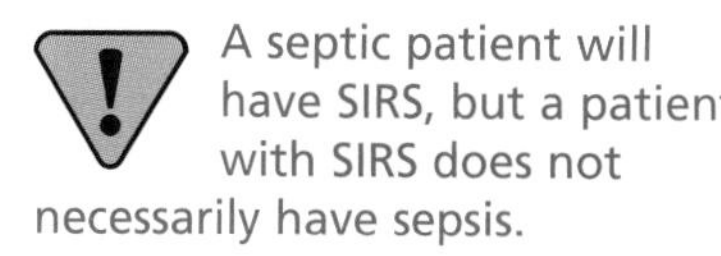

A septic patient will have SIRS, but a patient with SIRS does not necessarily have sepsis.

- Temperature > 38.3° or < 36° C; > 100.9 or < 96.8° F
- Tachypnea
- Tachycardia
- Altered mental status
- Positive fluid balance (>20 mL/kg over 24 hours)
- Hyperglycemia (>120 mg/dl) in the absence of diabetes)
- Hypotension (SBP < 90 mm Hg, MAP < 70 mm Hg)
- SvO_2 > 70%
- Cardiac index > 3.5 L/min/m^2
- White blood cell count (WBC) > 12,000 cells/mm
- WBC < 4000 cells/mm, or differential > 10% bands
- Elevated C-reactive protein
- Elevated procalcitonin

Once sepsis is present, the stage is set for progression to septic shock. Therefore, diligence must be taken to identify sepsis early and begin early goal-directed treatment and monitoring.

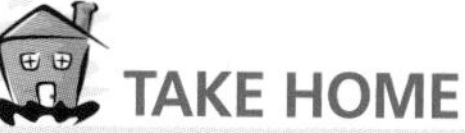

TAKE HOME POINTS

Patients at the greatest risk for septic shock include the following:
- Very young children
- Older adults
- Immunocompromised individuals
- Chronically ill patients
- Patients with malignancies

Acute sepsis patients have a microbial infection with a systemic response.

Bacteremia refers to a patient's blood cultures being positive for any type of bacteria.

A negative blood culture does not mean that someone does not have sepsis.

What You NEED TO KNOW

Septic shock is a distributive shock characterized by tachycardia, hyperthermia or hypothermia, and hypotension caused by decreased SVR. The blood volume is adequate but misplaced. Vasodilation occurs, capillary permeability increases, and fluid is lost in the interstitial space. A decline in SVR is one of the first indications of shock. In addition, the patient develops compromised CO and index as a result of decreased

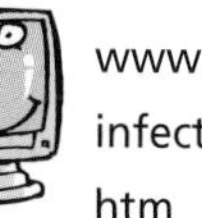

www.ccmtutorials.com/infection/sepsisrx/index.htm

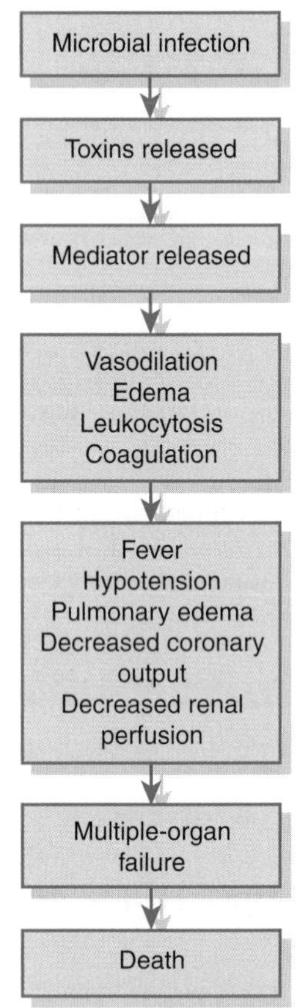

MODS due to infection as a result of septic shock. *(From Bucher L, Melander S:* Critical care nursing, *Philadelphia, 1999, WB Saunders.)*

Invasive monitoring lines, indwelling catheters, or venous access devices may predispose a patient to acquiring a nosocomial sepsis.

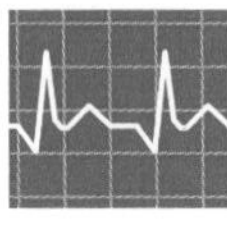

SVR decreases and CO increases.

vascular tone. Ascertaining this state without invasive hemodynamic monitoring may be difficult because the body compensates by increasing the heart rate. In this early preshock state, CO increases and the arterial pressures lower to typically a systolic pressure of less than 90 mm Hg or a decrease in 40 points from a previously hypertensive systolic pressure. Because of this compensation and vasodilation, the patient will have pink, warm skin with rapid capillary refill and a bounding pulse.

Compensatory mechanisms include baroreceptor reflex, which causes an increased heart rate and vasomotor tone. The SNS is stimulated, which results in the release of epinephrine and norepinephrine, which causes systemic vasoconstriction. This release causes blood to be shunted to the vital organs. Because of a decrease in blood flow to the kidneys, a decrease in glomerular filtration rate occurs, which activates the renin-angiotensin (I and II) and aldosterone system and results in sodium and water retention. The retention of sodium and water is the body's attempt to compensate for the decrease in blood flow by increasing the venous return to the heart and possibly increasing the patient's BP. Progression of the shock state causes the compensatory mechanisms to become ineffective, resulting in hemodynamic instability.

Continued decrease in blood flow to the vital organs ultimately causes tissue ischemia and acidosis from anaerobic metabolism. Anaerobic metabolism leads to depletion of cellular ATP and the failure of the sodium-potassium pump, which results in further hemodynamic compromise and an inability to maintain BP.

Respiratory failure is another complication and occurs in 30% to 80% of patients in septic shock. Tachypnea is observed in patients with and without fever and may be a result of endotoxins released by the invading microorganisms or by defense mechanisms mediated by the body in an attempt to maintain tissue oxygenation. With the progression of sepsis comes increased fluid in the lungs from the higher alveolar capillary permeability; the result is an even higher respiratory rate and hypoxia. Fatigue of breathing may ensue as the body attempts to maintain oxygenation. This fatigue leads to more shallow, less effective respirations that cause hypocarbia (decreased carbon dioxide), which triggers the CNS to further increase the respiratory rate, eventually causing exhaustion. The patient may progress into acute respiratory distress syndrome (ARDS).

The effect of septic shock on the kidneys can be profound. Renal involvement during sepsis can vary from a minor proteinuria to acute tubular necrosis (ATN) in septic shock. It is unknown whether the ATN is due to the decreased blood supply to the kidneys as a result of the hypotension or by the endotoxins released by the offending microorganism. Regardless of the cause, ATN can lead to renal failure. (For more information about ATN, refer to the discussion in Chapter 8.)

The patient in septic shock can exhibit skin lesions that are most often located on the lower extremities. These lesions can be associated with the development of disseminated intravascular coagulation (DIC), which is another complication of septic shock; the lesions can also be associated with the causative bacteria. Toxic shock syndrome (TSS) can produce a profound septic shock and has a very distinctive cutaneous component. *Staphylococcus aureus* or a severe streptococcal infection causes TSS. The rash can be localized or generalized and appears in the form of a macular erythema that blanches with pressure.

Serum glucose increases with septic shock as a result of gluconeogenesis and insulin resistance. Hyperglycemia can be the first indicator of sepsis in the patient with diabetes. Control of the hyperglycemia may be difficult until the infection is under control. Hypoglycemia is relatively uncommon in sepsis, but it occasionally occurs in patients with other underlying problems.

Septic encephalopathy occurs in 70% of patients in septic shock. The patient may be agitated, confused, lethargic, disoriented, or even unarousable, but seizures are rare. Infection of the CNS may be considered; however, most patients in septic shock do not have infections of the CNS. Recovery from septic encephalopathy hinges on the control of the underlying septic shock.

MODS can develop in patients with septic shock and involves two or more organ systems. The release of endotoxins causes a massive inflammatory response, which leads to microvascular injury to various organs. To complicate matters further, hypotension leads to tissue hypoperfusion and end-organ damage. Early intervention and the identification and treatment of the underlying infection are imperative in halting this destructive event (see Chapter 12 for more information).

What You DO

Maintaining a patent airway is the first and foremost intervention with the critically ill patient. An assistive device, such as an oral or a nasal airway, may be needed. In the event of respiratory failure, the nurse

One of the first signs of inadequate tissue perfusion is a decreased level of consciousness that can be exhibited as confusion.

TAKE HOME POINTS

- Respiratory failure in septic shock is associated with a higher mortality rate than in patients without respiratory failure.
- A common cause of TSS is the use of tampons.
- Prolonged hypotension causes tissue hypoperfusion and results in ischemia and end-organ damage.

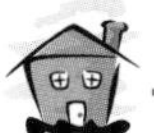

TAKE HOME POINTS

- According to the Surviving Sepsis Campaign, early goal-directed therapy within the first 6 hours improves survival.
- If mixed venous oxygenation is less than 70%, it is recommended that packed red blood cells be administered to achieve a hematocrit of at least 30%.
- A nasogastric tube might be needed in an intubated patient to prevent aspiration of gastric contents and to decompress the stomach.
- The blood volume is adequate in the patient in septic shock, but it is misplaced.

should be prepared to assist with intubation, which is usually performed by the attending physician, nurse anesthetist, or other qualified professional. Initial intervention is oxygen delivery at 5 to 6 L via nasal cannula. To assess the adequacy of oxygenation, pulse oximeter readings, arterial blood gases, and mixed venous gases should be monitored. Higher concentrations of oxygen may become necessary, depending on arterial oxygen saturation (SaO_2) and arterial blood gas values. Mechanical ventilation may become necessary as a result of respiratory muscle fatigue. Frequent assessment of breath sounds for rate, character, and quality indicate adequacy of the patient's ventilation.

FIRST-LINE AND INITIAL TREATMENTS FOR SEPSIS AND SEPTIC SHOCK

- Eradicate the offending organism.
- Provide supplemental oxygen (O_2).
- Administer intravenous (IV) fluids (crystalloids or colloids).
- Administer appropriate medications (vasopressors, inotropes).
- Immunotherapy (control the excessive host inflammatory response)
- Recombinant human activated protein C
- Glucose control (target <150 mg/dl)

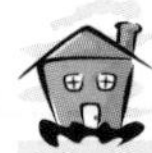

TAKE HOME POINTS

- Administration of IV fluids should achieve a CVP reading between 8 and 12 mm Hg in a nonventilated patient and between 12 and 15 mm Hg in a ventilated patient.
- Administration of vasopressors should be used to maintain MAP ≥ 65 mm Hg.
- Hypoglycemia is relatively uncommon in sepsis but does occasionally occur in patients with other underlying problems.
- SVR will be decreased in shock resulting in ↓ BP.

Optimal cardiac contractility and output is necessary to provide blood, which is rich in oxygen and nutrients, to the tissues. This can be accomplished by administering prescribed IV fluids and pharmacologic agents. Careful monitoring of the patient's BP, pulses, and cardiovascular and hemodynamic status is essential. If the patient becomes hemodynamically unstable, the critical care nurse should anticipate the use of inotropic agents and vasoactive drugs. If hemodynamic monitoring is available, the patient's filling pressures (CVP) should be monitored to assess adequacy of fluid replacement and pulmonary wedge pressures. Fluid replacement is an important step in the treatment of the patient in septic shock. In sepsis, massive vasodilation and increased capillary permeability occurs, which results in fluid moving into the interstitial space. Because the patient requires IV fluids and possible pharmacologic agents, a good IV access site is essential; furthermore, the patient often needs central venous access.

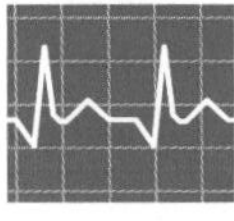

Close monitoring of the BP and cardiovascular status of the septic patient is essential.

Frequent vital sign monitoring helps the nurse assess the patient's response to therapy. Monitoring BP by means of an arterial line should be anticipated. MAP should be closely monitored because of the variable pressures in the patient in septic shock. A MAP of less than 60 mm Hg negatively affects perfusion of the brain and kidneys and should be immediately addressed. The nurse should promptly notify the physician if a trend of a decreasing MAP develops. PAPs and CVPs enable the nurse to assess the effectiveness of the patient's treatment and to help prevent fluid overload by monitoring the patient's intravascular fluid status. Urinary output is imperative to monitor as an indicator of renal perfusion.

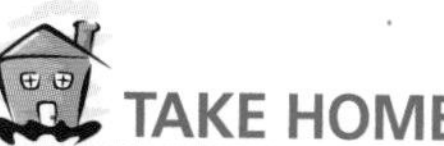

TAKE HOME POINTS

During hypotensive states, an arterial line measurement of BP is more precise than a manual or automatic cuff pressure.

Some debate continues over the management and treatment of fever for the patient in septic shock. Few studies exist relating the control of temperature to the mortality or morbidity rate. Fever is usually treated because of the increased demands that the hypermetabolic state of septic shock places on the body. Some studies show that decreasing fever also decreases oxygen demand for organs and tissues and promotes patient comfort; others suggest that fever itself may provide some protection from the microbial pathogens. Fever, however, is always treated in the immunosuppressed patient.

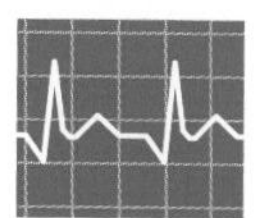

Observe the patient for changes in LOC because it may indicate hypoxia or decreased cerebral perfusion. Assessing nutritional adequacy requires close monitoring of serum electrolytes, blood glucose, serum albumin, weight, and fluid volume status. Trace elements, vitamins, and glucose are added as prescribed.

FIRST-LINE AND INITIAL TREATMENT FOR FEVER

- Administer an antipyretic agent such as acetaminophen.

Another major aim in the treatment of septic shock is to maintain blood glucose levels of less than 150 mg/dl. By maintaining blood glucose levels, patient outcomes are improved. A patient's nutritional status is also critical. The use of enteral nutrition is indicated unless contraindicated by the presence of acute pancreatitis, which requires parenteral nutrition. The patient needs increased nutrition because of the hypermetabolic state superimposed by the infection or disease state.

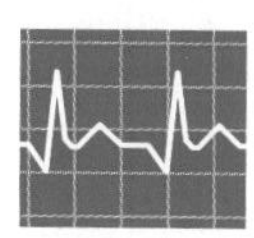

The desired urinary output is 0.5 mL/kg/hr for an adult.

Maintaining renal perfusion is a priority and is monitored by urine output. A urine output greater than 30 mL/hr or more than 0.5 mL/kg/hr indicates adequate renal perfusion. Indwelling urinary catheters are usually used to monitor hourly outputs. Catheter care is essential because the catheter can be a direct entry point for microorganisms. Therefore, catheter output must be closely monitored for change in color, consistency or odor of urine, which may indicate myoglobinuria, hemoglobinuria, or possible urinary tract infection.

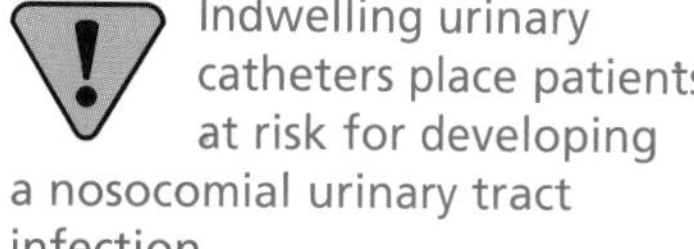

Indwelling urinary catheters place patients at risk for developing a nosocomial urinary tract infection.

Proper isolation of the infective organisms is usually identified by blood, urine, sputum, or other cultures. For this reason, obtaining these

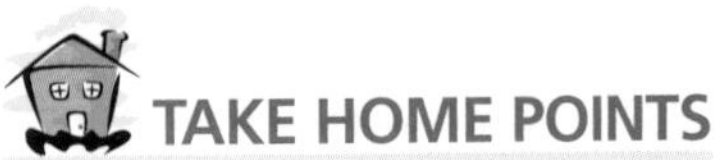

TAKE HOME POINTS

Because prompt identification of the infecting organisms is essential, blood cultures can sometimes be simultaneously drawn while initiating IV access.

cultures before initiating prescribed antibiotic therapy is important. The patient's outcome hinges on rapid identification and proper treatment of the infecting organism.

Do You UNDERSTAND?

DIRECTIONS: **Using the words listed below, fill in the blanks to complete the sentences below. Words are used only once, and some words are not used at all.**

>30 mL/hr
>60 mm Hg
<60 mm Hg
distributive shock
hypovolemic shock
invasive monitoring lines
less precise
mechanical ventilation
more precise
proper antibiotic treatment
rapid identification
urinary catheterization

1. ______________________ can predispose a patient to acquiring a nosocomial sepsis.
2. Septic shock is a ______________________.
3. A MAP of ______________________ leads to decreased renal and cerebral perfusion.
4. ______________________ may become necessary for respiratory muscle fatigue.
5. Arterial line BP monitoring is ______________________ than cuff pressures during hypotensive states.
6. The outcome of the patient in septic shock often depends on ______________________ and ______________________ of the infectious organism.

Answers: **1. invasive monitoring lines; 2. distributive shock; 3. <60 mm Hg; 4. mechanical ventilation; 5. more precise; 6. rapid identification, proper antibiotic treatment.**

References

Baird MS, Keen JH, Swearingen PL: *Manual of critical care nursing: nursing interventions and collaborative management,* ed 5, St Louis, 2005, Mosby.

Barker E: *Neuroscience nursing: a spectrum of care,* ed 3, St Louis, 2008, Mosby.

Bench S: Clinical skills: assessing and treating shock: a nursing perspective, *Br J Nurs* 13(12):715-721, 2004.

Bryant H: Anaphylaxis: recognition, treatment and education, *Emerg Nurse* 15(2): 24-28, 2007.

Dellinger RP, Levy MM, Carlet, JM, et al: Surviving sepsis campaign: international guidelines for management of severe sepsis and septic shock: 2008, *Crit Care Med* 36(1):296-327, 2008.

Ferns T, Chojnacka I: The causes of anaphylaxis and its management in adults, *Br J Nurs* 12(17):1006-1012, 2003.

Garretson S, Malbert, S: Understanding hypovolaemic, cardiogenic and septic shock, *Nursing Standard* 21(50):45-55, 2007.

Guly HR, Bouamra O, Lecky FE: The incidence of neurogenic shock in patients with isolated spinal cord injury in the emergency department, *Resuscitation* 76:57-62, 2008.

Jones GJ: Anaphylactic shock, *Emerg Nurse* 9(10):29-35, 2002.

Nobre V, Sarasin FP, Pugin J: Prompt antibiotic administration and goal-directed hemodynamic support in patients with severe sepsis and septic shock, *Curr Opin Crit Care* 13:586-591, 2007.

Reynolds HR, Hochman JS: Cardiogenic shock: current concepts and improving outcomes, *Circulation* 117:686-697, 2008.

Rivers EP, Coba V, Whitmill M: Early goal-directed therapy in severe sepsis and septic shock: a contemporary review of the literature, *Curr Opin Anesthesiol* 21:128-140, 2008.

Sole M, Lamborn M, Hartshorn J: *Introduction to critical care nursing,* ed 4, Philadelphia, 2005, WB Saunders.

Spaniol JR, Knight AR, Zebley JL, Anderson D, Pierce JD: Fluid resuscitation therapy for hemorrhagic shock, *J Trauma Nurs* 14(3):152-160, 2007.

Topalian S, Ginsberg F, Parrillo JE: Cardiogenic shock. *Crit Care Med* 36(1): S66-S74, 2008.

Urden L, Stacey K, Lough M: *Thelan's critical care nursing: diagnosis and management,* ed 5, St Louis, 2006, Mosby.

Wheeler AP: Recent developments in the diagnosis and management of severe sepsis, *Chest* 132:1967-1976, 2007.

NCLEX® Review

1. You are caring for a patient who has been admitted for a gastrointestinal (GI) bleed. On the second day of hospitalization, the physician prescribed 2 units of packed red blood cells (RBCs) to be given over 4 hours each. You hang the first unit of blood at 9 am. At 9:25 the patient is complaining that her hands are itching and she cannot get her wedding ring off. Your first priority should be to:
   1 Remind the patient that she should not be wearing her wedding ring in the hospital and that if it should get lost or stolen, the hospital would not be responsible.
   2 Run and get a syringe of epinephrine to administer subcutaneously because the patient is having an anaphylactic reaction.
   3 Stop the blood transfusion immediately because you suspect that it may be the cause of the patient's itching and swollen hands.
   4 Notify the physician about the patient's complaints and request an order for diphenhydramine or Benadryl to help with the itching.

2. You are the nurse taking care of a 55-year-old man who has been hospitalized for cellulitis of the left calf. You are about to go to lunch but decide to hang the patient's newly ordered antibiotic early so it will be finished when you return. You hang 1 piperacillin (PCN) 1 g in the IV piggyback and start the infusion to go over 1 hour. You tell the patient that you will return when it is finished to flush his IV. On your way to lunch you hear another nurse yell, "He's not breathing" from your patient's room. You then recall that your patient stated that he was allergic to PCN on his admission assessment. You immediately:
   1 Go to the room to see what the commotion is all about.
   2 Bring a syringe of epinephrine into the room and administer 0.3 to 0.5 mL of a 1:1000 solution subcutaneously (SC).
   3 Go to lunch because if you do not go now, you will probably not be able to eat later.
   4 Call the physician and tell him what has happened and that he prescribed the wrong antibiotic for your patient.

3. The major, immediate risk associated with the use of a left ventricular assist device (LVAD) is:
   1 Infection.
   2 Embolus.
   3 Pump failure.
   4 Immobility.

4. How is cardiogenic shock different from hypovolemic shock?
   1 No difference exists between cardiogenic shock and hypovolemic shock.
   2 The BP is increased in cardiogenic shock and lowered in hypovolemic shock.
   3 An increase of fluid exists in the heart during cardiogenic shock but not during hypovolemic shock.
   4 The pulse rate is decreased in cardiogenic shock and increased in hypovolemic shock.

5. What is the underlying pathophysiology of all forms of shock?
   1 Inadequate tissue perfusion.
   2 Respiratory alkalosis.
   3 Decreased SVR.
   4 Increased basal metabolic rate.

6. Hypovolemic shock causes:
   1 A decrease in CO and pulmonary capillary wedge pressure.
   2 Alkalosis.
   3 The release of nosocomial infection mediators.
   4 The release of antiplatelet factor (APF).

7. A patient arrives at the emergency department with the chief complaint of a temperature of 102° F, as well as nausea and vomiting for 3 days. The patient is experiencing tachycardia with a sustained HR of 120 bpm, BP of 95/60 mm Hg, tachypneic at 26 bpm. The nurse starts an IV knowing that the patient has deficient volume and is going to need a bolus of IV fluids. The initial treatment is with:
   1 NS 4 to 5 L.
   2 Colloids such as hetastarch.
   3 Ringer's lactate (RL) 1 to 2 L.
   4 Mannitol 10%.
8. What would be an appropriate intervention for a patient in septic shock who has the following?
   pH: 7.29
   pCO_2: 69
   pO_2: 60
   HCO_3: 32
   SaO_2: 83
   RR: 36 breaths/min, obviously labored
   Diaphoretic and complains of being tired
   1 Deliver oxygen by 100% nonrebreather.
   2 Place patient in upright position, and give supplemental oxygen and the prescribed anxiolytic.
   3 Provide intubation and mechanical ventilation.
   4 Consult respiratory therapy for a breathing treatment, and give supplemental oxygen.
9. Which patient is at greatest risk for septic shock?
   1 A 45-year-old man who has had coronary artery bypass surgery with a sternal infection 2 weeks earlier.
   2 An 86-year-old insulin-dependent diabetic woman with stage 4 sacral decubitus who is incontinent with an indwelling Foley catheter.
   3 A 60-year-old man with pneumonia.
   4 A 35-year-old man who has tested positive for human immunodeficiency virus (HIV) and is being treated for cellulitis of his hand on an outpatient basis.
10. Positive inotropic agents are given during septic shock to:
   1 Decrease anxiety.
   2 Decrease BP.
   3 Increase contractility of the heart.
   4 Increase the calcium pump of the heart.

NCLEX® Review Answers

1.3 Although epinephrine is the hallmark of management for anaphylactic reactions, the first step in treating a suspected anaphylactic reaction is to discontinue the causative agent to prevent further degranulation of mast cells and the release of mediators. The priority should be placed on investigating the patient's complaint; you should never reprimand the patient. Your knowledge of the situation should make you think of an allergic reaction to the blood, and you should immediately discontinue the blood.

2.2 Another nurse is already in the room evaluating the situation. You know that the patient is allergic to PCN and the antibiotic previously hung was a PCN. You should immediately suspect an anaphylactic reaction, and epinephrine should be brought to the room while other personnel are taking care of the patient. Morbidity and mortality decrease with faster treatment. You should never leave your patient in the time of a crisis; it is your responsibility to provide rapid direct treatment. The patient needs immediate intervention now.

3.3 Infection and embolus are not immediate problems. The patient does not have much forward flow if the pump fails. The patient can move with the device in and is not immobilized.

4.3 In cardiogenic shock the pump is damaged and cannot maintain adequate flow. This causes an increase in fluid (or blood) left in the heart. Hypovolemic shock is due to the loss of blood or fluid (or both) from the vascular space. The BP measurement is lowered, and the pulse rate is increased in both.

5.1 The hallmark of all forms of shock is inadequate tissue perfusion. Respiratory alkalosis is a compensatory mechanism to correct the acidosis that occurs from anaerobic metabolism. SVR increases in shock in response to hypotension and the compensatory vasoconstriction of the arterial vascular bed. Although the basal metabolic rate (BMR) is increased, it is not the underlying pathologic result.

6.1 A decrease in venous return to the right side of the heart, which leads to a decrease in filling pressure and volume, occurs with hypovolemic shock. Therefore, the result is a decrease in CO and PCWP. This decrease in volume is sensed by the baroreceptors that stimulate the sympathetic nervous system (SNS) to release epinephrine and norepinephrine. The posterior pituitary responds to the shock state by releasing ADH to conserve water. Acidosis is a result of inadequate tissue perfusion, which causes the cells to resort to anaerobic metabolism. Release of nosocomial infection mediators and APF are not related to hypovolemic shock.

7.3 Volume load with crystalloids is the first-line and most important treatment of hypovolemia. Initial treatment is with a bolus of 1 to 2 L Ringer's lactate and evaluation of the patient's response. NS is used for blood and blood-product administration. Too much NS can contribute to hyperchloremic acidosis. Colloids are not a first-line treatment. Colloids are expensive compared with crystalloids and are effective once the patient has had fluid replacement with crystalloids. Mannitol 10% is an osmotic diuretic.

8.3 A patient with an already severely compromised respiratory status who is complaining of tiredness may have ensuing respiratory collapse. Although oxygen by 100% nonrebreather may increase the arterial oxygen content, it does not help increase ventilation. A breathing treatment may be a first-line choice in a patient with respiratory compromise; however, the patient in septic shock with the same arterial blood gases has depleted the patient's reserve. A breathing treatment does not maintain the airway and intubation. Placing the patient in an upright position and administering supplemental oxygen and anxiolytics can support both oxygenation and ventilation, but the patient's compensatory mechanisms have already failed.

9.2 The patient in choice 2 is older, chronically ill, and has multiple sites for entry of microorganisms. Although patients in choices 1, 3, and 4 are at risk for sepsis, they are not as much at risk as the patient in choice 2.

10.3 Administration of positive inotropes increases the contractility of the heart, which counteracts the myocardial depression that occurs during septic shock. Positive inotropes increase contractility of the heart and thus increase the force of contraction, which leads to an elevation of BP; they do not have anxiolytic properties. An increase in the calcium pump of the heart does not occur.

Trauma and Emergency Care

Chapter 3

What You WILL LEARN

After reading this chapter, you will know how to do the following:

- ✔ Describe prevention approaches that can be instituted in the critical care environment.
- ✔ Describe relevant patient education topics.

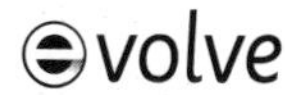

See http://evolve.elsevier.com/Schumacher/criticalcare for additional NCLEX® review questions.

What IS Rapid Sequence Intubation?

Rapid sequence intubation (RSI) is a specialized form of placing an endotracheal tube (ETT) in a patient to provide ventilation via a secure airway. Patients in respiratory distress or those unable to maintain a patent airway often require the placement of an ETT to allow some form of assisted or controlled ventilation. When the potential for gastric content regurgitation exists, an RSI is used to reduce the risk of aspiration. An RSI is designed to ensure that no gastric contents are aspirated into the tracheal tree, which could result in pneumonia or acute respiratory distress syndrome (ARDS).

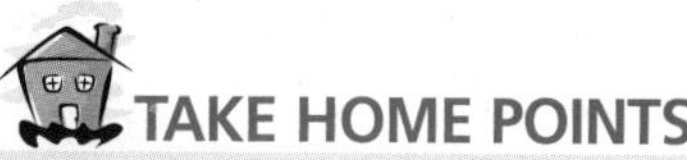

TAKE HOME POINTS

Securing the airway by intubating the trachea is an essential component of the resuscitation process in the emergency department for patients with compromised airways or ventilatory failure.

An aspirated volume as small as 25 mL may have disasterous consequences.

At-Risk Populations

Although prescribed most frequently for emergency and trauma patient populations, RSI is also used in any case in which there is a potential for aspiration or when the patient is assumed to have a "full stomach" (e.g., obstetrics [OB] and labor and delivery).

What You NEED TO KNOW

Clinical Technique

RSI differs from normal intubations in several key ways. Similar to all intubations, the patient should first be preoxygenated to fill the functional residual capacity (FRC) with 100% oxygen. However, unlike standard intubation procedure, RSI calls for the use of the Sellick maneuver (**cricoid pressure**) while the patient is induced with anesthetic medications. Once induced, the patient with RSI is **not** ventilated before administering neuromuscular-blocking agents or before attempting direct laryngoscopy. A period of apnea is intentionally instituted to prevent forcing air into the stomach via positive-pressure ventilation, which would increase intragastric pressure and potentiate regurgitation and aspiration. During a normal intubation, at least one attempt is made at controlled positive-pressure mask ventilation (**test breath**) between the administration of the anesthetic induction agent and the neuromuscular-blocking agent. This ventilation

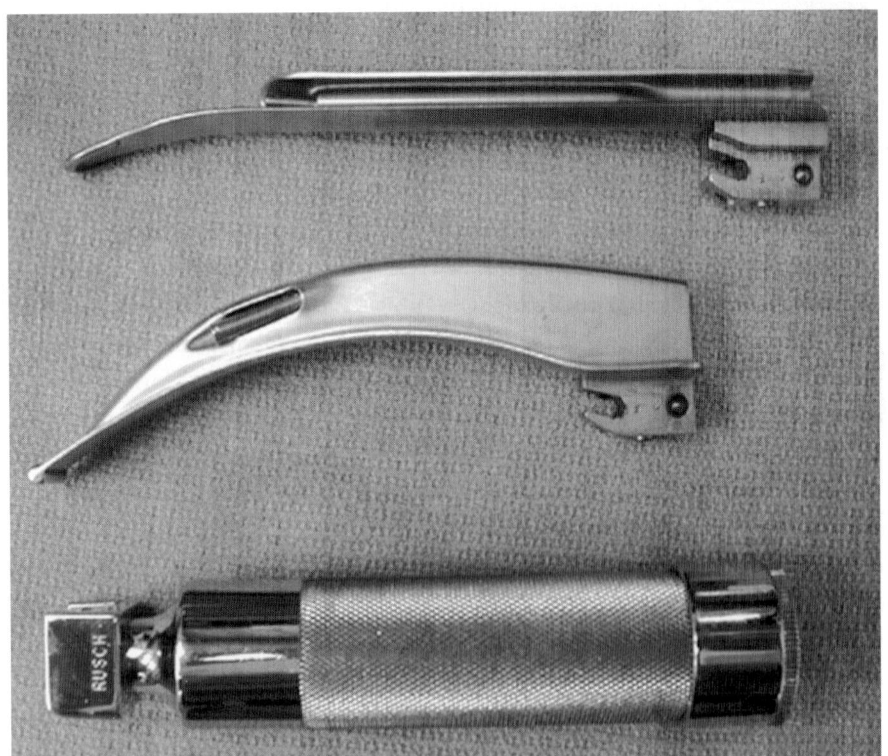

Bottom to top: laryngoscope handle and two blades (Macintosh 3, Miller 2). *(Courtesy of Matthew W. Kervin, RN, BS, BSN, CRNA, Medical College of Georgia, Augusta, Georgia.)*

provides the health care provider with the knowledge that the patient can be mask-ventilated in case intubation attempts are not successful. RSI does not allow for this ventilatory check, which increases the risk for hypoxia in the apneic patient. Thus, the major risk involved in performing an RSI is the inability to ventilate the patient in case intubation fails.

Assembly of all required equipment is essential before attempting any intubation. Suction must always be available to remove secretions, blood, and regurgitated materials from the oropharynx. One or more laryngoscope handles with charged batteries and at least two laryngoscope blades (Miller 2 and Macintosh 3 are recommended), as well as multiple sizes of ETTs should be at the bedside. At least one ETT should have a semirigid stylet inserted. A method for delivering positive-pressure ventilation must be at hand before intubating the patient (e.g., bag-valve-mask). A patent intravenous (IV) line is imperative, and all appropriate medications should be immediately available.

Hypoxia, hypercarbia, and airway trauma are also potential hazards with any RSI attempt.

Common Endotracheal Tube Sizes

Age and Sex	Appropriate Sizes	Most Common Size	Depth of Insertion as Measured at Teeth
Children	Age + $\frac{16}{4}$ (age = 4 + 4)	Variable	Age + 10 cm
Adult men	7.5 to 8.5	8.0	23 cm
Adult women	6.5 to 7.5	7.0	21 cm

Common Medications Used in Rapid Sequence Intubation

Medications	Uses	Doses (mg/kg)	Advantages	Considerations
Sodium thiopental (Pentothal)	Induction of anesthesia	4 to 6	Rapid onset, short duration	Hypotension, apnea
Etomidate (Amidate)	Induction of anesthesia	0.2 to 0.3	Rapid onset, short duration Cardiovascular stable May allow spontaneous ventilations	Myoclonus, nausea, vomiting, painful on injection
Propofol (Dipivan)	Induction of anesthesia	2.0 to 2.5	Rapid onset, short duration	Hypotension, apnea
Ketamine (Ketalar)	Induction of anesthesia	1.0 to 2.0	Increased sympathetic tone bronchodilation	Tachycardia, increased sympathetic tone, salivation
Succinylcholine (Anectine)	Depolarizing neuromuscular blockade	1.0 to 1.5	Rapid onset, 5- to 7-min duration "Gold standard" for RSI	Muscular fasciculations, malignant hyperthermia, muscle rigidity Hyperkalemia, bradycardia, and dysrhythmias
Rocuronium (Zemuron)	Nondepolarizing neuromuscular blockade	0.9 to 1.2	Rapid onset; no risk of hyperkalemia	Extended duration (45 to 90 min) Potential for IV precipitation
Vecuronium (Norcuron)	Nondepolarizing neuromuscular blockade	0.2	Cardiovascular stable	"Slow" onset (>2 to 3 min) Extended duration (>60 min)

RSI, Rapid sequence intubation; *IV*, intravenous.

If the patient is alert and cooperative, then 30 mL of sodium citrate (Bicitra) can be administered to decrease stomach acidity. If time permits, 50 mg of IV ranitidine (Zantac), 20 mg famotidine (Pepcid), or 10 mg of IV metoclopramide (Reglan) may be administered to decrease regurgitation and aspiration. Since most RSIs are attempted in emergent conditions, this precludes premedications.

Preoxygenation is recommended before attempting intubation. Despite differences in how preoxygenation is performed, its use is universal. Traditional methods include spontaneous ventilation of 100% oxygen for 3 to 5 minutes or three to five vital capacity breaths of 100% oxygen. The latter method demands that the patient be cooperative. Preoxygenation allows the patient's FRC to be filled with oxygen. FRC is that portion of the total lung volume that is not normally expired during spontaneous ventilation. By filling these areas of the lung with oxygen, the patient is provided with a small *reserve* of oxygen. In a young, healthy man, filling the FRC with 100% oxygen allows up to a 5- to 7-minute reserve of oxygen if the patient becomes apneic. Significantly, the duration of apnea caused by an induction dose of succinylcholine (Anectine) (1.0 to 1.5 mg/kg) is close to 5 to 7 minutes. Both obesity and pregnancy can significantly reduce the physical volume of the FRC, whereas tachycardia, sepsis, and other hyperdynamic states cause a more rapid use of the oxygen in the FRC. Additionally, both obesity and pregnancy increase the cephalad movement of the diaphragm on induction of anesthesia, further decreasing the FRC considerably.

When the oropharynx is filled with blood, secretions, or foreign material, these should be suctioned and an attempt should be made at preoxygenation in all but the direst situations. Unconscious and trauma patients who have lost their normal protective airway reflexes and who are not spontaneously ventilating pose a unique problem. Any positive-pressure breaths administered via a bag-valve-mask increase the chances for regurgitation and aspiration of gastric contents. In such cases, many practitioners choose to skip preoxygenation and establish a controlled airway via immediate tracheal intubation.

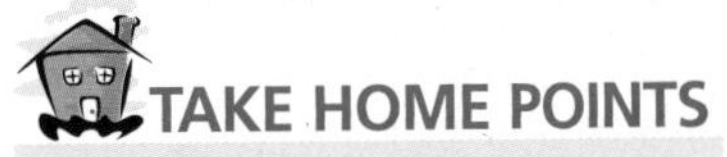

- *Vital capacity* is defined as a maximum inspiration immediately after a maximum expiration.

The next distinguishing technique in RSI is the use of cricoid pressure or the Sellick maneuver. The cricoid cartilage is the first tracheal cartilage ring below the larynx. More importantly, the cricoid cartilage is the **only** continuous cartilaginous ring below the larynx.

Application of pressure (from 0.5 to 8.0 lb/ft) to this cartilage ring results in compression of the esophagus, which lies immediately posterior to the trachea. Firm pressure helps prevent the chances of gastric content regurgitation, but excessive pressure can actually hinder intubation attempts.

Many disease states can significantly alter both the physical amount of the FRC and the amount of time the body takes to use this oxygen reserve.

An acronym that has been used to aid those applying cricoid pressure is B-U-R-P. **B** stands for *backward* or posterior displacement. **U** stands

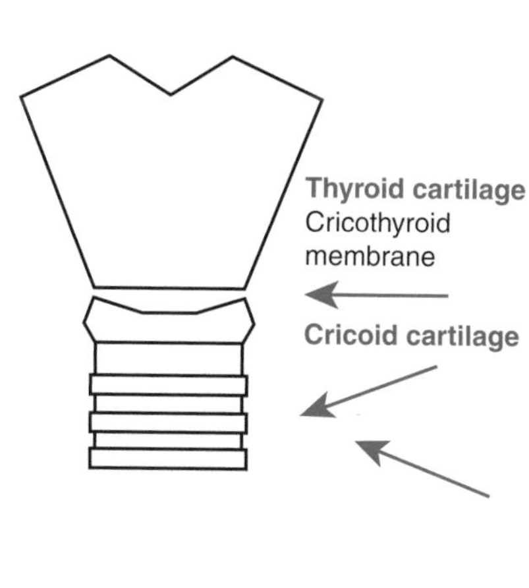

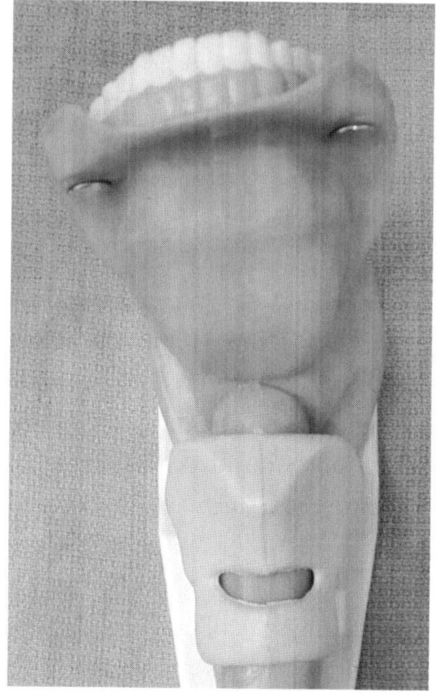

Anatomy for application of cricoid pressure. *(Courtesy of Matthew W. Kervin, RN, BS, BSN, CRNA, Medical College of Georgia, Augusta, Georgia.)*

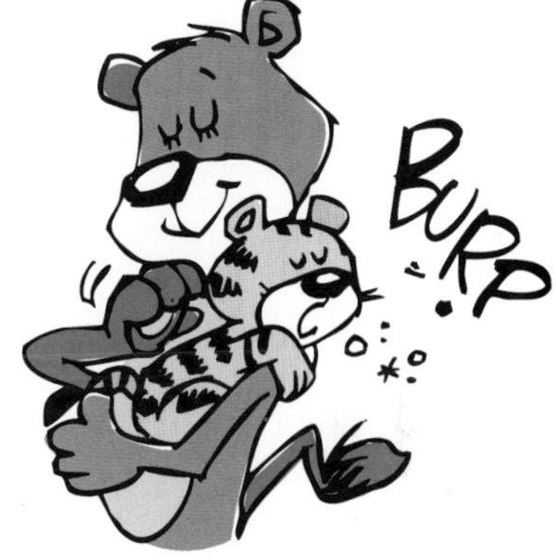

Acronym to aid in applying cricoid pressure (B-U-R-P).

for a slightly *upward* or cephalad movement. **R** stands for a slight *right* displacement of the larynx. **P** stands for the *pressure* used to occlude the esophagus. The person assisting with the intubation must correctly identify the cricoid cartilage before applying pressure. From the prominence of the *Adam's apple* **(thyroid cartilage)**, the nurse slides the fingers down the anterior aspect of the patient's neck until the first depression is felt, which marks the *cricothyroid membrane.* The next cartilage ring is the cricoid cartilage. Pressure is applied by the use of the thumb and first two fingers on opposite sides of the cricoid cartilage. The assistant's hand should not be on the larynx or thyroid cartilage (see Color Plate 3).

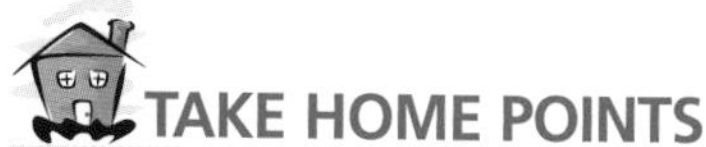

Suction should always be available when intubating a patient.

The application of cricoid pressure does have risks. Complications range from interference with tracheal intubation, to esophageal rupture, to fracturing the cricoid cartilage. Once pressure to the cricoid cartilage has been applied, it is not removed until placement of the ETT has been confirmed by end-tidal carbon dioxide ($ETCO_2$) and bilateral breath sounds (BBS). Cricoid pressure may be lessened if it interferes with endotracheal intubation.

Practitioners are split in their opinions of the best time to apply cricoid pressure. Slight pressure may be applied before administering any medications, increasing the pressure as the patient loses consciousness. Alternatively, cricoid pressure may be applied just as or immediately after the

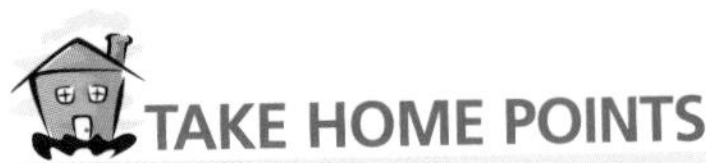

TAKE HOME POINTS

To apply cricoid pressure, remember **B-U-R-P**:

- **B**ackward
- **U**pward (slight)
- **R**ight displacement (slight)
- **P**ressure to occlude the esophagus

Do not remove cricoid pressure until intubation has been successful.

A long-acting neuromuscular-blocking agent should be administered with extreme caution and in consideration of the potential consequences.

patient loses consciousness. Excessive pressure is quite uncomfortable in an awake patient; however, patients lose their protective airway reflexes within one *arm-brain* circulation (10 to 15 seconds), predisposing them to regurgitation and aspiration. Informing conscious patients of the actions and goals before applying any pressure is reassuring.

As previously stated, an RSI does not allow for a test-breath ventilation after the patient is induced. Once preoxygenation is completed and cricoid pressure is applied, an appropriate induction drug is administered, which is followed by a neuromuscular-blocking agent. Succinylcholine (Anectine) is the "gold standard" for RSI because of its rapid onset and short duration of action. However, succinylcholine causes an increase in serum potassium levels of up to 0.5 to 1.0 mEq/L, making it contraindicated in patients with, most notably, burns and neurologic disorders (e.g., denervation injuries, spinal cord injuries, stroke, Guillain-Barré syndrome). These patient groups are potentially susceptible to cardiac-arresting hyperkalemia induced by succinylcholine (Anectine).

In search of a safe alternative for RSI in the patient who cannot take succinylcholine (Anectine), practitioners have traditionally used higher doses of a nondepolarizing neuromuscular-blocking agent such as vecuronium (Norcuron) or the rapid onset nondepolarizer rocuronium (Zemuron). Both drugs may be given in doses that allow for rapid tracheal intubation; however, their duration of action is significantly increased. This increased duration can prove disastrous in cases where the trachea cannot be intubated and the patient cannot then be ventilated with a mask. Again, no test-breath procedure can assess the ability to mask ventilate a patient during an RSI.

Practitioners should also be aware that administering rocuronium (Zemuron) too rapidly after giving sodium thiopental (Pentothal) could lead to remarkable precipitation in the IV line, rendering it unusable. Precipitation can also occur in and adjacent to injection ports of *needleless* systems.

Unconscious patients may be safely intubated without the use of a neuromuscular-blocking agent. In emergency situations and in some elective intubations requiring RSI in which succinylcholine (Anectine) is or may be contraindicated, the use of etomidate (Amidate) can allow successful intubation without the risks involved with the nondepolarizing neuromuscular-blocking agents. A key benefit of etomidate (Amidate) is that many patients continue to ventilate spontaneously, even after receiving an induction dose. Before deciding to skip paralyzation, the person performing an RSI should assess the need for some form of muscle relaxation.

Patients with tightly clenched jaws may not be able to be intubated without some form of pharmacologic relaxation. Only personnel skilled in intubating patients should intubate a patient without some form of neuromuscular blockade.

The delay between the administration of induction medications and the direct laryngoscopy allows for the medications to circulate and have a therapeutic effect. Oxygen should be applied via a mask, whether or not preoxygenation took place before induction. Although no positive-pressure ventilation is applied during this time, the high concentration of oxygen at the mask allows for diffusion.

Most induction medications have an onset of one arm-brain circulation, or about 15 to 20 seconds in patients with normal cardiac outputs. Patients already receiving external cardiac compressions may have extended onset times. Different practitioners administer the neuromuscular-blocking agent (if used) at varying times for RSI. Many wait until the induction agent has had an effect (i.e., loss of eyelid reflex), whereas others administer the paralytic agent immediately after inducing the drug. Still others give the neuromuscular-blocking agent before administering the induction agent to reduce the time delay of an unconscious, apneic patient. This last method may result in an awake but paralyzed patient.

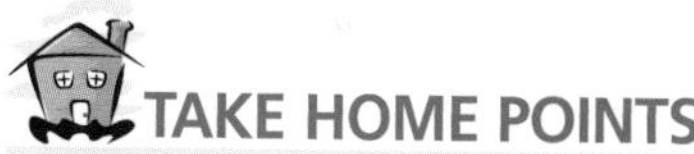

It is crucial to verify the placement of the ETT.

Usually, patients may be safely intubated approximately 1 minute after administering neuromuscular-blocking agents in RSI. Alternatively, the patient may be intubated once muscle fasciculations have ceased if succinylcholine (Anectine) is used. Suction must be immediately available because direct vocal cord visualization can be dramatically hindered by even small amounts of foreign matter in the oropharynx.

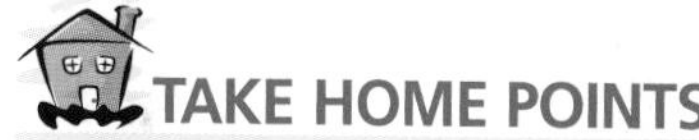

Cricoid pressure may be released only after the ETT placement has been verified. Although the laryngoscopist may ask for changes in the manner of applying cricoid pressure, it should never be completely removed.

Either BBS or $ETCO_2$, or a combination of the two, must be used to verify the placement of the ETT. The definitive standard for ETT placement is an anteroposterior chest x-ray study, which should be obtained as soon as possible.

Prognosis

Up to 40% of emergent intubations are unsuccessful on the first attempt. Any repeated attempts at intubation require some change in technique or current situation. The oropharynx may require deep suctioning, a different laryngoscope blade may be used, or the patient's airway may need to be repositioned.

What You DO

The ability to secure a patent airway in an emergency depends on being prepared. A feared complication of rapid sequence intubation is the inability to intubate and subsequently ventilate the patient. Personnel and equipment preparation are essential components in the management of a failed intubation. Essential equipment should be stored in the resuscitation area and be clearly identified as "difficult airway" equipment. The immediate availability of the following items is imperative:

Standard Intubating Equipment

- Laryngoscope handles with functioning light source
- Multiple laryngoscope blades (Macintosh 3 or 4/Miller 2 or 3)
- Oral endotracheal tubes or various sizes (5.0 to 8.0 mm)
- Stylet
- Ambu-bag with mask
- Oxygen source
- Suction, suction catheter, and Yankauer tip
- Induction and paralytic medications
- Easy cap CO_2 detector
- Stethoscope

Alternative airway equipment should be kept available in case an intubation should become difficult:

Minimum Essential Equipment

- Laryngeal mask airways (LMAs)
- Airways (nasal and oral)
- Tube exchangers (bougies)
- Tracheostomy tubes
- Needle cricothyroidotomy
- Lighted stylet
- Fiberoptic bronchoscope

Meticulous attention to detail, including the proper labeling of the medications used in the induction and intubation of patients, is essential.

The nurse's role may also involve moving the patient and applying cricoid pressure. If the professional performing the intubation uses a flexible stylet in the ETT, then he or she may ask the nurse to remove the stylet once the ETT is past the vocal cords. Only the stylet should be grasped and removed. Too vigorous removal or grasping the ETT may result in accidental extubation.

FIRST-LINE AND INITIAL TREATMENT FOR RSI

- Preoxygenate the patient (may be omitted if airway reflexes are lost or foreign material is observed in the oropharynx).
- Apply cricoid pressure.
- Administer medications (induction without ventilation).
- Provide intubation.
- Check placement of ETT.
- Release cricoid pressure (only after proof of endotracheal intubation [via BBS or $ETCO_2$]).

Do You UNDERSTAND?

DIRECTIONS: Fill in the blanks to complete the following statements.

1. The cricoid cartilage lies ______________________ the thyroid cartilage.
2. Aspiration of as little as __________ mL of gastric contents may result in significant injury to the patient.
3. Mrs. Smith is coming to the labor and delivery department for a scheduled full-term cesarean delivery. She has ingested nothing by mouth for 9 hours. Will she still require an RSI? __________ ______________________________ Why or why not? ______________________________ ______________________________

DIRECTIONS: Select the best answer, and place the appropriate letter in the space provided.

______4. One of the critical dangers of an RSI is:
   a. Increased chance of gastric content aspiration
   b. Inability to preoxygenate conscious patient
   c. Use of fiberoptic scopes
   d. Lack of a test-breath to assess airway patency

______5. Nurses administrating the medications for RSI should watch for which possible problem(s)?
   a. Bovine plasma reactions from administration of succinylcholine (Anectine)

b. Precipitation in the IV line with the use of certain combinations of induction and neuromuscular-blocking agents
c. Ultrashort duration of action of drugs such as rocuronium (Zemuron) and vecuronium (Norcuron)
d. Rapid-eye movements resulting in corneal abrasions

What IS Increased Intracranial Pressure?

Intracranial pressure (ICP) is a dynamic state that **reflects** the pressure of cerebrospinal fluid (CSF) within the skull. Increased ICP is described as pressures $\geq$ 20 mm Hg.

Normal ICP ranges according to age:

- Adults and older children: <10 to 15 mm Hg
- Young children: 3 to 7 mm Hg
- Infants: 1.5 to 6.0 mm Hg

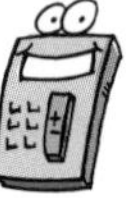

ICP is a dynamic physiologic process that is well regulated and maintained. To understand the pathophysiologic characteristics of increased ICP, certain neurologic concepts must become familiar. These include intracranial compliance, intracranial elastance, the Monro-Kellie hypothesis, cerebral blood flow (CBF), and cerebral perfusion pressure (CPP).

Intracranial compliance is the ability of the brain to tolerate increases in intracranial volume without adversely increasing ICP.

Intracranial compliance:

$$\text{Compliance} = \frac{\text{Volume}}{\text{Pressure}}$$

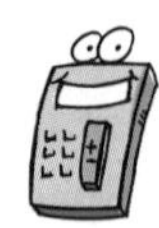

The ability of the brain to respond to intracranial volume changes with no increase in ICP indicates normal and adequate compliance. In contrast, a low compliance indicates that a small volume increase exists, which will cause an elevation in ICP.

Answers: **1. below; 2. 25; 3. Yes, All obstetric deliveries require an RSI; 4. d; 5. b.**

Intracranial elastance is the ability of the brain to tolerate and compensate for an increase in intracranial volume through distention or displacement.

Intracranial elastance:

$$\text{Elastance} = \frac{\text{Pressure}}{\text{Volume}}$$

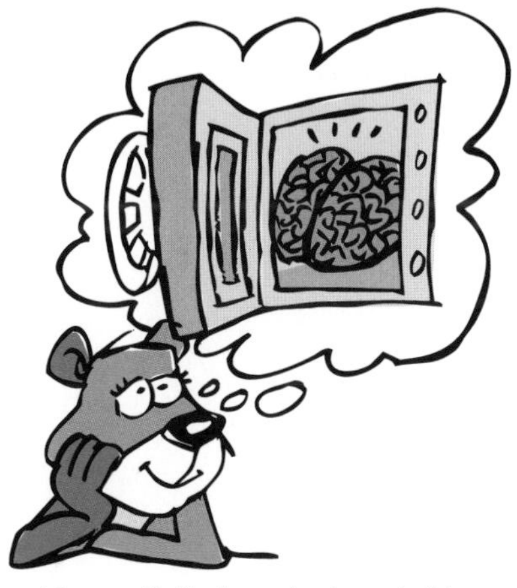

Monroe-Kellie hypothesis = skull is a closed, rigid vault containing brain tissue, blood, and CSF.

High elastance means that the brain is tight because the intracranial volume and the ability to distend and displace intracranial components is at its limit, resulting in a significant elevation of ICP.

The *Monro-Kellie hypothesis* states that the skull acts as a closed, rigid vault containing the intracranial components of brain tissue (84%), blood (4%), and CSF (12%) under which the total brain volume remains fixed.

When any one of the three components increases in volume, another must decrease to maintain the overall volume.

Normal intracranial values:

$$\text{Normal Intracranial Values} = \text{1700 to 1900 mL intracranial contents}$$

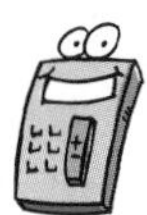

CBF delivers oxygen to the tissues in the brain and maintains cerebral perfusion through the compensatory mechanism of autoregulation. When changes in the blood pressure (BP) occur, cerebral blood vessels automatically constrict or dilate to maintain perfusion and deliver oxygen to the tissues. Autoregulation is maintained with a mean arterial pressure (MAP) of 50 to 70 mm Hg.

CPP is defined as a pressure gradient across the brain and is the difference between the arterial blood entering and the return of venous blood exiting the neurovascular system. It is viewed as an estimated pressure and is calculated as the difference between the incoming MAP and the opposing ICP on the arteries, which is affected by the ability of the venous volume to exit.

Cerebral perfusion pressure:

$$\text{CPP} = \text{MAP} - \text{ICP}$$

$$\text{MAP} = \frac{\text{Systolic BP (SBP)} + 2(\text{Diastolic BP [DPB]})}{3}$$

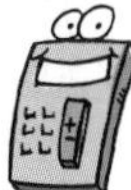

What You NEED TO KNOW

Monitoring ICP and recognizing increased ICP is crucial when caring for patients with neurologic diseases. ICP is a dynamic physiologic process. In the uninjured brain, mild transient elevations and fluctuations occur in everyday activities such as coughing or sneezing. During these periods of mild elevations, the process of autoregulation makes adjustments to accommodate the transient elevation in ICP. However, with the loss of autoregulation (i.e., an injured brain), the mild, transient increases in ICP cause the cell membrane to become more permeable, which disrupts the normal sodium and potassium pump. This loss also allows for the leakage of proteins and fluids into the brain tissue, which causes cerebral edema. Cerebral edema increases the tissue volume of the brain, which increases ICP and decreases CPP. Patients who are considered to be at risk for increased ICP include those with:

- Head injury
- Intracranial hematoma
- Glasgow Coma Scale (GCS) score < 8
- Decorticate or decerebrate (or both) posturing
- Space-occupying lesion (tumor, abscess, infection)
- Hypoxia
- Hypercarbia
- Cerebral edema (secondary to surgery, trauma, aneurysm, hemorrhage)
- Hydrocephalus

Elevations in ICP produce changes in the patient's neurologic assessment. These changes may be subtle or occur rapidly.

Early Signs and Symptoms of Increased Intracranial Pressure

- Changes in level of consciousness
- Restlessness
- Irritability
- Mild confusion
- Decreased Glasgow Coma Scale score
- Changes in personality
- Changes in pupil size or reactivity
- Motor or sensory deficits (e.g., paresthesia, weakness of extremities)
- Changes in speech (slurred, inappropriate, aphasia)
- Headache (early morning, especially upon waking)
- Vomiting (frequently without nausea)

Late Signs and Symptoms of Increased Intracranial Pressure

- Abnormal posturing
- Absent Babinski reflex
- Arm drift
- Changes in level of consciousness
  - Decreased level of arousal
  - Decreased GCS score
- Changes in respiratory patterns (irregular to apnea)
- Changes in speech (slurred, inappropriate, none)
- Changes in vital signs (Cushing triad: bradycardia, hypertension, irregular respirations)
- Cranial nerve dysfunction (cough, gag, corneal reflexes)
- Decreased reaction or no response to painful stimuli
- Flaccidity of extremities
- Hemiparesis
- Hemiplegia on opposite side of brain affected
- Loss of protective reflexes
- Motor deficits
- Possible seizure activity
- Pupil changes (unilateral or bilateral dilation)
- Weakness
- ECG changes (Q waves with ST depression, elevated T waves, supraventricular tachycardia, sinus bradycardia, AV blocks, preventricular contractions, agonal rhythm) leading to cardiac arrest

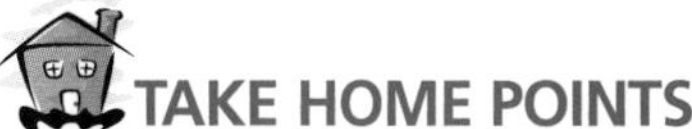

In the injured brain, the compliance is low and the degree of elastance is high; thus, the brain is unable to accommodate the fluctuations in the volume (fluid, blood, tissue) that can cause dangerous elevations of ICP.

Dangerous, sustained elevations in ICP can lead to brainstem compression and herniation of brain tissue, resulting in coma and ultimately death.

What You DO

Monitoring and identifying increased ICP is achieved through the use of various ICP monitoring devices: ventricular catheters, subarachnoid screws and bolts, parenchymal implanted devices, and epidural sensors. Each device has its own advantages and disadvantages. The monitoring device of choice is often dependent on the type of injury or the anticipated intervention or both.

Continuous ICP monitoring is routine in evaluating and managing intracranial disorders. The process of monitoring ICP requires a monitoring device sensor that may be inserted in the operating department or at the patient's bedside. Once the sensor is in place, the device is connected to a transducer cable, which goes to the bedside monitor. The pressure signal is conducted through the transducer, which translates the pressure to a visual image (waveform) and a numeric value.

Although ICP is monitored with a transducer, a fluid-coupled system is not connected to heparinized or saline-flush solution. Nothing should be infused into intracranial contents.

The purposes of ICP and CPP monitoring are to diagnose increased ICP, enable interventions, and provide tools for predicting the level of injury and patient outcome. The goals of monitoring ICP and CPP are to (1) restore them to normal values, (2) prevent serious and prolonged elevations in ICP, (3) prevent serious and prolonged decreases in CPP, (4) provide a means to reduce ICP, and (5) provide a means to maintain CPP.

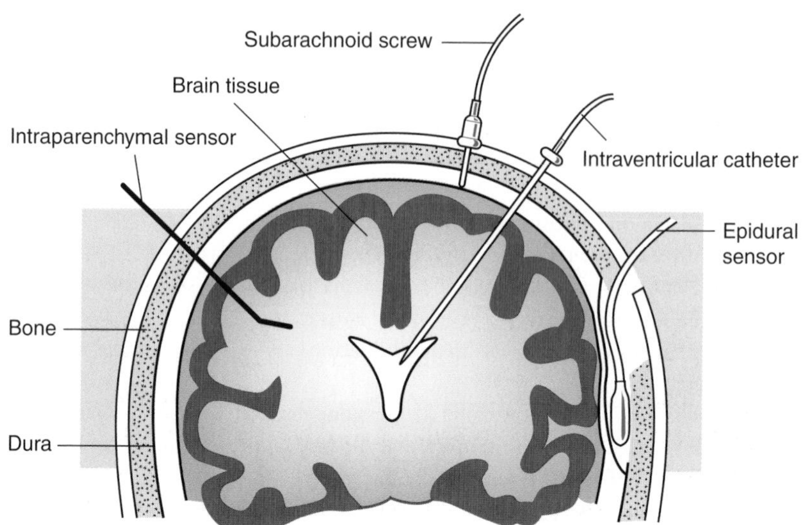

Four ICP monitoring devices. *(From Bucher L, Melander S:* Critical care nursing, *Philadelphia, 1999, WB Saunders.)*

ICP Monitoring Devices: Advantages and Disadvantages

ICP Monitoring Device	Advantages	Disadvantages
Subarachnoid bolt and screw	Less invasive	Unable to drain CSF
Parenchymal sensor	Decreased infection Not dependent on ventricular placement Provides wave and numeric value Does not require set-up and maintenance of fluid-coupled system	Can be unreliable with excessive (high) values Risk for leaks Risk for hemorrhage Risk for hematoma
Intraventricular catheter	Most reliable Ability to drain CSF Ability to sample and observe CSF Ability to administer intrathecal medications	Increases chance of infection (indwelling device) May become clogged with debris (tissue, blood) Difficult to place (especially with swollen brain) Values and drainage are level-dependent (depending on positioning and calibration)
Epidural	Lowest risk of infection Easy to insert Can be used in the neonate	Unable to drain or sample CSF May provide false readings

CSF, Cerebrospinal fluid.

Interventions used in the treatment of increased ICP and the manipulation of ICP and CPP include the following:

- Body positioning (head in straight alignment—care should be taken to avoid slight flexion caused by pillows)
- Elevation of head of bed ≤30 degrees
- Prone position and extreme flexion of hips, avoiding the Trendelenburg position
- Staggered timing and sequence of nursing care
- Controlled environmental conditions (quiet, darkened room)
- Temperature controlled to maintain normal or mild hypothermia (≤37° C [≤98.6° F])
- BP control, maintaining CBF and CPP
- CSF drainage
- Fluid restriction
- Ventilation and airway management
- Medications: osmotic diuretics, steroids, anticonvulsants, barbiturates, vasoactive drugs (to increase or decrease BP), sedatives, analgesics

Because of its potent effects on cerebral blood vessels, the ability to control and manipulate ventilation management is an important intervention for decreasing and maintaining ICP. Preventing hypoxia and monitoring oxygen and carbon dioxide (CO_2) levels are critical skills. Preventing hypoxia (oxygen tension in the arterial blood [PaO_2] at < 60 mm Hg) is achieved through administering oxygen and monitoring pulse oximetry readings and blood gas values. Monitoring arterial CO_2 is vital because of its potent vasoconstrictive properties with cerebral blood vessels. Hyperventilation works by decreasing the arterial level of CO_2 ($PaCO_2$), which causes vasoconstriction of the cerebral arteries that result in reducing CBF and decreasing ICP. Controlled hyperventilation means that the $PaCO_2$ is kept at the low-to-normal range. To control acute ICP elevations, hyperventilation is an immediate and key intervention that should be instituted by manually hyperventilating the patient for a brief period.

Recently, advanced invasive techniques for monitoring brain tissue oxygen ($PbtO_2$) have been instituted. Hypoxia at the brain tissue level has been linked to poor outcomes, so monitoring efforts are being aimed at early detection and intervention to prevent secondary brain injury. Brain tissue oxygen is monitored by inserting a catheter into the white matter of the brain, and the catheter is connected to a device calibrated to measure brain tissue oxygenation. Another useful technique for measuring cerebral oxygenation is jugular venous oxygen saturation ($SjvO_2$)

Prolonged hyperventilation can reduce cerebral perfusion, cause shifts in the intracranial dynamics, and result in cerebral ischemia or infarction.

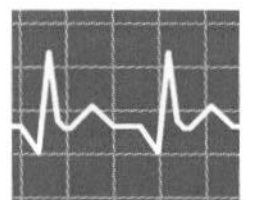

Intracranial dynamic monitoring levels:
Desired CPP levels: 60 to 70 mm Hg,
Desired MAP levels: >60 mm Hg

Osmotic diuretics can cause hypotension and tachycardia, which can compromise CBF and CPP. In addition, rapid fluid shifts from healthy to injured brain tissue can result in increased swelling and increased ICP.

monitoring, which is performed through a fiberoptic catheter positioned in the bulb of the jugular vein.

Positive end-expiratory pressure (PEEP) should be used with caution because it can decrease venous drainage and outflow, which increases ICP and CPP.

Monitoring and maintaining BP within desired limits is critical to maintaining ICP, CPP, and CBF. Physicians designate MAPs and systolic parameters that are to be maintained. MAP and CPP values can be manipulated through the use of various IV vasoactive agents such as dopamine (Intropin) and sodium nitroprusside (Nipride).

Osmotic diuretics such as mannitol (Osmitrol) are also an effective management strategy for reducing ICP. Mannitol (Osmitrol) has a rapid effect on ICP, and its onset is 10 to 15 minutes.

The placement of a ventricular catheter allows for CSF to be drained. Physician prescriptions and protocols usually allow for the drainage of CSF to maintain certain ICP levels.

Intracranial dynamics and increased ICP are important concepts to master to adequately assess, intervene, and monitor a patient in trauma.

Do You UNDERSTAND?

DIRECTIONS: **Fill in the blanks to complete each of the following statements with the appropriate words provided in the list below.**

aphasia
blood pressure
cerebral blood flow
cerebral edema
cerebral perfusion pressure
cerebral spinal fluid
compliance
decorticate
elastance
epidural
hyperventilation
intraventricular catheter
Monro-Kellie hypothesis
parenchymal sensor
pressure
pupil changes
restlessness
Trendelenburg
vasoconstriction
vasodilation
volume

1. Intracranial ______________________ is the ability of the brain to tolerate intracranial volume increases without increasing ICP.

2. ______________________________ is calculated by subtracting the ICP reading from the MAP and estimating the pressure gradient across the brain.
3. ______________________________ (unilateral or bilateral dilation) are a late sign of increased ICP.
4. Using a(n) ______________________________ is the most reliable means of monitoring ICP.
5. ______________________________ is an early sign of increased ICP.
6. The ______________________________ position should be avoided because it can actually increase ICP.
7. ______________________________ is used to keep $PaCO_2$ low, which causes ______________________________ of the cerebral arteries and decreases CBF and ICP.
8. To maintain ICP, CPP, and CBF, the patient's ______________________________ must be frequently monitored.

What IS Traumatic Brain Injury?

Traumatic brain injury (TBI) is a collective term describing a wide range of pathologic conditions and types of trauma involving the brain. TBI occurs when a substantial force—which can be blunt, penetrating, or a combination of the two—strikes the skull. The result is a brain injury. TBI is one of the leading causes of trauma death, and is responsible for nearly 50% of the 150,000 injury-related deaths in the United States yearly. Not only is TBI the most lethal of all trauma-related injuries, but its survivors also suffer the greatest disability with long-term effects and deficits.

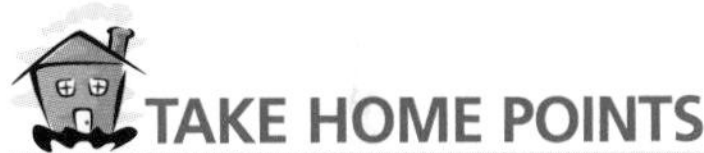

The mechanism of injury (MOI) or the extent of the injury—its effects and survivability—has many factors and is ultimately unique to each individual patient.

The contributory causes of TBI are customarily associated with motor vehicle crashes (MVCs), sports injuries, falls, and violence. Head trauma occurs when the generated force is greater than the cranial vault can absorb, transferring the kinetic injury to the delicate neural tissues beneath. The specific categories of TBI are discussed later in this chapter.

Initial assessment may be deceiving. For example, in the patient with a closed-head injury, brain damage may not be obvious because of an absence of external blood.

Understanding the basic anatomy, physiology, types of injury, and effects of trauma on the brain, as well as the rapid recognition of these signs and

Answers: 1. compliance; 2. cerebral perfusion pressure; 3. pupil changes; 4. intraventricular catheter; 5. restlessness; 6. Trendelenburg; 7. Hyperventilation, vasoconstriction; 8. blood pressure.

symptoms, is imperative in treating patients with brain trauma. Even a basic comprehension of TBI and its mechanisms can assist in the delivery of quality nursing care. The study and management of the central nervous system (CNS) can be intimidating and complex; however, it can be easily learned with the knowledge of a few simple facts and treatment principles.

What You NEED TO KNOW

Types of Trauma Brain Injury

Five major types of primary TBI have been established: (1) skull fractures, (2) concussion, (3) contusion, (4) diffuse axonal injury, and (5) hematomas.

When a patient suffers a *skull fracture,* approximately two out of every three patients acquire a mild-to-severe brain injury. A single blunt strike, which usually fractures along a fissure line in the cranium, is called a *linear fracture.* The linear fracture is most common, accounting for 75% to 80% of all skull fractures. The linear fracture is highly associated with subdural and epidural bleeds. A backward fall that is significant enough to cause a fracture to the skull usually involves the occiput, which is a *basal skull fracture.* These fractures can involve a shifting of bone articulations (e.g., break away or opening of the occipitosphenoidal fissure). These fractures are not usually life threatening but may disrupt the meningeal layers and allow leakage of CSF and blood from the ears and nose. A closer assessment finding of a basal skull fracture includes ecchymosis at the site of the mastoid process (battle signs) or around the periorbital area (raccoon eyes) or both.

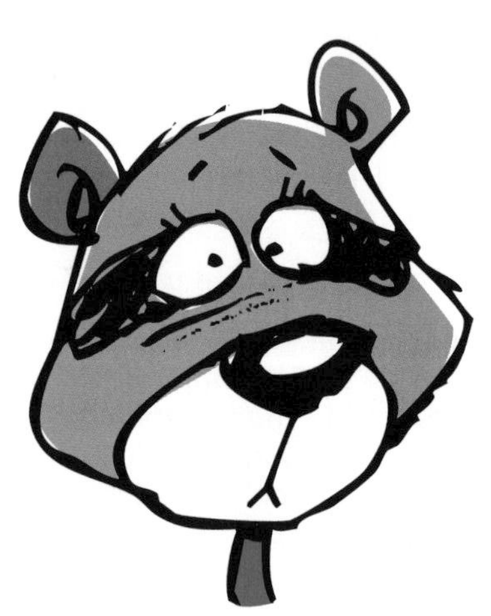

Raccoon eyes is a sign of basal skull fracture.

This injury often exposes the brain to the exterior environment with disruption of the *cribriform plate,* which is a small, thin bone that is separated by tissue in the nasal cavity. The patient with this type of fracture is at risk for encephalitis and meningitis. Another type of cranial bone injury is a *depressed skull fracture,* which may cause contusion or laceration to the brain tissue. If a fracture with a perforated scalp is observed, then it is an *open fracture.* The patient with this type of fracture is also at risk for developing an infection. The disruption of bones can damage brain tissue, vessels, and cranial nerves as they pass through the skull, requiring diligent and ongoing neurologic assessments.

A *concussion* is a direct brain injury involving neural tissue (**neural parenchyma**); it is generally mild but may have underlying pathologic consequences such as slow subdural bleed that is not observed until days after the injury. The MOI involving concussion is usually associated with a blunt trauma from a blow to the head or from a fall. The injury is traditionally diagnosed by the patient's manifestation of symptoms because obvious physical injury is not always present. In cases of concussion, a complete recovery usually occurs; however, many patients suffer amnesia involving events surrounding the trauma. In moderate-to-severe concussions, the symptoms may include a loss of consciousness, a diminished or complete loss of deep tendon reflexes (DTRs), and an apneic episode in some patients. The energy absorbed through the cranium is believed to stun the brain to the point of momentarily ceasing neurologic function; similar to the use of a defibrillator on the myocardium.

The edema and extent of the bleeding from a contusion are an immediate clinical concern.

Contusions occur when the head suffers a direct impact with a rigid object. The MOI is similar to that of a concussion but more severe. When the tissue damage occurs directly at the site of impact, it is categorized as a *coup injury*. A more involved contusion is often a result of an acceleration-deceleration event. This MOI causes the brain to shift rapidly and strike one side and then the opposing side of the cranium, causing lesions in two areas of the brain, known as a *coup-contrecoup injury*. The cerebral contusion is most often seen in temporal and frontal lobes of the brain. The contusion produces tissue edema and capillary hemorrhage.

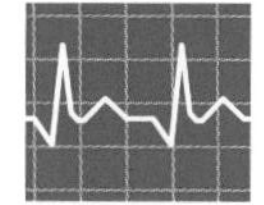

The degree and progression of the injury requires close monitoring and frequent neurologic testing to track the onset of subtle changes in neurologic status that indicate increased ICP.

Diffuse axonal injury (DAI) describes extensive damage involving a wide area of neural tissues throughout the cerebrum and brainstem. Up to this point, the injuries discussed primarily involved localized lesions in the outer neural gray matter. Diffuse axonal injury refers to damage that involves the innermost centroaxial areas of the neural white matter. These injuries disrupt the neural network fibers and tracts that facilitate communication among the brainstem, cerebellum, and hemispheres of the cerebrum. This type of injury is associated with MOI involving mechanical sheering forces generated by an MVC or other similar events. Diffuse axonal injuries occur in approximately one-half of all trauma-related comas and are responsible for long-term neural deficits in the recovering patient with a TBI.

Symptoms of TBI may be progressive, which requires vigilant monitoring of neurologic functions, ensuring the patient's subtle changes are appropriately tracked.

An *epidural hematoma* develops under the arterial pressure of the bleed, which tears the periosteal layer (a part of the dura mater) from the cranium as the hematoma expands, resulting in the compression of brain tissue. The symptoms may involve a rapid onset of neurologic signs, or the patient may remain lucid many hours after the TBI and then suddenly deteriorate. An epidural hematoma is an emergency condition that requires the hematoma to be drained quickly to prevent permanent brain damage.

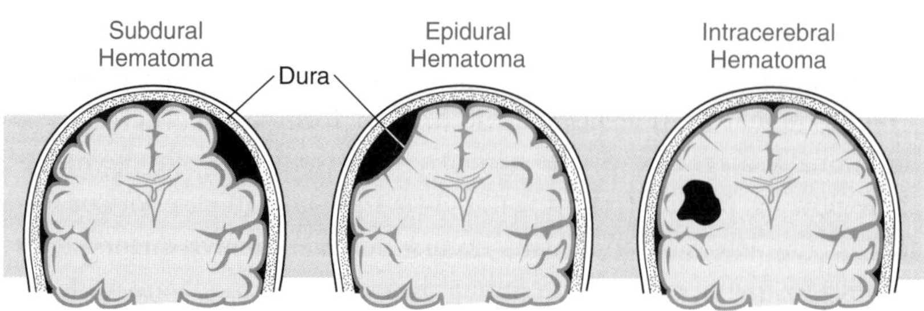

(*From Urden L, Stacy K, Lough M:* Thelan's critical care nursing: diagnosis and management, *ed 4, St Louis, 2002, Mosby.)*

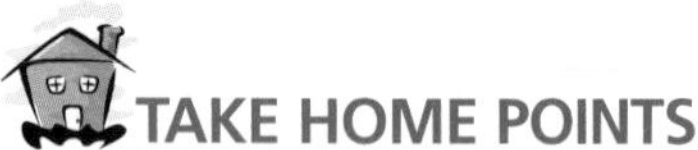

TAKE HOME POINTS

An epidural hematoma is an arterial bleed and develops quickly; a subdural hematoma is a venous bleed and develops slowly.

A *subdural hematoma* is an intracranial venous bleed involving the space between the dura meningeal layer and the arachnoid layer. A subdural hematoma often involves the bridging veins that transverse the dura mater, occurring commonly on the lateral aspects of the hemispheres of the cerebrum. Subdural hematomas expand as a result of venous bleeding (low pressure bleed), and the onset of symptoms are slow in developing—beginning from as early as 48 hours to as long as 2 weeks after head injury. Characteristic symptoms include increased drowsiness, confusion, and nonlocalizing headache directly related to the increase of ICP. A minor head injury can initially cause similar signs and symptoms observed in the subdural bleed.

Without a solid knowledge base and understanding of TBI, a serious injury could be easily overlooked.

Other traumatic intracranial hematomas that may occur include bleeding into the ventricles, subarachnoid space, and superior sagittal sinus. Any of these bleeds can occur together and may involve any combination of the previously mentioned TBIs. Patients with intracranial hemorrhage quickly lose their ability to physiologically compensate, and this development can occur with less than 100 mL of blood.

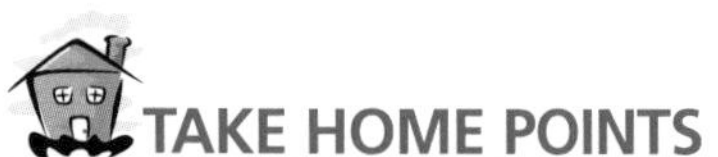

TAKE HOME POINTS

Survivability is low in the patient with a catastrophic brain injury.

A catastrophic brain injury is a severe injury in which the cranium is exposed to extraordinary force involving MVCs, falls from significant heights, mechanical crushing, and missile penetration. The brain's direct or indirect absorption of this momentous kinetic energy (KE) lacerates or tears the parenchymal tissue, causing a disruption of the meninges, neural tissue, nerve tracts, and blood vessels. A TBI caused by a projectile that forcefully enters the cranium creates a cavitation that displaces tissue in the brain, delivering direct and extensive damage as it travels through the cranium and possibly exits the skull. This patient often has a terminal prognosis; if only the brain is involved, the patient becomes a prime candidate for organ donation.

Secondary Brain Injuries

A *secondary brain injury* consists of neurologic tissue damage that occurs after the initial injury and increases the morbidity and mortality of the patient, a result of the brain's reduced ability to maintain a homeostatic environment. Most often, MAP, CBF, ICP, and CPP are adversely affected. As the symptoms and damage progress, hypoventilation and hypoperfusion states lead to acid-base issues, causing the accumulation of cellular toxins and decreasing the autoregulation ability. Once the blood flow to the brain becomes compromised, the brain tissue does not receive oxygen or essential nutrients (e.g., glucose) that are carried in the blood, resulting in further injury. A late sign of severe cerebral ischemia is the *Cushing response,* a feedback mechanism that attempts to reduce the ischemia by increasing CBF. If the rising ICP is not treated, death ultimately occurs as the brainstem herniates through the foramen magnum, ceasing all cardiopulmonary function and causing brain death. Understanding the intracranial perfusion principles is of paramount importance in managing complications caused by TBI. (Refer to the discussion on increased ICP on p. 62).

If secondary brain injury goes uncontrolled, the risk of mortality doubles.

What You DO

When acutely impaired patients arrive in the emergency department or trauma center, basic standardized steps are initiated. Without a uniform approach, patients with horrific wounds can easily distract care team members and crucial resuscitative steps can be omitted. The operational tenet of the ABC algorithm is to "keep it simple," which allows the care team to function in an orchestrated manner during stressful, time-sensitive events involving TBI.

The first and most important step is airway evaluation. Patients with extensive brain injury usually arrive at the hospital via the emergency medical service (EMS), often with initial airway measures accomplished. In TBI cases, other than obvious foreign body obstruction or traumatic injury to the oral pharynx, an accepted threshold for initiating RSI is based on the patient's GCS score (usually GCS < 8) and the patient's inability to protect his or her airway. Adhering to cervical spine precautions at all times is imperative because of the increased risk of cervical spine fracture, which is four to six times more likely in a patient with a TBI. As the assessment begins, key questions are asked to treat and anticipate the immediate needs of the patient (refer to the discussion on RSI on p. 53).

Assessment Question 1

Is the patient's GCS score at 9 or above?

Yes	No
Use supplemental oxygen. Continue assessment.	Prepare to implement RSI protocol. Intubate. Securely fasten ETT. Set up appropriate oxygen delivery system. Limit ETT movement (manipulation can irritate the vagus nerve and therefore increase ICP). Suction equipment available (increased ICP can cause projectile emesis and posttraumatic seizures).

When evaluating the respiratory status of a patient with a TBI, hypoxia along with the TBI can further increase the ICP, decreasing both MAP and CBF and further injuring the brain by increasing ischemia. Aggressive hyperventilation is not recommended; however, maintaining a $PaCO_2$ of approximately 35 mm Hg should be the therapeutic goal for ventilation management.

Assessment Question 2

Is the patient able to ventilate adequately with a spontaneous regular rate and effort?

Yes	No
Continue assessment: Rate and depth of respirations Saturations (pulse oximeter > 97%) Satisfactory arterial blood gas results	Assist with breathing (high-flow oxygen and airway delivery systems). Consider intubation, if not already intubated. Maintain normocapnia ($PaCO_2$ of ~35 mm Hg); may require hyperventilation of patient. Elevate head of the bed if not contraindicated.

The degree of injury and the brain's ability to compensate are reflected in the circulatory system's response. Assessing the patient's circulatory status involves distinguishing the rate, rhythm, and intensity of the pulse. Next, assess for secondary signs of hypoxia, such as cool, clammy skin and cyanosis of the nail beds and oral membranes. Treating hypotension is a priority over other interventions for the brain injury: Problems must be corrected early to maintain CBF and CPP. Hemodynamic monitoring protocols must be initiated and therapeutic modalities need to be used to help keep the patient's circulation within normal or acceptable parameters.

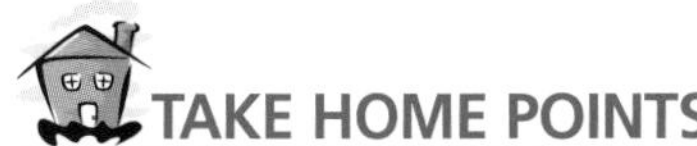

The identification of low BP and rapid reversal of this deficit provides positive outcomes in managing TBI.

Assessment Question 3

Is the patient's systolic blood pressure (SBP) above 90 mm Hg, and are there strong peripheral pulses?

Yes	No
Obtain 1 or 2 IV sites (preferably 18-gauge). Continue assessment. Await fluid and medication orders.	Obtain two large-bore (16-gauge) IV sites; may need to assist in central line placement if one is not in existance. Prepare to deliver crystalloid rapidly or other colloid IV fluids. Obtain rapid fluid infuser. Closely monitor cardiovascular status. Anticipate the use of emergency medications. Place urinary catheter. Closely monitor fluid status (intake and output).

If a nasogastric (NG) tube is needed, extreme caution must be taken during placement. An undiagnosed skull fracture could allow the NG tube to perforate the parenchyma of the brain.

The *ABCs* **(airway, breathing, circulation)** of trauma resuscitation are the primary life-saving measures used in stabilizing the patient, but **D** for *disability* is the treatment step that collectively takes the brain injury into account. This step incorporates ABC management to help reduce secondary brain injury and thus improves the patient's chance of recovery. The "tools of the trade" are used to obtain a baseline neurologic examination to help determine the primary injury, anticipate urgent care needs, and further monitor the stabilization process. In addition, the nurse needs to anticipate using therapeutic medications to help in stabilize the patient with TBI.

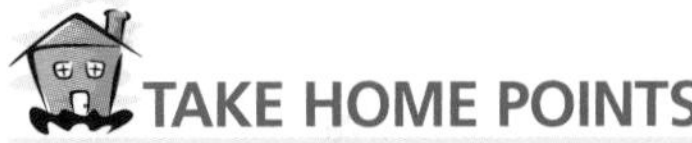

The early hours after brain injury, intervention is critical but the at the same time the brain is fragile and vulnerable. During this time continuous monitoring of vital signs and the neurologic status an essential task for the nurse.

The nursing objective in caring for the patient with TBI is vigilant, accurate, and objective monitoring. This objective is achieved with a strong knowledge base of anatomy, physiology, and keen observational skills. Regardless of the skill level, a standardized tool or instrument needs to be used properly to quantify the patient's assessments and to make comparative assessments.

The most prominent and widely used tool for tracking a patient's neurologic baseline and injury progression is the GCS. The GCS uses a number system to describe level of consciousness (LOC). The GCS ranges from 3 (poor, no response) to 15 (normal). The GCS rates (1) eye opening, (2) motor movement of the arms and legs, and (3) verbal response. Adding the scores from the three parts of the scale produces an overall score. Importantly, the GCS does not determine or predict the patient's final outcome.

A complete neurologic examination requires assessment of the pupils and extremities. These assessment components are completed in the mental status, motor movement, and cranial nerve assessments along with pupil responses. Neurologic changes and trends are best observed by conducting serial assessments, using a standardized format, and ensuring that all elements are approached in the similar manner. These standardized serial assessments ensure that each examiner encounters less variation and can thus provide a more objective clinical record.

Glasgow Coma Scale

Eye Opening

4 = Spontaneous
3 = Response to voice
2 = Response to pain
1 = No response

Best Motor Response

6 = Follows commands
5 = Localizes to pain
4 = Withdrawal to pain
3 = Decorticate (flexion to pain)
2 = Decerebrate (extension to pain)
1 = No response

Best Verbal Response

5 = Oriented and converses
4 = Disoriented and converses
3 = Inappropriate words
2 = Incomprehensible sounds
1 = No response

Note: Best score is 15; the lowest score is 3.

Components of Neurologic Assessment

Mental Status

- Level of consciousness (GCS score)
- Orientation (time, person, place)
- Memory (ability to recall three items)
- Judgment (process of forming an opinion that is accurate and reasonable)
- Cognition (serial 7s)

Motor Testing

- Flex and extend all extremity joints against resistance
- Grading:
  - 5/5: Movement against gravity with full resistance
  - 4/5: Movement against gravity with some resistance
  - 3/5: Movement against gravity only
  - 2/5: Movement with gravity eliminated
  - 1/5: Visible and palpable muscle contraction; no movement
  - 0/5: No contraction

Cranial Nerves

- Olfactory—assessment of ability to smell
- Optic—assessment of vision; document pupils—equal, round, reactive to light and accommodation (PERRLA)
- Oculomotor—assessment of eye movement and tracking
- Trochlear—assessment of eye movement
- Trigeminal—assessment of bilateral facial sensation and ability to chew
- Abducens—assessment of lateral eye movement
- Facial—assessment of whether smile is symmetric
- Auditory—assessment of hearing and balance
- Glossopharyngeal—assessment of gag reflex and ability to feel ears
- Vagus—observe the soft palate and check to see whether arch is symmetric (the "aahh" test)
- Accessory—assessment of shoulder muscle resistance as patient shrugs shoulders
- Hypoglossal—assessment of tongue position

GCS, Glasgow Coma Scale.

The recurring theme in managing the patient with TBI is the importance of monitoring and managing the ICP. The immediate treatment goal in the acute phase of brain injury is to keep the patient's environment quiet to avoid agitating the patient further and inadvertently increasing the ICP. Equally important in reducing elevated ICP are medications designed to manage and reduce the fluid (blood or obstructed CSF) and edema collecting on the brain. Only a few medications are available for use in the

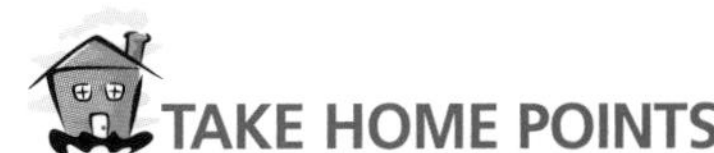

The GCS provides a common language and quickly communicates the patient's neurologic status to other health care providers.

A drop of more than 2 points in the total GCS score is a sign of dangerous neurologic deterioration.

TAKE HOME POINTS

Pupil changes will be on the same side **(ipsilateral)** as the brain injury; extremity symptoms (weakness) will be in the opposite side **(contralateral)**.

Corticosteroid therapy—current research indicates that the use of steroids is not beneficial in the treatment of ICP. In addition, they suppress immune response, placing the patient at increased risk for infection. The drug is not contraindicated and may still be used in some hospital settings.

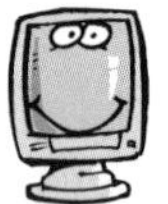

Website Information

Brain Injury Association www.biausa.org

Brain Trauma Foundation www.braintrauma.org

American Association of Neuroscience Nurses www.aann.org

treatment of TBI; when these agents fail or require augmentation, invasive procedures are then used to relieve pressure on the brain. (Refer to the discussion on increased ICP on p. 64.)

The pharmacologic agents discussed in this chapter and the box that follows offer a brief overview of the pharmacologic treatments in managing TBI. The dosing information provided is only an example, and an approved drug reference should always be consulted when administering medications to patients.

Pharmacologic Treatments

Modality 1: Sedation

Benzodiazepines

- Midazolam (Versed)—used most often to prevent agitation
  Adults: Titrate slowly to achieve desired effect. Usual dose range is between 1 and 5 mg IV administered over a 2-minute period.

Opiates

- Morphine sulfate used to treat pain
  Adults: 4 to 10 mg IV; with appropriate dose titration, there is no maximum dose of morphine.

Modality 2: Fluid Reduction

Osmotic diuretics

- Mannitol (Osmitrol)—predominate drug used in the United States*
  Adults: Initially, 1.0 to 2.0 g/kg IV, followed by 0.25 to 1.00 g/kg IV q4h

*The mechanism of action mannitol (Osmitrol) remains unclear; however, it reduces ICP, draws water off the brain, can affect cardiac preload, and, in turn, increases CBF.

At this point in the patient's treatment, assessment and reassessment continues with a goal of obtaining radiologic studies (e.g., computed tomography [CT], x-ray series, and possibly a magnetic resonance image [MRI], depending on availability and condition of the patient). Baseline blood work is prescribed with close attention to arterial blood gas (ABG) results, hemoglobin, hematocrit, and other values based on the complete patient history. The extent of the patient's TBI and resultant deficits is determined during the first hours or days after the initial care is received.

Although TBI is usually presented as a singular injury, approximately 75% of patients with brain trauma have significant injuries to other body systems. The actual resuscitation is more complex, but the basics for the resuscitation are the same.

Do You UNDERSTAND?

DIRECTIONS: **Provide the spelled out meaning of each of the following acronyms.**

1. MVC: ____________________
2. CPP: ____________________
3. GCS: ____________________
4. MOI: ____________________

DIRECTIONS: **Identify the following statements as *true* (T) or *false* (F).**

_____5. When skull fractures result from a TBI, the most common fracture is a linear (single fissure) fracture.

_____6. The most at-risk demographic for suffering TBIs is the adult woman younger than 30 years of age.

DIRECTIONS: **Match the types of TBIs in Column A with the most appropriate descriptions in Column B.**

Column A	Column B
_____7. Depressed skull fracture	a. Localized lesion on the brain; predominantly limited to the area of impact on the skull
_____8. Brain contusion	b. May cause a contusion or laceration to the brain tissue. This injury may or may not be associated with a perforated scalp.
_____9. Epidural hematoma	c. Venous bleed under the dura mater
	d. Deep-tissue injury in the brain, disrupting neural paths and involving white matter
	e. Arterial bleed between the cranium and dura mater

DIRECTIONS: **Provide short answers to the following questions.**

10. What classification of pharmaceuticals is used to sedate patients with severe TBI?

____

11. Why is mannitol used to treat some patients with TBI?

____

12. Which cranial nerve is tested to assess the gag reflex?

____

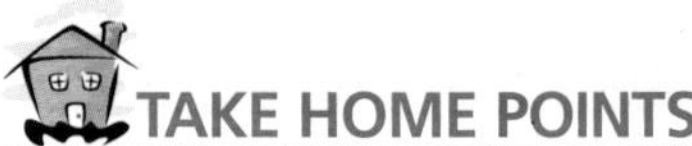
TAKE HOME POINTS

Kinetic energy, which is carried by the bullet and subsequently transferred into the tissues, causes the damage in a gunshot victim.

What IS Acute Hemorrhage Related to Gunshot Wound?

Penetrating trauma is one of the leading causes of hemorrhage, and gunshot wounds are the leading source of high-velocity penetrating trauma. These injuries are often treatment challenges, particularly because only a small hole may be observed externally; however, internal injuries may be massive and life threatening.

What You NEED TO KNOW

Once a bullet penetrates the skin, it meets resistance as it travels at a high velocity through the tissues, creating an enlarged, cone-shaped path that results in significant damage to tissues. The bullet either exits or comes to rest within the body. According to the *American Trauma Life Support (ATLS) Manual,* the important indicators for determining the extent of injuries include the gun caliber, the presumed path and velocity of the bullet, and the distance from the weapon to the victim's entrance point. Suicides are usually single shot intraoral wounds whereas homicides are multiple shots to the temporoparietal region.

Many sources describe the entrance wound (inlet velocity) (V_1) as the maximal point of energy. If the bullet never exits the body, the exit wound (**outlet velocity**) (V_2) is said to be zero. One bullet can cause tremendous damage by deflecting off bone and traveling across the body, damaging many structures in its path. As the projectile of the bullet travels, it meets resistance of the tissues, which is known as *retardation.* The high V_1 creates

Answers: **1. motor vehicle crash; 2. cerebral perfusion pressure; 3. Glasgow Coma Scale; 4. mechanism of injury; 5. True; 6. False; 7. B; 8. A; 9. E; 10. benzodiazepines; 11. decreased ICP by drawing water off the brain; 12. glossopharyngeal.**

an inward path along which the bullet travels, but a negative pressure also exists behind the bullet, which pulls debris and bacteria into the wound.

The path subsequently collapses as all energy is expended into the tissues. The bullet and its path is nondiscriminatory and destroys or damages muscle, vascular tissue, nerves, and bone tissue. Different tissues have varying degrees of specific gravity or density that determine how much energy can be transferred from the bullet to the tissues.

Tissue that is dense has a tendency to take up more energy, resulting in greater damage. For example, ribs have a specific gravity of 1.11 and lungs have a specific gravity of only 0.5 to 0.4. As expected, if a bullet strikes a rib, the rib shatters, creating more projectiles and the possibility of significant damage to surrounding structures and tissues. However, if a bullet strikes a lung, damage to the lung may cause tremendous detriment to the patient secondary to oxygenation issues, but damage to the surrounding tissues is not directly affected by the damage to lung tissue.

Physics offers a description of a gunshot injury for consideration. Handguns shoot a single bullet that contains powder encased in metal, whereas shotgun shells are metal encasements containing multiple smaller pellets—as few as six or as many as 200, depending on the gauge of the shotgun. In addition, a small piece of material, usually paper, separates the pellets from the gunpowder. The mechanisms and extent of injury vary because of these differences. Broadly, what happens when a gun is fired is that a dart-shaped projectile (bullet) is launched at significant speed through the bore of a gun. The bullet may deviate slightly from its path and begin to slow, secondary to the air force encountered once it leaves the gun and enters the atmosphere. The speed at which the bullet meets the skin is V_1, where most of the energy is expended into the tissues. It may penetrate as a direct hit or on an angle, which affects how the bullet will travel as it progresses through the layers of tissue. Some bullets travel in a slightly upward and downward motion as they push forward; this is known as *yawing*. Other bullets tumble end-over-end through the tissues. Either way, the extent of damage is directly related to the transference of energy from the bullet into the tissues. Some manufacturers manipulate bullets to create more devastation on impact; the hollow-point bullet is an example.

V_2 is the velocity at which the bullet exits the body. As previously mentioned, if the bullet fails to exit the body, V_2 is equal to zero. The calculation describing this concept is the "law of energy" output.

TAKE HOME POINTS

- Contamination of the wound may result from the debris and bacteria that has been pulled into the wound.
- The bullet easily lodges in or travels through organs with the end result being organ or hemodynamic compromise (or both), dysfunction, or even death.

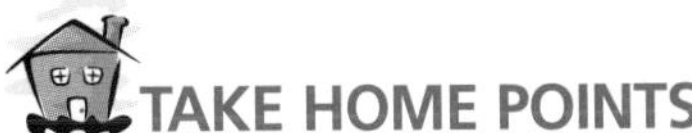

TAKE HOME POINTS

Tissues that are elastic sustain less damage.

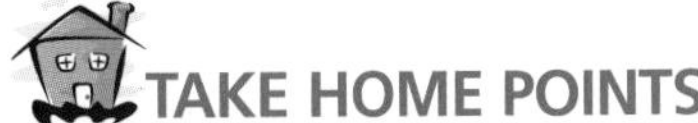

TAKE HOME POINTS

Hollow-point bullets tend to flatten and implode on impact and transfer a great amount of KE. In contrast, smaller-diameter or lower-caliber bullets tend to produce less damage.

Calculation of KE:

$$KE = 1/2\ mv^2 \text{ or } KE = \frac{Mass \times (V_1^2 - V_2^2)}{2 \times g}$$

An increased V_1 and decreased V_2 result in significant internal damage. In addition, if the mass is doubled, then the energy is doubled; if the velocity is doubled, the energy is quadrupled.

Some degree of hemorrhage is frequently involved with the victim of a gunshot wound. *Hemorrhage* refers to a rapid loss of circulating intravascular volume. Various stages of hemorrhage are characterized by the amount of blood lost, in relation to the total blood volume. Unfortunately, no one at the scene can collect the blood that has been lost and then inform the emergency department personnel of the need for fluid resuscitation and/or blood transfusion. Another concern is that the patient's bleeding may be primarily internal. Even when a significant amount of blood has not been identified at the scene, the patient can exhibit symptoms of intravascular depletion, which may indicate that he or she is hemorrhaging internally.

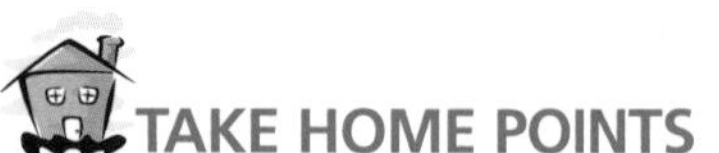

The average person weighs 70 kg and has approximately 5000 mL of total blood volume.

The attending nurse must be alert for signs of internal bleeding and remember that certain body compartments are capable of holding significant amounts of blood.

The abdomen, chest, and thighs are quite capacious and can retain a large volume of blood. In some cases, the skin may become taut, distended, and shiny or the patient may exhibit signs and symptoms of compromise from organs in the body compartment involved. However, sometimes the bleed is more insidious and more difficult to detect, such as a retroperitoneal bleed. The methods of estimating fluid loss in the next section may be very helpful in treating the trauma patient. However, aggressive resuscitative measures should be implemented the minute that blood loss is apparent.

What You DO

Patients with class I and II blood loss can be managed with crystalloid replacement at a rate of 3 mL for every 1 mL of blood loss. Patients with class III and IV blood lost, however, require blood replacement therapy in addition to crystalloids. Patients with class IV hemorrhage usually die if immediate emergency intervention is not implemented because compensatory mechanisms are short term and inadequate to handle a blood loss of this volume.

Classification of Fluid and Blood Losses*

	Class I	Class II	Class III	Class IV
Blood loss (mL)	≤750	750 to 1500	1500 to 2000	>2000
Blood loss (% blood volume)	≤15%	15% to 30%	30% to 40%	>40%
Pulse rate	<100	>100	>120	>140
Blood pressure	Normal	Normal	Decreased	Decreased
Capillary refill	Normal	Delayed	Delayed	Delayed
Respiratory rate	14 to 20	20 to 30	30 to 40	>35
Urine output (mL/hr)	>30	20 to 30	5 to 15	Negligible
Mental status	Slightly anxious	Mildly anxious	Anxious and confused	Confused, lethargic
Fluid replacement (3:1 rule)	Crystalloid	Crystalloid	Crystalloid and blood	Crystalloid and blood

*Amounts are based on the patient's initial presentation.
From American College of Surgeons Committee on Trauma: *The advanced trauma life support student manual*, Chicago, 1993, American College of Surgeons.

Identifying the classification of blood loss and administering the appropriate treatment needed to stabilize the patient are important.

The main treatment goals are to decrease blood loss and increase intravascular volume. These goals can be accomplished by instituting specific interventions to control bleeding and to replenish intravascular volume with crystalloids and/or blood products. If the patient continues to bleed despite resuscitative measures, surgical intervention may be necessary.

FIRST-LINE AND INITIAL TREATMENTS FOR ACUTE HEMORRHAGING

- Secure or support a patent airway (cervical spine precautions).
- Optimize breathing.
- Maintain circulation.
- Establish intravascular access with large bore catheters.
- Replace intravascular volume (blood products or crystalloids).
- Manage bleeding by applying direct pressure on a compressible site.

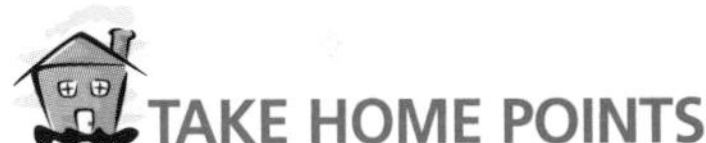

The patient who is hemorrhaging—internally or externally—exhibits the pathophysiologic signs and symptoms of hypovolemic shock. (Refer to the discussion on hypovolemic shock in Chapter 2.)

The usual ABCs should be followed in the management of the patient with hemorrhage. The airway should be assessed, oxygen should be applied, and, if necessary, the patient should be intubated. The goal is to maintain tissue perfusion. The patient has already lost some oxygen-carrying capacity secondary to the bleeding; therefore, it is important to saturate the hemoglobin that remains with as much oxygen as possible to enhance tissue perfusion.

Vasopressors, steroids, and sodium bicarbonate should not be considered in the initial treatment of the bleeding patient. Patients must have their intravascular volume replenished first.

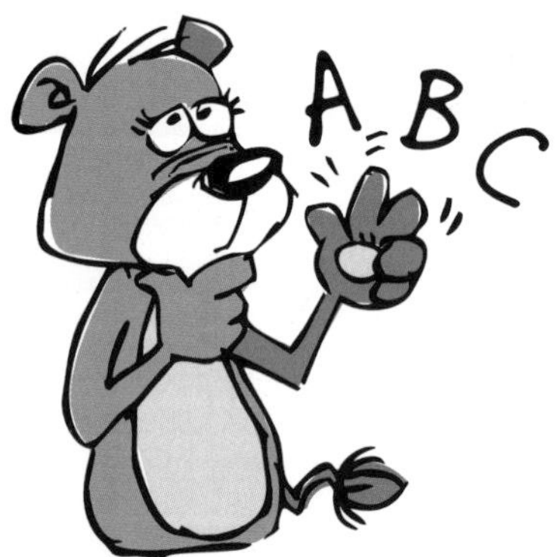

Airway, breathing, circulation.

Careful assessment of breathing and assisting or managing ventilation as necessary are required. Circulation should be assessed by both physical examination and vital signs. Estimating the patient's SBP is accomplished by palpating the pulses and assessing the pulse characteristics (i.e., rate, rhythm, strength).

Pulse Site	Approximate SBP Value
Radial	80 mm Hg
Femoral	70 mm Hg
Carotid	60 mm Hg

TAKE HOME POINTS

Cervical spine precautions are included in the A of the ABCs of all trauma patients. Without proper stabilization, securing a patent airway may not be possible without compromising the integrity of the cervical spine.

At this time, two IV accesses should be obtained with large-bore (16- or 18-gauge) IV catheters, preferably in the upper extremities; antecubital is preferred. The prudent practitioner should also collect blood to be sent for baseline testing that includes complete blood count, basic metabolic panel, prothrombin time, partial thromboplastin time with international normalized ratio (INR), type and cross match, ABGs, and beta human chorionic gonadotropin (hCG) in women of childbearing age to determine whether the patient is pregnant. Fluid resuscitation should be initiated with crystalloid solutions, normal saline (NS), or lactated Ringer's solution.

A urinary catheter should also be placed to assess the patient's fluid status and the adequacy of renal perfusion.

FIRST-LINE AND INITIAL TREATMENT FOR BLOOD LOSS

- Infuse lactated Ringer's solution.

Crystalloids are administered at a rate of 3 mL for every 1 mL of blood loss. All fluids should be warmed, and a rapid infusing device may be necessary.

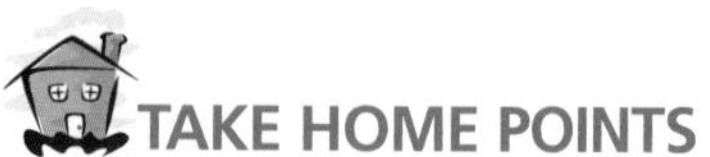

TAKE HOME POINTS

It is reasonable to have lactated Ringer's solution infusing on one body side and NS infusing on the other body side in preparation for possible blood transfusion.

Blood transfusions should be considered when the intravascular requirements are not being met by crystalloid infusion. Initially, O-negative packed red blood cells (PRBCs) may be given; however, once the type and cross have been completed, patient-specific blood should be transfused. Whole blood is rarely administered, although it would provide all the blood components that the patient has lost and decrease the exposure to the number of donors.

Whole blood is not usually given because most patients do not need all the components. Further, most blood banks cannot store whole blood cost effectively. Autotransfusion is another option; however, certain restrictions and contraindications apply. Injuries that result in the contamination of blood at the site of injury (e.g., perforation of the colon) are usually not ideal for the use of the cell-saver device. The reason for this is that bacteria from the colon is now present in the blood; this same blood would be subsequently transfused to the patient and could result in the development of sepsis. In addition, certain chemicals used during orthopedic surgery, such as methylmethacrylate, may not be appropriate for autotransfusion.

When the patient's blood volume has become significantly depleted, additional transfusions with other blood components may be indicated.

Devices may be used to assist in attaining hemostasis from an actively bleeding wound in addition to increasing venous return. One such device is the pneumatic antishock garment (PASG), formerly known as medical antishock trousers (MAST). Current indications for the use of PASG or MAST devices include the treatment of hypotension (SBP $<$ 80 or $<$ 100 mm Hg if symptoms of shock are present) to help stabilize lower extremity or pelvic fractures and to control bleeding anywhere under the device. The use of these devices is sometimes controversial. Absolute contraindications include pulmonary edema, left ventricular dysfunction, or known diaphragmatic rupture. Controversial uses include injuries to the head, thorax, and cardiac tamponade. Relative contraindications are pregnancy (regarding inflation of the abdominal apparatus), abdominal evisceration, impalement of the abdomen, compartment syndrome, lumbar spine instability, or inability to control bleeding outside of the garment. Tourniquets are no longer indicated in the treatment of hemorrhage because they cause ischemia to tissues distal to the injury. The only time the application of tourniquets is used is in the event of traumatic amputation.

Prevention of hypothermia in the hemorrhaging patient is another very important intervention. Although it is important to expose the patient to assess for injuries, maintenance of body temperature is critical and all fluids and blood should be warmed either before or during administration. Patients with hypothermia who are bleeding have less ability to tolerate the loss in blood volume.

The end result of massive blood loss is hypovolemic shock. Rapid and aggressive intervention is critical in the hemorrhaging patient to prevent the deterioration and possible hemodynamic instability of the patient. The nurses' role in the management of the patient who is hemorrhaging from a gunshot wound is of utmost importance, and the information gathered or missed can significantly influence patient outcomes.

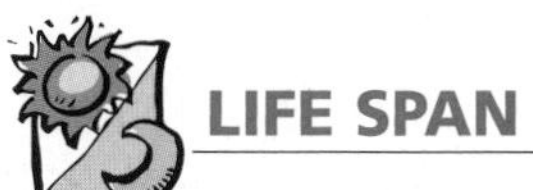

LIFE SPAN

The American College of Surgeons recommends fluid replacement with 1 to 2 L of fluid administered rapidly for the adult patient and 20 mL/kg for the pediatric patient.

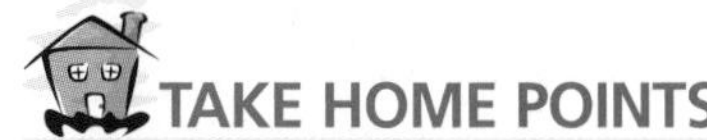

TAKE HOME POINTS

O-negative blood is usually transfused in the emergent patient without a type and cross match. O-positive blood may be substituted in life-threatening situations if O-negative blood is not available.

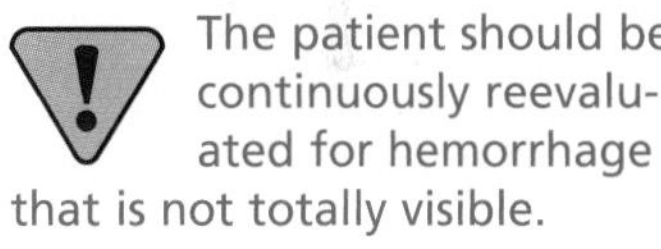

The patient should be continuously reevaluated for hemorrhage that is not totally visible.

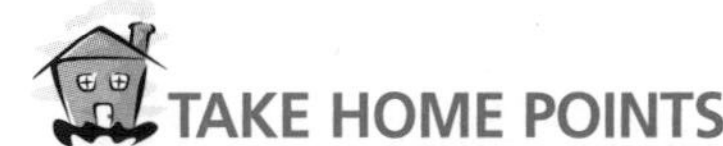

TAKE HOME POINTS

Ongoing, careful assessments of the patient and response to interventions is crucial.

Do You UNDERSTAND?

DIRECTIONS: Fill in the blanks to complete each of the following statements.

1. One of the most common causes of high-velocity penetrating trauma is a ______________ ______________ ______________.
2. V_1 refers to energy transferred from bullet to tissue when ______________ the wound.
3. V_2 refers to energy transferred from bullet to tissue when ______________ the wound.
4. The loss of 15% of the blood volume describes class ______________ hemorrhage.
5. Class II hemorrhage is the loss of ______________ to ______________ mL of blood.
6. The patient with a class III hemorrhage has a(n) ______________ BP and a(n) ______________ heart rate.
7. The patient with a class IV hemorrhage has a(n) ______________ pulse pressure.
8. The patient with a class IV hemorrhage usually requires ______________ ______________ ______________ and ______________ ______________ to survive.
9. Blood is replaced with crystalloids at a rate of ______________ mL for every ______________ mL of blood loss.
10. Palpation of a radial pulse usually indicates the patient's systolic pressure is at least ______________ mm Hg.
11. Palpation of a femoral pulse usually indicates the SBP to be about ______________ mm Hg.
12. Palpation of the carotid pulse usually indicates the SBP is ______________ mm Hg.
13. Primary goals for treating the victim with a hemorrhaging gunshot wound include control of ______________ and ______________ replacement.

DIRECTIONS: Identify the following statements as *true* (T) or *false* (F).

_____ 14. Vasopressors are beneficial as initial treatment for the hypotensive patient with a gunshot wound.

_____ 15. Tourniquets are routinely used to control bleeding in most patients with trauma.

_____ 16. $D_5\frac{1}{2}$ NS is the intravascular fluid (IVF) of choice and is rapidly transfused into the patient with trauma on arrival to the emergency department.

_____ 17. MAST or PASG devices are beneficial to patients with pulmonary edema, left ventricular dysfunction, or diaphragmatic rupture.

What IS Cardiac Tamponade?

Cardiac tamponade is a life-threatening condition where no blood is ejected from the heart, resulting in cardiac arrest. It requires immediate intervention. Cardiac tamponade is defined as major compression of all four chambers of the heart caused by an accumulation of one or more of the following: blood, clots, pus, other fluid, or gas. The fluid accumulates in the pericardial sac that surrounds the heart, almost completely obstructing venous return, causing hypotension and jugular venous distention. The amount of fluid necessary to cause cardiac tamponade in an adult varies. As little as 150 mL of rapidly accumulating fluid to 1 L of slowly accumulating fluid in the pericardial sac can cause cardiac tamponade.

This fluid accumulation increases the pressure in the pericardial sac. This rising pressure results in an equalization of the diastolic pressure in all four chambers of the heart. This change in pressure leads to a decrease in cardiac filling, resulting in a decrease in stroke volume. Cardiac tamponade becomes fatal when the pericardial pressure increases to the point that the heart cannot effectively pump to maintain circulation.

Many diseases may result in cardiac tamponade. These include acute and chronic pericarditis, cancer, renal disease, HIV-TB coinfected patients, and systemic lupus erythematosus. Cardiac tamponade may also occur as the result of certain procedures: for example, cardiac catheterization, balloon angioplasty, pacemaker insertion, central line insertion, transmyocardial revascularization, fine-needle biopsy of the chest, coronary artery bypass surgery, and heart transplantation. Certain medications also predispose patients to tamponade. These medications include anticoagulants,

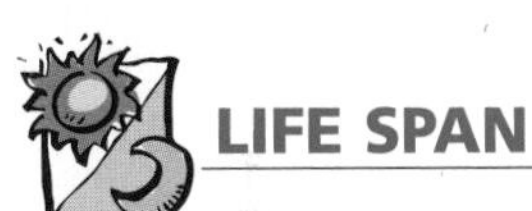

- Premature infants are at the greatest risk of tamponade associated with central lines. Central lines can be in place as long as 48 hours before causing tamponade in premature infants.
- Women and older adults are at the greatest risk for tamponade after revascularization procedures.

Answers: 1. gunshot wound; 2. entering; 3. exiting; 4. I; 5. 750, 1500; 6. decreased, increased; 7. decreased; 8. transfusion of blood, blood components; 9. 3, 1; 10. 80; 11. 70; 12. 60; 13. bleeding, fluid; 14. F; 15. F; 16. F; 17. F.

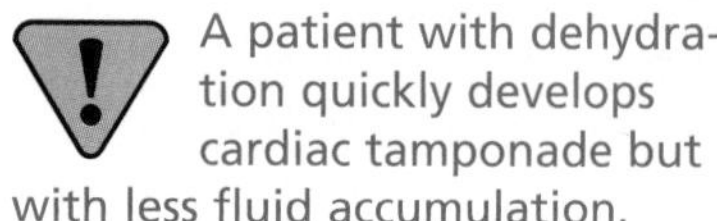
A patient with dehydration quickly develops cardiac tamponade but with less fluid accumulation.

chemotherapeutic agents (i.e., abciximab), and thrombolytic agents. Acute cardiac tamponade may also occur as the result of chest trauma or rupture of the heart after a myocardial infarction (MI).

What You NEED TO KNOW

The clinical manifestations of cardiac tamponade vary. The signs and symptoms can be similar to the signs and symptoms of other conditions such as heart failure and pulmonary embolism. The patient may report chest tightness, dizziness, shortness of breath, vague discomfort, dysphagia, and dysphoria including restlessness and statements of impending death. Clinical signs include tachycardia, edema, a positive hepatojugular reflex, reduced extremity pulses, rising central venous pressure, a decrease in the difference between the SBP and diastolic blood pressure (DBP) (narrowing of the pulse pressure), shocklike symptoms, and pulsus paradoxus. *Pulsus paradoxus* is defined as a greater than 10–mm Hg drop in SBP occurring on inspiration. The condition indicates high thoracic pressure. Pulsus paradoxus can be observed on arterial line tracing or measured using a sphygmomanometer. It is more pronounced in patients with lung masses or in those profusely dehydrated.

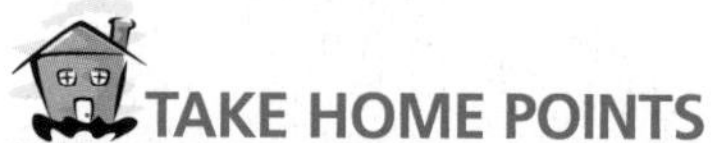
TAKE HOME POINTS

Cardiac tamponade is a serious, life-threatening condition requiring immediate intervention.

How to Measure Pulsus Paradoxus

1. Inflate the BP cuff 15 mm Hg above the highest systolic measurement.
2. Deflate the BP cuff slowly until the first Korotkoff sounds are heard (Step 1). Initially, the sounds will only be heard during expiration in the presence of cardiac tamponade.
3. Continue to deflate the BP cuff until the Korotkoff sounds are heard throughout the respiratory cycle (i.e., inspiratory and expiratory).
4. The difference between the first measurement obtained (Step 1) and the last measurement is the pulsus paradoxus.

An electrocardiographic (ECG) tracing may show a decrease in the amplitude of the QRS complex, an alternating high and low voltage where the R wave alternates between upward and downward deflections (electrical alternans), and other T-wave abnormalities. However, ECG changes are observed in only about 20% of patients with tamponade.

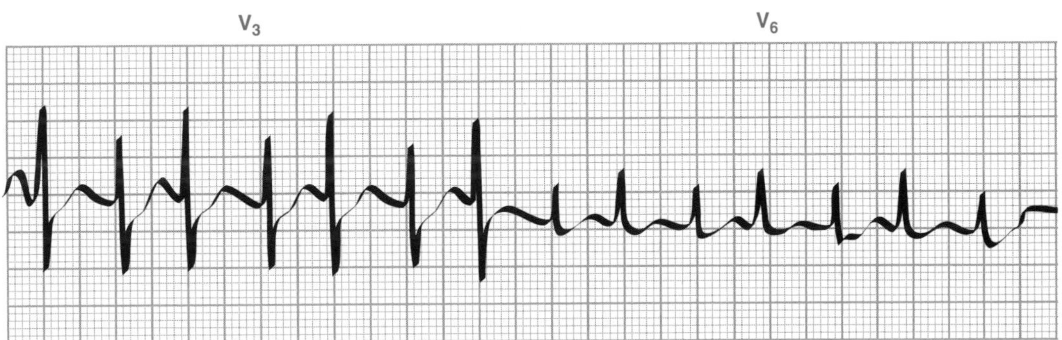

ECG alternating high-low voltage.
V_3 = decreased amplitude in QRS complex.
V_6 = t-wave abnormalities.
(From Conover M: Understanding electrocardiography, *ed 8, St Louis, 2003, Mosby.)*

Hypotension, muffled heart tones, and severe jugular vein distention (JVD) are considered classic signs of cardiac tamponade and are referred to as Beck's triad.

When an underlying disease is causing the tamponade, the symptoms reported by the patient may be similar to the disease.

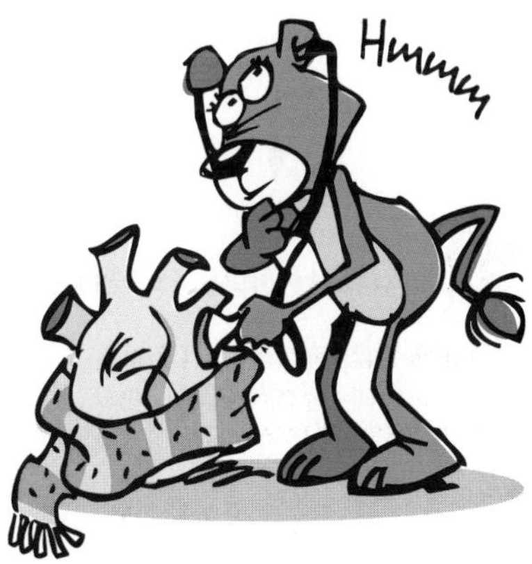

Muffled heart tones, a classic sign of tamponade.

What You DO

Heart catheterization and echocardiography can confirm cardiac tamponade. An echocardiogram is the safest method for detecting cardiac tamponade and is used more frequently because of the time required to prepare the client for a heart catheterization. An echocardiogram shows increasing tricuspid and pulmonary flow velocities and decreasing mitral and aortic valve flow velocities during inspiration. A heart catheterization shows that the right atrial, pulmonary capillary wedge, and pulmonary artery DBPs are elevated and are all equal to each other (within 5 mm Hg). Cardiac output is also decreased, whereas systemic vascular resistance is elevated. A chest x-ray shows an enlarged heart, which can indicate tamponade when compared with previous x-ray studies.

Once the diagnosis of tamponade has been confirmed, a physician needs to remove the excess fluid in the pericardial space by needle aspiration, needle pericardiocentesis, or open surgical drainage. Needle pericardiocentesis can be performed at the bedside using a local anesthetic; it involves the insertion of a needle through the chest wall into the pericardial sac. The fluid is gently aspirated.

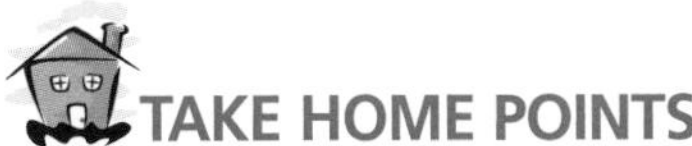

TAKE HOME POINTS

Beck's triad consists of hypotension, muffled heart sounds, and JVD.

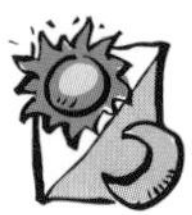

LIFE SPAN

Although many of the symptoms in infants and children are similar to those in adults, infants develop bradycardia instead of tachycardia. The possibility of cardiac tamponade should be investigated in any infant who has a central line catheter and in whom bradycardia and hypotension develop.

Although Beck's triad is a classic sign of cardiac tamponade, it is frequently a late development; other symptoms may occur earlier.

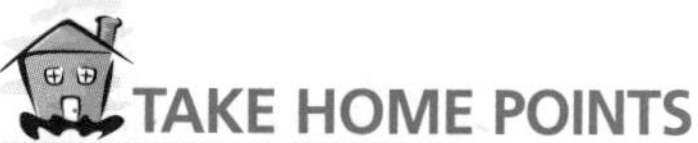

TAKE HOME POINTS

Pericardiocentesis is safer when guided by a two-dimensional echocardiogram.

The removal of as little as 10 mL of pericardial fluid can mean the difference between life and death for the patient.

The use of nitroglycerin should be avoided because the patient's preload is already reduced.

The characteristics of the fluid aspirated will vary with the cause of the tamponade. For example, the fluid appears bloody if the tamponade is the result of bleeding, but it may appear purulent if the cause is infection. A sample of the fluid should be sent to the laboratory for smear, culture, and cytologic studies. Open surgical drainage may be performed when the cause of the tamponade is unknown.

While the patient is awaiting drainage of the pericardial fluid, IV fluids may be given to expand the intravascular blood volume. Dobutamine, dopamine, or nitroprusside may be administered to increase cardiac output and maintain BP; these are only temporary measures.

The goal of most nursing interventions is early detection of cardiac tamponade. Any patient undergoing a procedure that places him or her at high risk for cardiac tamponade should be closely monitored for at least 24 hours after the procedure. The patient is observed for symptoms associated with cardiac tamponade (e.g., shortness of breath, vague discomfort, anxiety, dizziness, JVD, chest tightness or discomfort). Heart tones and breath sounds are assessed, paying particular attention for muffled heart tones (possibly indicative of cardiac tamponade) or adventitious breath sounds (possibly indicative of other problems). Vital signs are monitored for tachycardia (adults) or bradycardia (infants), for changes in BP, and for narrowing of pulse pressures and pulsus alternans.

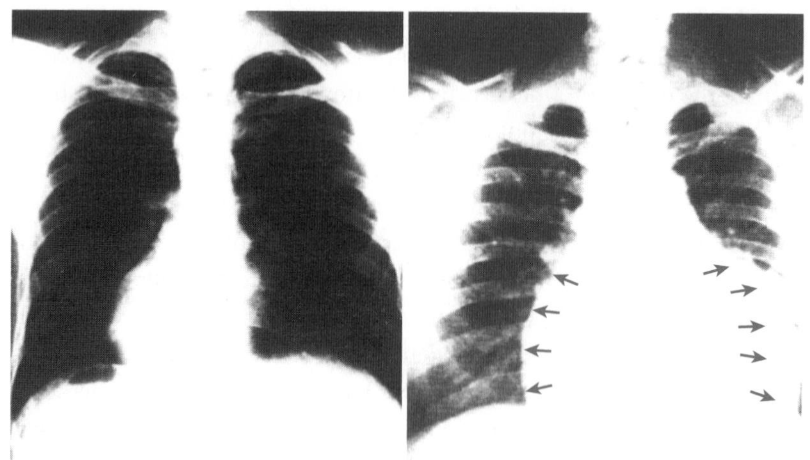

Normal Chest X-Ray **Enlarged Cardiac Silhouette on Chest X-Ray**

(*From Lewis SM, Heitkemper MM, Dirksen SR:* Medical-surgical nursing: assessment and management of clinical problems, *ed 5, St Louis, 2000, Mosby.*)

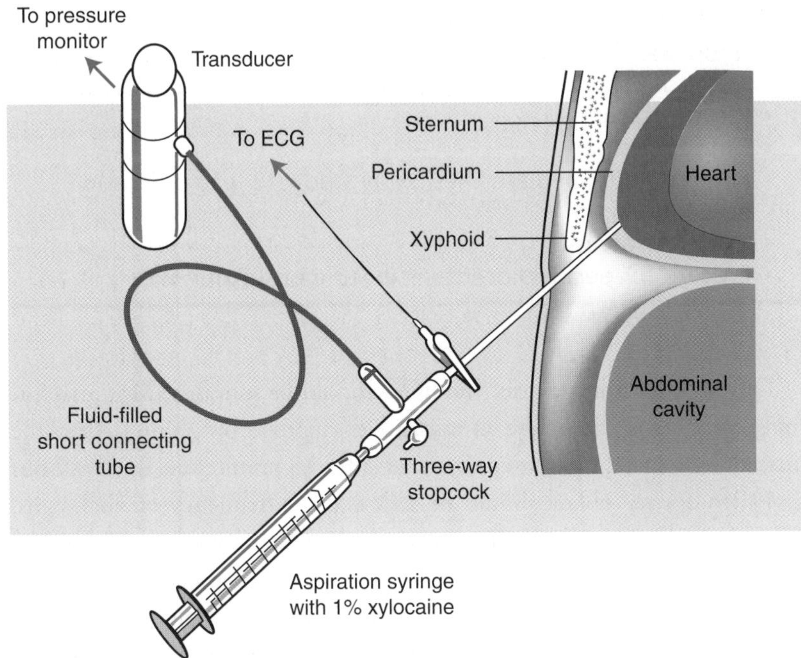

Needle pericardiocentesis. *(From Lewis SM, Heitkemper MM, Dirksen SR:* Medical-surgical nursing: assessment and management of clinical problems, *ed 5, St Louis, 2000, Mosby.)*

If the patient has a pulmonary artery catheter in place, central venous pressure, pulmonary capillary wedge pressure, and cardiac output are monitored. An ECG is assessed for changes in voltage and alternating patterns of high and low voltage. Laboratory values are monitored for signs of dehydration and hypokalemia. Hypokalemia can precipitate arrhythmias during pericardiocentesis. Intake and output levels are monitored to assess for dehydration. Chest tube drainage of a patient who has had open-heart surgery is closely monitored because blocked or kinked chest tubes can result in cardiac tamponade. A sudden decrease in chest tube drainage should be investigated.

When cardiac tamponade is suggested, oxygen is administered. The physician is immediately notified, and an immediate request for a chest x-ray, 12-lead ECG, and echocardiogram is prescribed. If the patient does not already have an IV in place, one should be started. If time allows, a blood sample is sent to the laboratory for type and cross match and for an assessment of the potassium level. Hypokalemia can increase the occurrence of arrhythmias during pericardiocentesis.

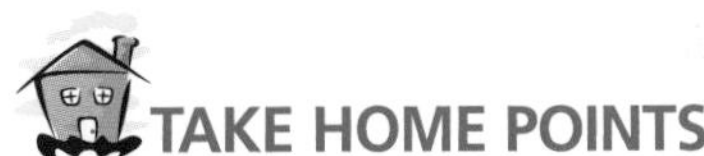

Cardiac tamponade can be detected early with careful assessment, such as a blocked or kinked chest tube.

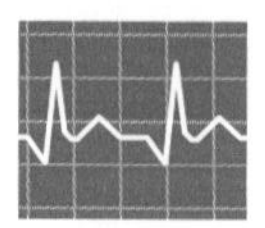

Signs and symptoms of cardiac tamponade can be similar to other conditions, making additional careful assessment necessary.

FIRST-LINE AND INITIAL TREATMENT FOR CARDIAC TAMPONADE

- Provide oxygen.
- Notify physician.
- Request an immediate chest x-ray study, 12-lead ECG, and echocardiogram.
- Obtain IV access.
- Prepare for pericardiocentesis (needle or subxiphoid).

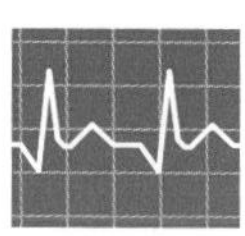

Continuous ECG monitoring for arrhythmias and frequent assessment of vital signs are necessary during pericardiocentesis.

During pericardiocentesis, the ECG should be monitored for arrhythmias; vital signs should be monitored during the procedure. After the procedure the vital signs are monitored every 15 minutes for the first hour and then agency policy should be followed for frequency of vital signs. After the procedure, the dressing over the needle insertion site should be monitored. Any excessive drainage (>200 mL/day) should be reported to the physician. Drainage is usually serous or serosanguineous.

Emotional support and patient teaching are necessary to help decrease anxiety. A calm and consistent demeanor can also help decrease anxiety. The patient should be encouraged to report all symptoms. Diagnostic tests such as echocardiogram should be provided. If needle pericardiocentesis is to be performed, the patient should be provided with information. Staying with the patient before the procedure should also provide reassurance and emotional support. If possible, the nurse should stay with the patient during the needle pericardiocentesis. Preoperative teaching should be provided to the patient having open surgical drainage.

Do You UNDERSTAND?

DIRECTIONS: **Fill in the blanks to complete each of the following statements.**

1. Cardiac tamponade occurs when ________________ accumulates in the ________________ ________________ around the heart.
2. The fluid accumulation in the pericardial sac causes the pressure in the sac to ________________________ ; this leads to a ________________________ in cardiac filling.
3. ____ ________________________ are at the greatest risk for tamponade resulting from central line placement.

DIRECTIONS: Provide a short answer to each of the following questions.

4. What is pulsus paradoxus?

____

____

5. What are the signs of cardiac tamponade that are referred to as Beck's triad?

____

____

6. What sign of cardiac tamponade is different in infants?

____

____

DIRECTIONS: Identify the following statements as *true* (T) or *false* (F).

______ 7. A cardiac catheterization is the safest method for diagnosing cardiac tamponade.

______ 8. If possible, a potassium level should be checked before performing pericardiocentesis.

______ 9. An ECG tracing can be used to detect pulsus paradoxus.

______ 10. If cardiac tamponade is suspected, the nurse should notify the physician immediately.

What IS Hypothermia?

Hypothermia can be defined as a fall in the core body temperature to below 35° C (95° F). The temperature reading must be obtained from a source that measures core temperature, preferably from two such sources. Hypothermia can be classified as primary (accidental) or secondary (deliberate).

Environmental exposure or prolonged surgical tissue exposure, especially during surgery of the thoracic or abdominal cavities, are the causes of primary or accidental hypothermia. Deliberate, mild hypothermia is used during neurosurgical procedures to provide protection of the brain and spinal cord during periods of interrupted perfusion. Profound hypothermia (as low as 28° C or 82.4° F) is often used during cardiopulmonary bypass.

Primary or accidental hypothermia occurs as a result of cold exposure. Secondary or deliberate hypothermia may be observed in patients with

Answers: **1. fluid, pericardial sac; 2. increase, decrease; 3. premature infants; 4.** > 10 mm Hg drop in BP occurring on inspiration; 5. hypotension, muffled heart tones, and severe JVD; 6. They develop bradycardia; 7. False; 8. True; 9. False; 10. True.

decreased heat production, such as hypoadrenalism and hypothyroidism, or abnormal temperature regulation, such as occurs with brain injuries involving the hypothalamus. Many mental or physical disease states or medications may interfere with the body's heat-balancing mechanisms. Some of the risk factors for developing hypothermia are listed in the following box.

Risk Factors for Hypothermia

- Extremes of age
- Trauma, especially CNS trauma
- CVA
- Hypothyroidism
- Hypoadrenalism
- Parkinson's disease
- Multiple sclerosis
- Burns
- Extensive skin diseases
- Vasodilation induced by alcohol or prescription or "street" drugs
- Malnutrition
- Sepsis
- Shock
- Renal or hepatic failure
- Alzheimer's disease and psychiatric problems that alter ability to respond to hypothermia
- Paraplegia or quadriplegia
- Trauma

CNS, Central nervous system; *CVA,* cerebrovascular accident.

In the United States, hypothermia is responsible for more than 700 deaths per year, and half of these deaths occur in patients who are 65 years old and older. The older patient has age-related impairment of homeostatic mechanisms affecting thermoregulation, cultural and economic factors that increase the likelihood of exposure to cold, and diseases and drugs that can impair thermoregulation, interfere with heat generation, or impair conservation of body heat. With advanced age comes a progressive weakening of the shivering response; the vasoconstrictor response develops, and a progressive reduction in the ability to detect and respond to changes in environmental temperature occurs.

What You NEED TO KNOW

The physiologic effects of hypothermia are summarized in the following table.

Physiologic Effects of Hypothermia

Hypothermia Stage	Core Temperature	Signs and Symptoms
Impending hypothermia	36° C (96.8°F)	• Skin: pale, numb, waxy • Shivering • Fatigue • Weakness
Mild hypothermia	32° to 35° C (89.6° to 95° F)	• Uncontrolled, intense shivering • Movement less coordinated • Coldness creates pain and discomfort • Tachycardia • Vasoconstriction • Increased BP • Increased CO • Increased CVP (from shivering) • Increase in oxygen consumption • Myocardial ischemia, pulmonary edema, CHF (in patients with impaired cardiac function) • Metabolic acidosis
Moderate hypothermia	28° to 32° C (82.4° to 89.6° F)	• Absence of shivering (stops below 32° C) • Muscles stiffen • Mental confusion • Apathy • Slowed, vague, slurred speech • Slow, shallow breathing • Drowsiness • Strange behavior • No complaints of being cold (occurs below 35° C)
	28° to 32° C (82.4° to 89.6° F)	• Decreased heart rate • Decreased cardiac output • Increased risk of atrial and ventricular arrhythmias • "J" or Osborne wave (hypothermia hump) may appear on ECG • Decreased respiratory rate • 50% reduction in oxygen consumption • Impaired insulin action • Hyperglycemia
Severe hypothermia	28° to 30° C (82.4° to 86° F)	• Skin cold, bluish gray in color • Weak • Lack of coordination • Decreased level of consciousness to coma • Absent tendon reflexes • Rigid extremities (may appear dead) • Decreased or absent respirations • Pupils dilated • Nonreactive pupils (29° to 30° C) (84.2° to 86° F) • Loss of cerebral autoregulation • Decreased cerebral blood flow • Decreased cardiac output • Decreased renal blood flow (oliguria)

BP, Blood pressure; *CO,* cardiac output; *CVP,* central venous pressure; *CHF,* congestive heart failure.

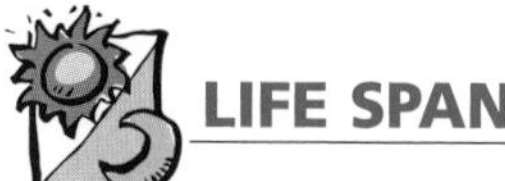

LIFE SPAN

- With advanced age, impairment of the compensatory mechanisms occurs, and the older adult is less able to detect and respond to changes in temperature.
- Neonates can generate heat, but they have a small body, a greater body surface–body weight ratio than adults, and a thin layer of subcutaneous fat; consequently, they become hypothermic more easily than adults do.

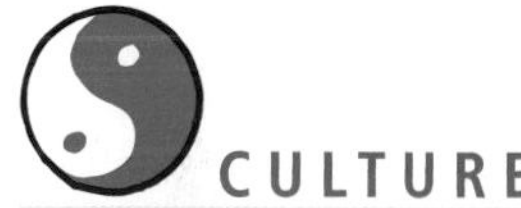

CULTURE

In the United States, most cases of hypothermia occur in urban areas and are caused by environmental exposure and alcohol abuse, street drug abuse, mental illness, or homelessness. However, some cases are a result of outdoor work or recreation.

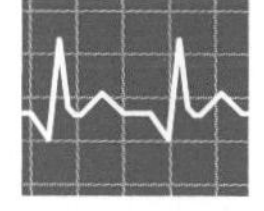

Bradycardia is due to slowed depolarization of pacemaker cells. A *J* or Osborne wave may appear on the downstroke of the QRS. This is best seen in an ECG and appears at the J point.

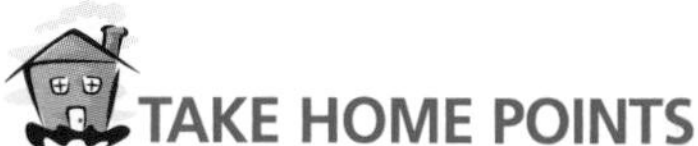

TAKE HOME POINTS

In impending hypothermia, shivering may be overcome by activity.

• Bradycardia during hypothermia may be unresponsive to atropine or pacing.
• A high risk of aspiration is due to altered mental status and ileus in hypothermia.
• If core body temperature falls below 26° C and is not corrected, then respirations stop and asystole occurs.

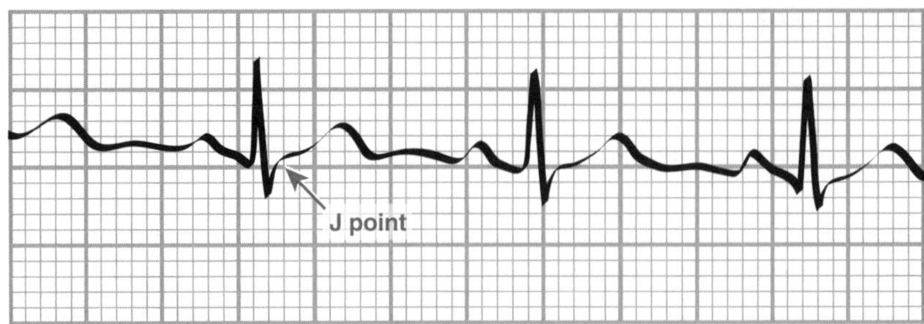

In hypothermia, the downstrike of QRS on an ECG is called the 'J' point. *(From Conover M:* Understanding electrocardiography, *ed 8, St Louis, 2003, Mosby.)*

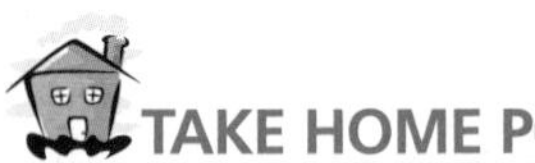

TAKE HOME POINTS

- The body's core compartment makes up approximately 50% to 60% of body mass.
- Approximately 90% of heat leaves the body through the skin and 10% leaves through the respiratory tract.

In addition, hypothermia impairs platelet function, the coagulation cascade, and fibrinolysis, all of which lead to increased bleeding, which is of great significance during trauma resuscitation and surgery. In the immune system, neutrophil and macrophage function is impaired. Vasoconstriction and increased blood viscosity and decreased tissue partial pressure for oxygen occur, all of which increase the risk of wound infection. Hypothermia impairs the response to catecholamines. Hypothermia also impairs drug metabolism by decreasing hepatic and renal blood flow. Hypothermia causes a "cold diuresis" that is a result of impaired renal tubular function, leading to increased urinary loss of sodium, potassium, and water. In addition, high-energy phosphates such as adenosine triphosphate (ATP) are depleted and the oxyhemoglobin dissociation curve shifts to the left, which impairs tissue oxygen delivery. Hypothermia can also cause hypokalemia because of a depression of the sodium-potassium-adenosinetriphosphatase (Na-K-ATPase) pump, as well as hyperglycemia because of the decreased release of insulin and peripheral use of glucose.

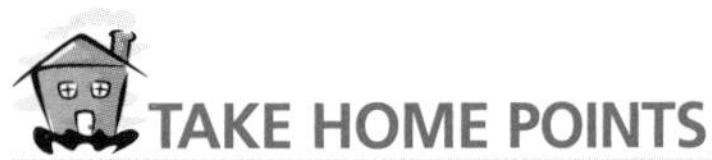

TAKE HOME POINTS

A normal white blood cell (WBC) count is necessary for hypothalamus temperature regulation.

Heat Balance

In humans, an internal thermoregulatory system maintains core body temperature within a narrow range, coordinating heat loss, heat production, and heat conservation. Many of the chemical processes necessary to maintain life can only take place within a specific temperature range.

Humans have both core and peripheral thermal compartments. The *core* is defined as the well-perfused central tissues; they include the brain, thorax, and abdomen. The temperature in the core compartment is kept constant within a narrow range. Heat is rapidly distributed, and most of the metabolic processes, which require energy and produce heat, take place in the core compartment. Heat generated by metabolic processes in the core must get to the external environment. The *peripheral* compartment consists of the extremities and skin.

Temperature in the peripheral compartment may be 1° to 3° C lower than the temperature in the core, depending on the thermal environment. Temperature gradients may occur between the superficial and deep structures within the compartment. Contraction of voluntary muscles, either by normal muscle activity or shivering, produces heat in the peripheral compartment.

Heat moves from the core to the peripheral compartment by both convection and conduction within the blood vessels and is influenced by the amount of blood flow to the peripheral tissues. (Conduction and convection are discussed in the section on heat loss mechanisms later in this chapter.)

The hypothalamus is the body's temperature regulation control center. It has both heat- and cold-sensitive neurons and receives afferent input from temperature sensors in the skin, spinal cord, abdominal viscera, and in or near the great vessels in the thorax. The sensory data are transmitted via the anterior spinothalamic tracts to the preoptic nuclei of the hypothalamus. The hypothalamus continuously maintains the core body temperature at the set point of approximately 37° C or 98.6° F. If the core temperature falls, heat production increases to maintain it at this set point. The efferent component of this temperature control system is the sympathetic nervous system, which initiates shivering to produce heat and vasoconstriction to conserve heat.

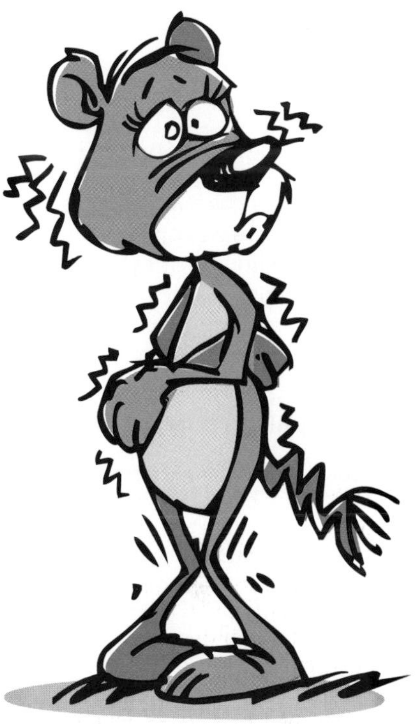

Voluntary muscle contractions lead to shivering, which produces heat.

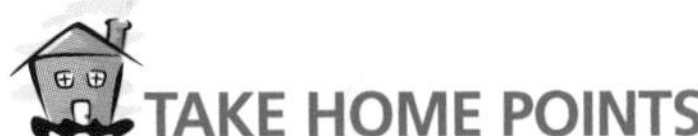

TAKE HOME POINTS

A daily variation in temperature (circadian rhythm) occurs, which can be influenced by food intake, exercise, infection, thyroid status, and medications.

Mechanisms of Heat Production and Loss

The body increases heat production by increasing muscle tone and by shivering. Shivering is a fairly effective method for heat production because most of the energy produced is retained as heat. Shivering can increase body heat production four to five times above normal levels. Shivering requires increased muscle blood flow, which reduces the effectiveness of vasoconstriction to maintain the core temperature.

Epinephrine is released and causes vasoconstriction, which shunts blood to the core compartment where heat cannot be lost by the usual mechanisms. Epinephrine also generates chemical thermogenesis by increasing the basal metabolic rate on a short-term basis. Prolonged cold exposure stimulates the release of thyroxine, which also increases the metabolic rate.

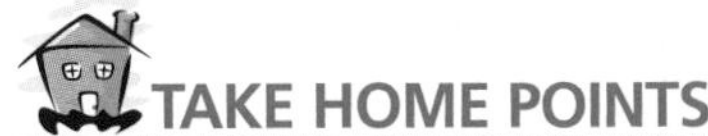

TAKE HOME POINTS

The core temperature at which shivering develops is usually between 34° C (93° F) and 37° C (98.6° F).

The body loses heat by four mechanisms: radiation, conduction, convection, and evaporation. *Radiation* is heat loss or gain in the form of infrared rays, which are a type of electromagnetic energy. Radiation is the most important source of heat loss, making up approximately 60% of its total. All objects with a temperature above absolute zero radiate heat waves. The warmth sensed when standing in direct sunlight or next to a hot stove is produced by radiation. If body temperature is higher than surrounding air or objects, then more heat is radiated away from the body than toward the body.

Conductive heat loss increases on contact with water, especially immersion.

Conduction is the transfer of heat to a solid object directly in contact with the skin, such as an operating room table, and is responsible for only about 3% of body heat loss. Hypothermia that results from administering cold IV fluids is an example of conduction because the fluids are warmed to body temperature by conduction from blood and tissues.

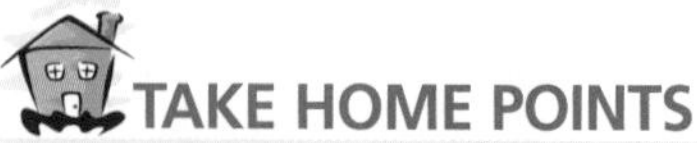

Convection is a more efficient method of heat loss than conduction.

Convection is responsible for about 15% of body heat loss. In convection, conduction of heat occurs into the air that surrounds the body; once that same air reaches body temperature, no more heat is lost until the air molecules move away from the body and are replaced with other molecules at a lower temperature. Convection is an important source of heat loss in operating rooms, where airflow should be 10 full-room air exchanges per hour and even higher in laminar-flow rooms. Convection is the basis for the well-known "wind-chill" factor.

TAKE HOME POINTS

- Increasing ambient airflow with a fan will increase both evaporative and convective heat loss.
- Perioperative heat loss is increased by evaporation from large surgical wounds, particularly in the thorax or abdomen, and by the use of cold-skin preparation solutions, particularly alcohol, which evaporate quickly.

Evaporation is heat lost as water leaves the respiratory tract and skin. It accounts for 22% of body heat loss. Even when there is no diaphoresis, 450 to 600 mL of water is lost per day from evaporation. This heat loss cannot be controlled because of the continuous loss of water by diffusion through the skin and respiratory mucosa. Heat loss is increased if more fluids are available at the skin surface, and fluid is then actively secreted through the sweat glands. Evaporative cooling occurs in response to sympathetic nervous system stimulation, and the amount of heat lost by sweating depends on the difference between the temperature of the body and the environment and the relative humidity of the air.

Clothing traps air next to the skin, creating a private air zone. Clothing decreases conductive, convective, and radiation heat losses. A typical suit of clothes can decrease heat loss by one half when compared with a nude body. Arctic-type or thermal-insulated clothing can also decrease the heat loss to one-sixth. When it is wet, even with perspiration, clothing does not help maintain body temperature. Water has a high thermal conductivity—32 times greater than air. Concrete has an even higher thermal conductivity than water, contributing to hypothermia in the older patient who falls on a concrete surface, becomes immobilized, and is not found for hours.

TAKE HOME POINTS

The body adapts over time to warm environments and high altitudes, but no significant physiologic adaptation to cold is apparent in the body.

Alcohol increases a patient's risk of becoming hypothermic because it causes vasodilation, suppresses the hypothalamic temperature regulating center, impairs shivering, and decreases the patient's awareness of and response to a cold environment.

What You DO

Diagnosis and Treatment of the Patient with Hypothermia

Early recognition of hypothermia is critical. A treatment facility must have thermometers able to measure core temperatures of 25° C or less, and temperature must be measured at two core sites.

Laboratory tests should include the following:

- **Blood glucose.** Both hyperglycemia and hypoglycemia (with prolonged hypothermia) can be observed.
- **Potassium.** Both hyperkalemia and hypokalemia can exist. Hyperkalemia is usually indicative of extensive tissue damage.
- **ABGs.** ABGs should not be corrected for temperature. Patients with hypothermia have a higher level of oxygen and CO_2 and a lower pH than normothermic patients.
- **Hemoglobin.** Hemoglobin rises 2% for each 1° C fall in temperature as a result of cold diuresis and subsequent hypovolemia.
- **Coagulation studies.** Hypothermia interferes with the enzymes needed to activate the coagulation process. Platelet function is also inhibited because platelet production of thromboxane B2 is impaired by cold. Transfused platelets also function poorly. However, the coagulation studies may not reflect these changes because the tests are performed at 37° C and the enzymes have been reactivated by warming the test tube.

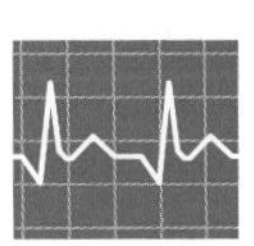

MONITORING: Temperature must be measured at two core sites.

- The cold heart is irritable, and diagnostic maneuvers such as central line insertion (which may be necessary because of peripheral vasoconstriction), intubation, or even patient movement may precipitate ventricular fibrillation.
- The very cold heart (core temperature of 30° C or 86° F or less) is not responsive to vasoactive drugs, defibrillation, or pacemaker activation to increase the heart rate.

Treatment

Airway and Breathing. Supplemental oxygen is indicated for the hypothermic patient because of the leftward shift of the oxyhemoglobin dissociation curve. Oxygen should be heated to 40° to 45° C (104° to 113° F) and humidified to return heat to the core compartment. If the patient's protective airway reflexes are impaired as a result of an altered mental status, then the patient should be given oxygen before intubation and intubated as gently as possible to avoid triggering ventricular arrhythmias.

Circulation. Hypothermic patients are usually volume depleted and need infusion of warm saline. The hypothermic liver cannot metabolize the lactate from lactated Ringer's solution. The saline solution should be heated to between 40° and 42° C, but it may not contribute significantly to core rewarming unless large volumes of crystalloid solution are used. Central lines may be needed not only to monitor intravascular volume but also because peripheral access is difficult as a result of peripheral

Heparinized solutions should not be used for maintaining line patency.

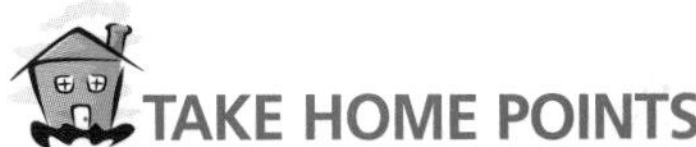

TAKE HOME POINTS

Intubation may be technically difficult because of muscle stiffness, with subsequent difficulty in opening the mouth or moving the neck.

vasoconstriction. If the patient is hypotensive and his or her BP remains low despite volume and rewarming, IV dopamine (Intropin) 2 to 5 mcg/kg/min may be considered. The patient should be carefully monitored for any cardiac arrhythmias. Atrial arrhythmias can usually be watched until rewarming because the ventricular rate will be slow as a result of hypothermia. If ventricular arrhythmias occur, then they must be treated. The patient having ventricular arrhythmias may not respond to conventional therapy, and resuscitation must continue until core temperature reaches at least 30° C.

Methods of Rewarming. Three methods of rewarming can be used: (1) passive, (2) active external rewarming, and (3) active internal rewarming.

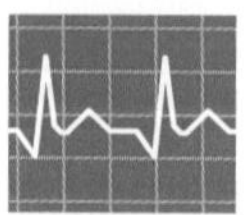

Esophageal temperatures will no longer be reliable once heated gasses are administered through the ETT.

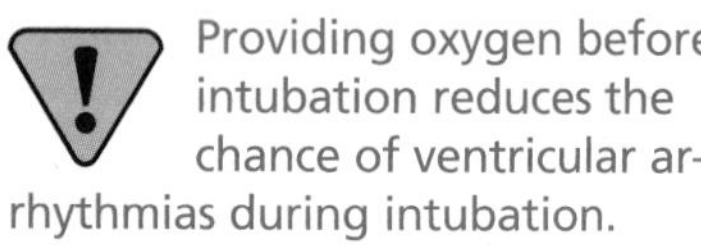

Providing oxygen before intubation reduces the chance of ventricular arrhythmias during intubation.

Methods of Rewarming with Interventions

Methods of Rewarming	Interventions
Passive	Remove wet clothing and items. Cover with blankets. Prevent convective loss from wind chill.
Active external	Provide: • Water baths (Hubbard tank) • Heat lamps • Circulating water blankets • Forced-air systems (Bair Hugger)

Active internal	Provide:
	• Lavage of numerous body cavities with warm saline
	  • Gastric
	  • Colonic
	  • Bladder
	  • Thoracic
	• Hemodialysis with potassium-free dialysate (warmed 40° to 45° C) (104° to 113° F)
	• Extracorporeal venovenous rewarming
	• Cardiopulmonary bypass

TAKE HOME POINTS

IV solutions should be warmed between 40° and 42° C (104° and 107.6° F) before infusing.

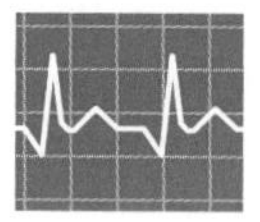

BP levels may fall during rewarming as a result of vasodilation or hypovolemia.

Care must be taken with warming extremities of moderate-to-severe hypothermic patients, especially patients who have been hypothermic for prolonged periods. Peripheral vasodilation from application of external heat can cause cold acidotic blood to return to the core compartment. The patient can develop hypotension, which can progress to shock, ventricular arrhythmias, and a sudden fall in core temperature called an *afterdrop.* Application of forced-air rewarming methods to the trunk alone may prevent afterdrop.

Active internal methods of rewarming will likely be needed for moderate-to-severe hypothermia and are definitely needed if the patient is in cardiac arrest because heat must be added to the core compartment.

- Vasoconstricting medications should be avoided because they will probably have minimal effect on the vasculature as a result of the ongoing vasoconstriction from hypothermia.
- Lidocaine (Xylocaine) should not be used as the antiarrhythmic medication for the patient in ventricular fibrillation because it is not usually effective below 30° C.
- Procainamide (Pronestyl) may increase the risk of ventricular fibrillation.

Complications subsequent to rewarming the severely hypothermic patient include rewarming shock because of a dilated vascular bed, a depressed myocardium, and hypovolemia. Complications also include pneumonia, gastrointestinal bleeding, cardiac arrhythmias, pulmonary edema, gangrene, myoglobinuria from rhabdomyolysis, intravascular thrombosis, and compartment syndrome.

Cardiopulmonary Resuscitation (CPR) in the Patient with Hypothermia. CPR should begin unless the patient has a documented "do not resuscitate" order, a fatal injury, or a chest wall that is frozen, making external cardiac massage impossible. A history of cardiac arrest before the onset of hypothermia most likely indicates a poor prognosis because the hypothermia probably had no protective effect on the brain before cardiac arrest. The American Heart Association's *Advanced Cardiac Life Support Provider Manual* (2001) states that severe hypothermia with a core temperature below 30° C reduces blood flow to the heart, brain, and all other vital organs and reduces BP. The patient needs to be kept horizontal because of impaired cardiovascular reflexes and resultant hypotension. In addition, the pulse and respiratory effort may be hard to detect. At least 30 to 45 seconds should be allowed to detect a pulse or respirations before starting chest compressions; if available, Doppler may be useful in detecting the pulse.

TAKE HOME POINTS

Forced-air rewarming systems (Bair Hugger) are practical and efficient, and can be used together with warmed IV fluids and warmed, humidified oxygen.

Hypotension can be worsened by catecholamine depletion from prolonged shivering and cold diuresis.

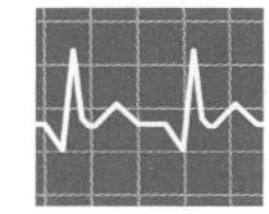

Continuous temperature monitoring is needed if active internal rewarming methods are used.

FIRST-LINE AND INITIAL TREATMENT FOR HYPOTHERMIA

- Maintain the patient's ABCs.
- Apply rewarming therapy.
- Consider underlying causes, and correct them.

Vasoactive drugs are not effective in the presence of hypothermia and are poorly metabolized by a cold liver. If repeated doses are given during the time the patient is hypothermic, drug toxicity from these repeated doses can occur during rewarming.

- The hypothermic heart is very irritable and prone to ventricular fibrillation. The patient should be given three shocks, per the basic life support (BLS) protocol, but the cold heart may not respond to defibrillation, and further shocks should not be given until the patient's core temperature is warmed above 30° C.
- Rewarming therapy should continue until the patient's core temperature is at least 32° C before any decision is made to terminate life support efforts.

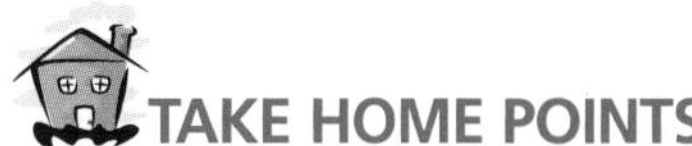

TAKE HOME POINTS

A serum potassium level of more than 10 mEq/L indicates extensive cell destruction and a poor prognosis.

Vasoconstricting medications should be avoided because they will probably have minimal effect on the vasculature as a result of the ongoing vasoconstriction from the hypothermia.

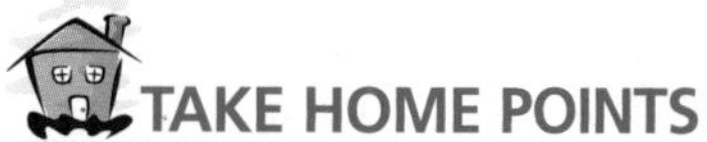

TAKE HOME POINTS

In hypothermia, expect an ↑ in hematocrit and BUN laboratory tests and either an ↑ or ↓ in K^+ and glucose.

Do You UNDERSTAND?

DIRECTIONS: **Fill in the blanks to complete each of the following statements.**

1. Hypothermia is caused by exposure to a cold environment, but it can also be the result of medical illnesses such as ____________________ and ____________.
2. The very ____________ and ____________ ____________ are especially susceptible to hypothermia.
3. With severe hypothermia, the patient may be ____________, with a fall in ____________ blood flow, ____________ blood flow, and ____________ output.
4. Body temperature is regulated by the ____________ and is carefully regulated to a ____________ ____________ of approximately 37° C.
5. The body is divided into ____________ and ____________ thermal compartments.
6. The four mechanisms of heat loss are ____________, ____________, ____________, and ____________.
7. ____________ accounts for most of the body's heat loss.
8. Mechanisms for heat production and conservation include ____________ and ____________.
9. "Wind chill" is a form of ____________ heat loss.
10. Both water exposure and alcohol consumption increase the risk for hypothermia. Water can absorb body heat much faster and better than ____________, and alcohol causes ________ which reduces the effectiveness of the ____________ and decreases ____________ of the cold environment.
11. When treating the patient with hypothermia, gentle movement is necessary; great care must be exercised when placing central lines to prevent triggering ____________ ____________ arrhythmias.
12. Laboratory abnormalities seen in hypothermia may include elevated ____________ and ____________ ____________ as a result of hemoconcentration and either high or low ____________ and ____________.

13. Active external rewarming includes forced-air ________________, which can add heat to both ________________ and ________________ compartments.
14. Airway assessment is always the first intervention, and supplemental ________________ heated to ________________ should be provided even to the mildly hypothermic patient because the oxyhemoglobin dissociation curve is shifted to the ________________.
15. Active internal rewarming may include ________________ via a Foley catheter, NG tube, and chest tubes.
16. ________________ bypass may also be needed, especially if the patient is in cardiac arrest as a result of hypothermia.
17. Warming of ________________ fluids and administering ________________ is important to help prevent heat loss from the core compartment.
18. Complications of rewarming may include rewarming ________________, pulmonary ________________, and myo- ________________.
19. CPR for the patient with hypothermia requires ________________ initial defibrillations, but further shocks should wait until ________________ is above 30° C.
20. The hypothermic patient in arrest may not respond to vasoactive ________________. On successful resuscitation, blood levels of those ________________ given during resuscitation can become ________________ after rewarming because of ________________ and because a cold ________________ metabolizes drugs poorly.

Answers: **1. hypoadrenalism, hypothyroidism; 2. young, old: 3. comatose, renal, cerebral, cardiac; 4. hypothalamus, set point; 5. core, peripheral; 6. conduction, convection, radiation, evaporation; 7. Radiation; 8. shivering, vasoconstriction; 9. convective; 10. air, vasodilation, hypothalamus, awareness; 11. ventricular; 12. hematocrit, blood urea nitrogen, potassium, glucose; 13. rewarming, peripheral, core; 14. oxygen, 40° C, left; 15. lavage; 16. cardiopulmonary; 17. IV, oxygen; 18. shock, pneumonia, globulinuria; 19. three, core temperature; 20. drugs, drugs, toxic, hypoperfusion, liver.**

What IS Overdose?

Various situations require emergent and critical care for patients. Among these is the presentation of a patient with a drug overdose. Intentional drug overdoses are the most common reported method for attempted suicide. Treatment includes stabilization, reducing further drug absorption, eliminating the drugs from the body, and ongoing monitoring.

TAKE HOME POINTS

All drugs, whether prescribed by a physician, purchased over the counter, or purchased "on the street," have the potential for detrimental outcomes.

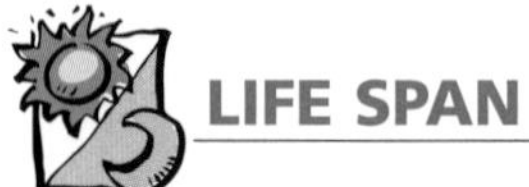

LIFE SPAN

The older adult is at greater risk for inadvertently overdosing or underdosing medications because of diminished eyesight.

A drug overdose can be a life-threatening situation, resulting in serious long-term consequences and even death. Overdose is defined as the accidental or intentional use of an illegal drug or legal medicine in an amount that is higher than prescribed. Any drug or medication has the potential to cause an overdose. Both legal and illegal drugs can be lethal when improperly used. The patient with a possible drug overdose requires emergent care and can be a challenge for the health care provider. A drug overdose can result in multisystem involvement that dictates the need for immediate attention to avoid further complications.

The nurse should also determine whether the overdose was accidental or an attempt to commit suicide. Until this issue is resolved, patients must be closely monitored to ensure no further attempts at self-harm are made. Stabilizing the patient's physical condition is the first and most crucial treatment step.

What You NEED TO KNOW

The initial evaluation of a patient with a possible drug overdose includes obtaining a complete and reliable history. The goal is to identify the drug or drugs taken alone or in combination with other drugs or substances. It is important to find out what drug has been taken, what amount has been taken, and the time of the intake. Any medical and psychiatric history, current medications, allergies, and any history of drug overdose should also be obtained. Next, a thorough physical examination is performed, which provides baseline information and identifies any physical symptoms. This examination must be completed as quickly as possible because time is of the essence. The initial physical evaluation must determine whether the patient's life is in immediate danger and identify any additional medical conditions or injuries that might become a concern while providing the necessary care for the overdose.

Obtaining a complete history may be difficult because the patient may be in a state of confusion, unconscious, or unable to provide information. In such cases, family members may be the main source of information. In other cases, the patient and family may find it embarrassing to provide information related to the addiction, or the patient may be found alone or he or she has been brought to the hospital for emergent care. In these cases, the emergency medical technicians may become the main source of information. Those providing patient information should be questioned about the circumstances in which the patient was found by asking the following questions:

- Was the patient conscious? Could he or she provide any information when initially found, including location and time?
- Were any prescription bottles present—with or without pills?
- Was any drug paraphernalia found?

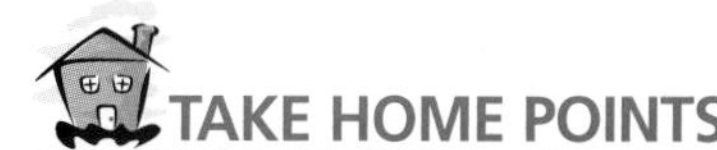

Questions help identify the drug, how much was taken, and when it was taken.

As previously mentioned, a physical evaluation must be completed as quickly as possible. If the history of the patient is unattainable, the physical evaluation becomes the only means of obtaining vital information in the search to identify the drugs of the overdose and to make decisions regarding appropriate care. The initial physical evaluation should include the review of vital signs, skin, breath (odor), ears, nose, throat, lungs, heart, abdomen, extremities, and neurologic (seizures) status. Each assessment finding will help identify the actual and possible systems affected by the drug overdose and will also provide clues as to the type of drug or drugs used and how each was introduced into the system. For example, the inspection of the skin may reveal fresh needle marks.

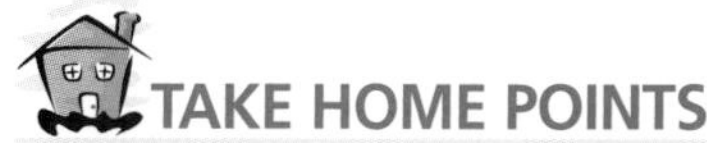

- An extensive physical examination is required because various drugs produce various symptoms.
- Common sites of IV drug entry include the arms, in between the toes, and the lower leg.

As an additional adjunct, laboratory tests can provide valuable information. Blood can be screened for drugs in the system, and ongoing monitoring can determine how fast the drug is being eliminated from the body. Urine tests can also be used to screen for some drugs and to detect changes in body chemistry. In addition, kidney and liver damage can be detected with blood and urine tests. If the evaluation eliminates the need for advanced life support efforts, supportive care becomes the choice of medical management for the patient who has overdosed.

What You DO

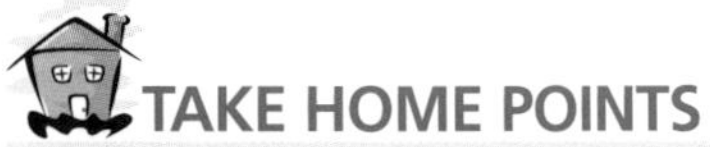

TAKE HOME POINTS

Know the telephone number of the Poison Control Center to aid in assessment and treatment: 1-800-922-1117.

The ideal first step is to obtain a complete history and physical evaluation; however, a critical patient requires immediate medical interventions. Assessment of the LOC is necessary to determine whether the patient is alert, arousable, or unresponsive. Sufficient ventilation and perfusion must be priorities. Airway and breathing assessment is performed to ascertain whether the patient's trachea is blocked. Correct positioning of the head (head tilt–chin lift or jaw thrust) prevents the posterior of the tongue from occluding the airway. This positioning may be all that is required to ensure that the patient can resume breathing on his or her own. Intubation may be necessary in the patient who is comatose, has lost the gag reflex, or is having seizures. Oropharyngeal airways can also assist. These airways are used in the patient who is spontaneously breathing but remains unconscious. These prevent the tongue from blocking the airway and provide for suction of secretions. If possible, oxygen should be administered after ABGs are obtained (refer to the discussion on RSI on p. 54).

FIRST-LINE AND INITIAL TREATMENT FOR THE PATIENT WHO HAS OVERDOSED

- Assess responsiveness.
- Establish an airway (head tilt–chin lift position, jaw thrust, oropharyngeal airway, intubation).
- Provide oxygen.
- Check pulse. If no pulse, initiate CPR.
- Initiate cardiac monitoring.
- Establish IV access (20- or 18-gauge for an adult).
- Provide fluid replacement.
- Determine substances taken; give appropriate reversal agent.

IV lines need to be initiated as soon as possible. Fluid replacement is necessary for patients who experience drug-induced hypotension. In addition, the IV route is preferable for administering medications. For the patient with cardiac compromise, a central venous line may also be indicated and an ECG may be prescribed to assist in determining the presence of any cardiac injury. The patient's cardiac status needs to be monitored until medically cleared.

If the patient exhibits an altered mental status, a trial dose of a therapeutic reversal agent may be administered. Naloxone (Narcan), dextrose, thiamine, and oxygen are all considered safe and innocuous agents. Glucose and thiamine may be life-saving measures to the patient who has hypoglycemia. Thiamine is also effective in preventing Wernicke-Korsakoff syndrome, which is associated with alcohol withdrawal.

Focus Areas for the Management of the Patient Experiencing an Overdose

- Supportive care
- Prevention of absorption
- Enhancement of excretion (if possible)
- Administration of an antidote (if available)

One of the more important elements in the management of the patient who has ingested an overdose is supportive care. This includes frequent monitoring of vital signs with particular focus on the temperature, which helps identify hypothermia or hyperthermia. It is necessary to monitor multiple systems as indicated to identify any system failure. Acute and subtle changes to the LOC must be detected quickly to avoid further complications such as aspiration. IV fluids are given for fluid maintenance and replacement or to provide forced diuresis. Frequent monitoring of ABGs is needed when using alkaline therapy or when the patient is on a ventilator. Lastly, the management of hypotension requires care based on patient needs and the drug ingested.

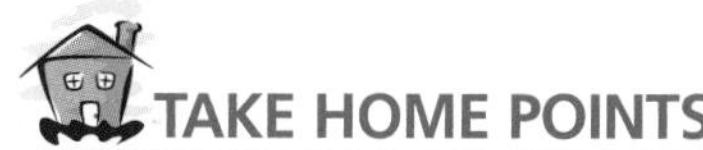

An oral slurry of 60-100 grams for adults and 15-30 grams for children of a mixture of activated charcoal and sorbitol is used in conscious patients with a gag reflex. This can be given in multiple doses as needed.

Most overdoses occur by way of the gastrointestinal tract. In these situations, it is most important that further gastrointestinal absorption be stopped. Several methods are available to remove the drug from the gastrointestinal tract. These include emesis, gastric lavage, cathartics, and absorbents.

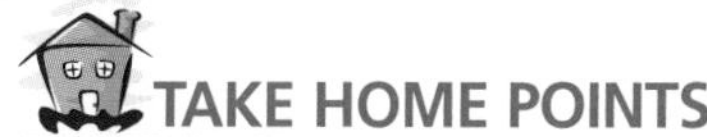

We no longer induce emesis in patients, so the use of ipecac syrup is no longer done.

Gastric lavage is another method for removing gastric contents. This procedure calls for the passage of the largest tube passable through the patient's oropharynx. A 32- to 40-French orogastric tube is used in an adult. The patient is placed in a left lateral decubitus Trendelenburg position with knees flexed. This position allows for the greatest abdominal relaxation and gastric emptying, and it reduces the risk for aspiration in case emesis occurs. Confirmation of proper tube placement is obtained before lavage and via an x-ray film. Tap water or saline, typically 10 to

Gastric lavage is no longer considered effective when the patient has taken medications in the last 45 minutes.

20 L, is induced into the stomach. The solution may be warmed, which hastens the dissolution of pills that remain in the stomach. The solution is then emptied from the stomach by way of lowering the tube to the floor and siphoning off the fluid or suctioning, which is known as *stomach pumping*. The patient is lavaged until the return is clear.

As a means to decrease drug absorption, activated charcoal and a cathartic are administered. Absorbents provide the means for decreasing any further absorption of the involved overdose drug into the system. Activated charcoal and cathartics are used for this purpose. Activated charcoal plays a major role in the treatment of the overdose patient. Activated charcoal is a residue of destructive distillation of burned organic materials such as wood, pulp, paper, bone, and sawdust—to name a few. Heating with CO_2, which increases the surface binding area and in turn increases the absorption ability of the materials, activates the charcoal. Activated charcoal is a fine, black powder, tasteless and odorless, with a gritty consistency. It is mixed with 60 to 90 mL of water to make a slurry. Between 30 and 100 g for an adult is then induced into the stomach by way of an NG or lavage tube. It can be administered orally if the patient is alert and cooperative. The recommended dose for an adult is 50 to 100 mg mixed in 8 ounces of water. Major prevention of further drug absorption occurs the sooner the activated charcoal is given after ingestion of the drug. No identifiable contraindications exist, but patients with ileus who have repeated charcoal doses are predisposed to vomiting. Vomiting has been documented in 10% to 15% of patients who are given charcoal alone.

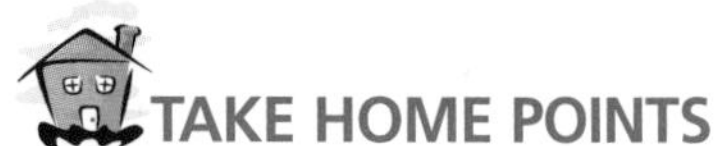

Sorbitol 33 cc and activated charcoal 50-75 grams via gastric tube is a common treatment for overdose in adults.

Cathartics are administered as a means of eliminating drugs from the gastrointestinal tract, as well as assisting with the passage of charcoal. They decrease the gastrointestinal transit time of the drug, thus decreasing the possibility for absorption. The cathartics include the following agents: sorbitol, magnesium sulfate (Epsom salt), magnesium citrate, sodium sulfate (Glauber's solution), and disodium phosphate (Fleet enema). The fastest and most potent cathartic is the osmotic agent sorbitol. Magnesium sulfate and magnesium citrate and hypertonic saline agents are slower acting, and magnesium levels need to be monitored. These agents should be avoided in patients with salt-intake restrictions and in those with a history of heart failure.

Multiple methods can be used to enhance the excretion of drugs from the body. These include forced diuresis, alteration of urine pH, hemodialysis, and hemoperfusion. Each has limited use and is instituted when an antidote is not available.

Forced diuresis involves the flow of urine at the rate of 3 to 5 mL/kg/hr, which may require a diuretic. This process should only be used when specifically indicated, such as an overdose with phenobarbital, bromides, lithium, salicylate, and amphetamines. It is not used frequently because of complications such as volume overload or electrolyte disturbances.

Alteration in urine pH involves the concept of ion trapping. Rapid movement across membranes is enhanced with low degrees of ionization and high lipid solubility. Weak acids are ionized in a more alkaline medium, and weak bases are ionized in a more acidic medium. If a pH difference exists across the membrane, ion trapping occurs. More total drug exists in the compartment where ionization is greater because the non-ionized form crosses the lipid cellar membrane more readily than does the ionized form.

Hemodialysis and *hemoperfusion* can be valuable adjuncts to treatment, although many drugs such as diazepam (Valium), digoxin (Lanoxin), and phenytoin (Dilantin) are not well removed with these invasive and complicated procedures. Similarities between hemoperfusion and hemodialysis exist. Both call for an extracorporeal means through which blood is passed. Hemoperfusion requires the blood to be delivered through a cartridge that contains an absorbent such as activated charcoal. The blood is then returned to venous circulation. Hemodialysis is similar except the blood is sent through a dialyzer, which helps separate diffusible substances from other, less diffusible substances.

Some patients who come to the emergency department with an overdose may respond to the administration of an antidote. Antidotes are divided into physiologic and specific. General or supportive antidotes are also available. General or supportive antidotes, which include activated charcoal and sodium bicarbonate, are not true antidotes but help treat overdose symptoms. Although numerous treatments are available, the following table lists the basic rules of supportive care that need to be instituted for all patients with a possible overdose.

Disodium phosphate (Fleet enema) must be used cautiously in children because of anatomic and physiologic factors. Absorption of the drug depends on the anatomic care of the rectum. Medications administered in the lower portion of the rectum bypass the liver circulation and metabolism. In addition, caution must be taken regarding possible fluid and electrolyte shifts that occur when an enema is administered.

TAKE HOME POINTS

- Peritoneal dialysis should not be used as the mode of dialysis because it is inefficient, and most overdose substances bind to plasma proteins.
- Hemodialysis is effective and essential in overdose cases with methanol, ethylene glycol, and salicylates.

Drug Antidotes and Antagonists

Drug	Antagonist	Dose
Acetaminophen (Tylenol)	Acetylcysteine (N-acetylcysteine)	Oral solution (5%) Adult loading dose 140 mg/kg, followed by maintenance dose 70 mg/kg, q4h, for 17 additional doses
Opioids	Nalmefene (Revex) Naloxone (Narcan) Naltrexone (ReVia)	Administered IV, IM, SQ, titrated individually Administered IV, IM, SQ Adults 0.4 to 2.0 mg Administered orally 50 mg/day or 100 qod

IV, Intravenously; *IM,* intramuscularly; *SQ,* subcutaneously; *q4h,* every 4 hours; *qod,* every other day.

Common Overdose Drugs and Their Symptoms

As previously mentioned, all drugs have the potential to be an agent of overdose. Accidental or intentional drug overdoses can result from drugs commonly prescribed, bought over the counter, or purchased on the street. Various symptoms of overdose are present, depending on the type of drug ingested. The following table lists some drugs commonly seen in overdose situations.

Common Drugs and the Symptoms of Overdose and Treatment

Drug	Symptoms of Overdose	Treatment
Anticholinergics (Atropine, scopolamine, belladonna, antihistamine, antidepressants, antipsychotics, OTC cough and cold medicines)	• Increased respirations • Increased or decreased BP • Increased heart rate (dysrhythmias) • Dry, hot skin and membranes • Dilated pupils • Decreased bowel sounds • Urinary retention • Seizures	Supportive care
Acetaminophen (Tylenol)	• Immediate symptoms: nausea, vomiting, diaphoresis, anorexia, fatigue, paleness • Advanced symptoms: nausea, vomiting, jaundice, right upper quadrant pain, lethargy, coma, bleeding, hypoglycemia, renal failure	Gastric lavage Administration of antidote (N-acetylcysteine, Naloxone, nalmefene, methadone) Supportive care
Salicylates (aspirin, muscle and joint pain creams)	• Increased respirations, respiratory alkalosis, hyperventilation • Nausea, vomiting, diaphoresis, gastrointestinal discomfort • Confusion, lethargy, seizures, tinnitus, irritability • Cardiovascular failure, increased heart rate, metabolic acidosis	Gastric lavage Activated charcoal Forced diuresis Supportive care
CNS stimulants (amphetamines, cocaine, methylphenidate)	• Increased heart rate, dysrhythmias, myocardial infarction, cardiac arrest, increased BP • Stroke, seizures, behavioral changes, headache	Gastric lavage Activated charcoal Supportive care
CNS depressants (sedatives, choral hydrate, meprobamate, hypnotics), benzodiazepines (Xanax, Ativan, Valium, Klonopin)	• Decreased BP, decreased heart rate, cardiac arrest • Decreased respirations, respiratory arrest • Drowsiness, stupor, coma	Gastric lavage Activated charcoal Forced diuresis Dialysis Hemoperfusion Supportive care
Barbiturates (phenobarbital, Nembutal, secobarbital)	• Decreased heart rate, decreased BP • Decreased respirations, respiratory depression, pulmonary edema	Gastric lavage Administration of antidote (Naloxone) Supportive care

Common Drugs and the Symptoms of Overdose and Treatment—cont'd

Drug	Symptoms of Overdose	Treatment
Narcotics and opioids (morphine, codeine, heroin, Percocet, methadone, clonidine, Lomotil)	• Decreased level of consciousness, pinpoint pupils	Narcan
Hallucinogens (LSD, MDMA [also known as Ecstasy], PCP)	• Increased heart rate, increased BP • Hyperreflexia • Stupor, coma (PCP)	Gastric lavage Activated charcoal Supportive care
Alcohol (Ethanol)	• Neurologic—visual impairment, headache, poor coordination, stupor • Cardiac—increased heart rate, cardiac collapse • Respirations—decreased respirations • Gastrointestinal—nausea, vomiting, abdominal pain, hypoglycemia	Gastric lavage Supportive care

OTC, Over the counter; *CNS,* central nervous system; *LSD,* lysergic acid diethylamide; *MCMA,* methylenedioxymethamphetamine; *PCP,* phencyclidine; *BP,* blood pressure.

Special Considerations

Once the overdose patient has been medically stabilized, the decision must be made whether ongoing observation is needed. Complications from treatments may require ongoing observation. The patient who experiences a drug overdose may require hospitalization for numerous reasons. In addition, those who have additional medical problems outside of the overdose may also require continued hospitalization. Finally, some drugs such as acetaminophen have a latent phase. In 24 to 72 hours, the patient who appears to be doing well may begin to decompensate.

Drug withdrawal may also necessitate the need for ongoing hospital observation. Withdrawal from some drugs can be life threatening and require medical management (see the table on the following page for a listing of drugs and signs of withdrawal). Once the patient has been through withdrawal, follow-up care such as rehabilitation should be obtained.

Patients who intentionally overdose require close monitoring while in the emergency department. Suicide precautions such as active listening and effective communication should be initiated to avoid further attempts. Depressed patients, those who have suicidal thoughts, and those who have attempted suicide in the past are at high risk for overdose. All patients who have overdosed should receive a psychiatric clearance before being discharged from the hospital.

Drug Withdrawal Syndromes

Drugs	Withdrawal Signs and Symptoms
CNS stimulants	Muscular aches, abdominal pain, chills, tremors, hunger, anxiety, prolonged sleep, lack of energy, profound depression, suicidal, exhaustion
CNS depressants	Dilated pupils, rapid pulse, gooseflesh, lacrimation, abdominal cramps, muscle jerks, "flu" syndrome, vomiting, diarrhea, tremors, yawning, anxiety

CNS, Central nervous system.

Do You UNDERSTAND?

DIRECTIONS: **Identify the following statements as *true* (T) or *false* (F).**

_____ 1. Physician-prescribed medications cannot produce drug overdoses.

_____ 2. The primary goal when dealing with an overdose patient is physical stabilization.

_____ 3. The four areas of focus for managing the overdose patient are providing supportive care, preventing absorption, enhancing excretion, and administering antidotes.

_____ 4. Activated charcoal and cathartics are used to enhance excretion.

_____ 5. Drug withdrawal may require ongoing hospitalization for the patient treated for a drug overdose.

What IS a Disaster?

A disaster is any situation or occurrence, natural or manmade, which causes human suffering, loss of property or infrastructure, and creates needs for the victims that cannot be alleviated without outside assistance.

At-Risk Populations

Many populated areas are located on fault lines, increasing the risks for earthquakes; low-lying areas are prone to flooding; and in sections of the Midwest known as "Tornado Alley," frequent and multiple tornados can

Answers: 1. F; 2. T; 3. T; 4. F; 5. T.

occur. Coastal regions are vulnerable to hurricanes and, as populations spread out from urban areas, homes become more susceptible to wildland fires. Manmade disasters such as chemical spills, industrial accidents, and terrorist acts can occur anywhere.

What ARE the Stages of Disaster Response?

1. *Non-disaster or inter-disaster stage*: When no disaster is occurring, but the threat or potential still exists. This is when community planning and preparation should take place.
2. *Pre-disaster stage*: There is an impending disaster, but it has not yet occurred. During this stage, warning, mobilization of resources, and evacuation should take place.
3. *Impact stage*: The disaster has occurred. Initial assessment of the disaster and its effects on the community takes place. Stage lasts until the threat of destruction has passed.
4. *Emergency stage or post-impact stage*: Begins immediately following the disaster impact stage. Rescue and relief efforts begin and continue until no threat of injury, illness, or destruction exists from the disaster.
5. *Recovery stage*: Time of rebuilding, reconstruction, and restoration of the community to restore normal order and function. This stage commonly lasts for months and may continue for years after a major disaster.

What IS Triage?

The term Triage comes from the French word "Trier" meaning "to sort, sift, or select." Traditional emergency room triage is based on the concept of providing the optimal and highest level of care for each patient. During a disaster, triage shifts to a system of evaluating casualties or patients in order to maximize effective use of available resources and to do the most good for the greatest number of people. During the Triage process, victims are rapidly evaluated, and each is assigned a treatment priority level based on the severity of their injuries and likelihood to survive with treatment. The principles of Disaster Triage are to quickly remove those who require minimal care or no care from the immediate area and then rapidly assess, stabilize, and evacuate those who require treatment by a medical provider. The United States Military utilizes a standardized triage system: Immediate (Priority 1), Delayed (Priority 2), Minimal (Priority 3), Expectant (Priority 4), and dead (not considered a triage category). Casualties categorized as Immediate are the highest priority. This category involves those who have an obvious threat to life or limb. Patients in this category will likely die without medical treatment but will likely survive with rapid intervention. Delayed casualties clearly need medical care but are likely to survive even if care is delayed by several hours to days. Common injuries in this group include open fractures, chest or abdominal injuries with stable vital signs, large or deep open wounds with controlled bleeding, and no airway instability or breathing compromise. Minimal will include all patients with minor injuries who are able to ambulate and have stable vital signs. Expectant casualties are those whose injuries are so severe that they are not expected to survive, even with extensive treatment.

The MASS Triage model provides a method for rapidly classifying large numbers of casualties during a Mass Casualty Incident. The first step is **M**ove; ask the casualties to move to a designated area (usually designated by color: green for *Minimal*, yellow for *Delayed*, red for *Immediate*, and blue or black for *Expectant*) if they need medical attention. Those who are able to move are categorized as *Minimal.* Next, ask for anyone who did not move with the first group and needs medical attention to raise an arm or a leg so someone can come to them and help. These patients are categorized as *Delayed.* Finally, identify those casualties who did not respond with one of the first two groups. These are seriously injured or dead, and will be classified as *Immediate, Expectant,* or *dead.*

The second step in MASS triage is **A**ssess; conduct a rapid assessment of all casualties in the Immediate category and determine those whose injuries are so severe that they are categorized as Expectant. Rapid assessment involves assessing the ABCs and treating any immediate life threatening conditions unless the casualty is expectant.

The third step in MASS triage is to **S**ort patients into each of the groups and to reclassify them as needed based on injuries and any changes in status. **S**end is the final step and here patients are evacuated to hospitals and other treatment facilities.

Where Do I Find Resources and Information for Disaster Response?

The Federal Emergency Management Agency (FEMA) website (www.fema.gov) serves as a primary resource for disaster information at all levels. It provides up-to-date information on current and potential disasters in the United States as well as online training for both citizens and responders, links to state and local disaster response and relief agencies, and detailed information on the different types of disasters. The American Red Cross website (www.redcross.org) provides information on both U.S. and international disasters and disaster response. Your local Emergency Management Agency is the best resource for information and volunteer opportunities in your community.

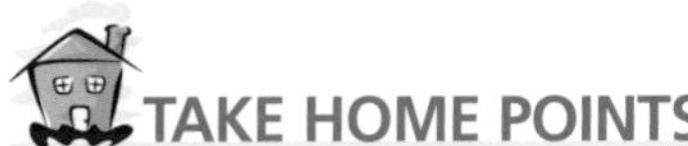

Rapid Casualty Assessment and Triage

- Go to the group of victims who were unable to move or follow simple commands first.

Rapid ABC assessment

- Open Airway? If not, attempt to open. If unable to open the airway, classify as Expectant and move to next patient.
- Uncontrolled bleeding? Apply tourniquet or direct pressure.
- Fatal injuries likely? Classify as Expectant and move to next patient.

References

AACN-AANN Protocols for Practice: *Monitoring technologies in critically ill neuroscience patients.* Sudbury, MA, 2009, Jones and Bartlett.

Alspach JG: *American Association of Critical Care Nurses certification and core review for high acuity,* ed 6, St. Louis, 2007, Saunders/Elsevier.

Baird MS, Keen JH, Swearingen PL: *Manual of critical care nursing: nursing interventions and collaborative management,* ed 5, St. Louis, 2005, Elsevier.

Barker E: *Neuroscience nursing: a spectrum of care,* ed 3, St. Louis, 2008, Mosby/Elsevier.

Carley SD, Cwinnutt C, Bulter J, Sammy I, Driscoll P: Rapid sequence induction in the emergency department: a strategy for failure, *Emergency Medicine Journal,* 19:109-113, 2002.

Chernecky C & Berger B: *Laboratory tests and diagnostic procedures,* ed 5, St. Louis, 2008, Elsevier.

Chulay M, Burns SM: *American Association of Critical Care Nurses essentials of critical care nursing,* New York, 2006, McGraw Hill.

Edelstein JA: Hypothermia. 2007, Retrieved May 23, 2008, from www.emedicine.com/emerg/TOPIC279.HTM.

Ikematsu, Yuko. Incidence and characteristics of dysphoria in patients with cardiac tamponade, *Heart & Lung,* 36(6): 440-449, 2007.

Kovacs G, Law A, Tallon J, Petrie D, Campbell S, Soder C: Acute airway management in the emergency department by non-anesthesiologists, *Canadian Journal of Anesthesia* 51:174-180, 2004.

Molina DK & DiMaio VJ. Rifle wounds: a review of range and location as pertaining to manner of death, *American Journal of Forensic Medicine and Pathology,* 29(3): 201-205, 2008.

Morton PG, Fontaine DK, Hudak CM, Gallo BM: *Critical care nursing: a holistic approach,* ed 8, Philadelphia, 2004, Lippincott Williams & Wilkins.

Perry JJ, Lee JS, Sillber VH, Wells GA:Rocuronium versus succinylcholine for rapid response induction intubation. *Cochrane Database of Systematic Reviews* 2003, *Issue 1.* No. CD002788. DOI: 10.1002/14651858.CD002788.pub2.

Phillips TG: 2008, Hypothermia. Retrieved May 23, 2008, from www.emedicine.com/MED/topic1144.htm.

Pousman R: Rapid sequence induction for prehospital providers. *Emergency and Intensive Care Medicine, 4(1).* Retrieved May 15, 2008, from www.ispub.com/ostia/index.php?xmlFilePath journals/ijeicm/vol4n1/rapid.xml.

Putza M, Casati A, Berti M, Pagliarini G, Fanelli G: Clinical complications, monitoring and management of perioperative mild hypothermia: anesthesiological features. *Acta Biomed* 78:163-169, 2007.

Reichman E, Simon R (eds): *Emergency medicine procedures,* New York, 2004, McGraw-Hill.

Urden LD, Stacy KM, Lough ME: *Thelan's critical care nursing diagnosis and management,* ed 5, St Louis, 2006, Elsevier.

NCLEX® Review

1. Mr. Jones, an 84-year-old quadriplegic patient with significant history of gastroesophageal reflux disease (GERD) and chronic renal failure (CRF), is exhibiting signs of respiratory distress. The decision has been made to provide intubation and, when assisting during RSI, you are aware that:
   1 Some of the medications used to intubate Mr. Jones will have a delayed onset because of the CRF.
   2 Mr. Jones will require a fiberoptic intubation because of his history of quadriplegia.
   3 Succinylcholine (Anectine) may induce a hyperkalemic response in Mr. Jones.
   4 Mr. Jones will need more induction medication because of upregulation of central nervous system (CNS) receptors secondary to quadriplegia.
2. The ability of the brain to tolerate increases in intracranial volume is called compliance. Compliance is based on which two concepts?
   1 RR and BP.
   2 Temperature and CO.
   3 Volume and pressure.
   4 Temperature and volume.
3. A pressure gradient across the brain defined as mean arterial pressure (MAP). CBF maintains:
   1 Cerebral blood flow.
   2 CO.
   3 Brain volume.
   4 Cerebral perfusion pressure.
4. Sustained increased ICP can lead to brainstem herniation. The outcome of brainstem herniation is:
   1 Cerebral stroke.
   2 Seizure.
   3 Death.
   4 Migraine headache.
5. A 21-year old male is admitted to the trauma ICU after falling 20 feet from a ladder with a head injury after being in an MVC. The nurse assesses a small amount of bloody drainage in the patient's nose. Using a 4- × 4-gauze pad to catch the blood the nurse notices a halo effect of blood and clear fluid on the gauze. The nurse also observes ecchymosis around the eyes. The nurse suspects:
   1 Basilar skull fracture.
   2 Depression fracture.
   3 Linear skull fracture.
   4 Increased ICP.
6. The appropriate drug for an agitated patient who requires a reduction in ICP based on reducing fluid on the brain is:
   1 Mannitol (Osmitrol).
   2 Morphine.
   3 Midazolam (Versed).
   4 Epinephrine (Adrenaline).
7. Which of the following is a contraindication for the use of medical antishock trousers (MAST) or pneumatic antishock garment (PASG)?
   1 Hypovolemic shock.
   2 Pelvic or lower extremity fractures.
   3 Septic shock.
   4 Left ventricular dysfunction.
8. Mr. JW, an 18-year-old man, is brought to your level 1 ED by car. His friends state he has been shot. You note multiple gunshot wounds. He is tachycardic, tachypneic, and lethargic. Vital signs are HR of 146 bpm, RR of 40 breaths/min, and BP at 60/40 mm Hg. He is bleeding profusely from a gaping abdominal wound. When considering care for this patient, what would you presume to be the most likely sequence of events?
   1 Start an IV, and administer vasopressors and IV fluids. Monitor vital signs in the ED until bleeding is controlled.

2 Secure airway and cervical spine, administer oxygen, support respirations, start two large-bore peripheral IVs, and administer crystalloids and blood while assessing and preparing the patient for immediate transport to the surgical department.
3 Transport the patient to an ED that is better equipped to manage a patient like this.
4 Stabilize the patient, and immediately transport for CAT scan evaluation.

9. A 65-year-old man has recently had a balloon angioplasty. Which of the following signs could indicate cardiac tamponade?
1 Crackles in both lung fields.
2 Bradycardia.
3 Muffled heart tones.
4 Hypertension.

10. Cardiac tamponade is caused by:
1 Excess fluid or clots collecting in the ventricles of the heart.
2 Decreased venous return.
3 Excess fluid accumulation of fluid in pericardial sac.
4 Increased CO.

NCLEX® Review Answers

1.3 Neuromuscular disorders such as spinal cord injuries predispose patients to dangerous hyperkalemia when succinylcholine (Anectine) is used. CRF has minimal effects on the onset times of the induction and paralytic medications. Many factors affect the need for fiberoptic intubation. Quadriplegia alone is not sufficient reason. Patients with spinal cord injuries do not routinely require more induction medications.

2.3 Volume divided by pressure is the concept for intracranial compliance. RR and BP might contribute to compensation; however, they are not directly involved with intracranial compliance. Temperature and CO are not directly involved with intracranial compliance.

3.4 Cerebral perfusion pressure (CPP) is a pressure gradient across the brain. CBF maintains cerebral perfusion; CO is stroke volume × HR, and brain volume is an intracranial component.

4.3 Herniation of the brainstem causes immediate death. Although some of the late signs of increased ICP mimic stroke, stroke is not the outcome of brainstem herniation. Possible seizure activity is a possible late sign of increased ICP; however, stroke is not the outcome of brainstem herniation. Headache is a possible early sign of increased ICP and is not the outcome of brainstem herniation.

5.1 The symptoms described are accurate for a classic presentation for a basilar skull fracture supported by the presence of CSF and bloody drainage from the nose in conjunction with the classic presentation of ecchymosis around the eyes (called raccoon eyes). There was no indication of a bony step-off on the cranium, which is associated with a depression skull fracture. The linear fracture is the most common skull fracture, but in this case, the additional findings indicate otherwise. The information discussed in the questions did not support or rule out an increase in ICP.

6.3 Versed is regularly used in TBI management to calm and/or sedate the agitated patient. This action helps reduce the patient's ICP by eliminating or reducing the agitation and movement of the patient. Mannitol can reduce ICP by drawing fluid off the brain but offers no sedating qualities. Morphine and epinephrine can be harmful in TBI patients because the mechanisms of action can exacerbate ICP.

7.4 Left ventricular dysfunction is a contraindication for MAST or PASG. Compression to the lower extremities and abdomen increases intrathoracic pressure and compression of lower body vasculature, causing increased work for the poorly functioning left ventricle. Hypovolemic shock and septic shock are both indications for MAST or PASG. They increase venous return and support BP. Pelvic or lower extremity fractures may also be indications for MAST or PASG.

8.2 The ABCs have been followed and you have recognized that the patient's injuries are too extensive to be controlled in the ED. The only chance for survival for this patient in a class IV hemorrhage is to control the bleeding and provide aggressive volume replacement, both of which may be accomplished in the surgical unit.

9.3 The increased fluid in the pericardial sac results in muffled heart tones. Crackles in lung fields do not indicate cardiac tamponade. Bradycardia is a sign of tamponade in infants, not in a 65-year-old patient. Hypotension is more commonly associated with tamponade.

10.3 Tamponade is caused by the accumulation of fluid, clots, gas, or pus in the pericardial sac. The ability of the ventricles of the heart to fill and contract is diminished in cardiac tamponade. Decreased venous return can be a sign of cardiac tamponade, but it is not a cause. CO decreases as a result of cardiac tamponade.

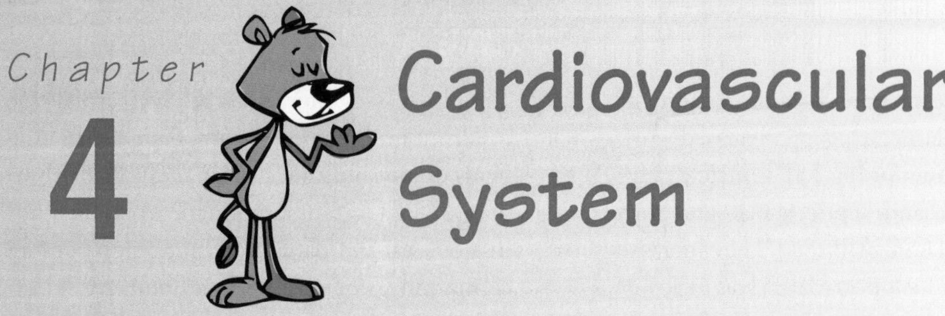

Chapter 4 Cardiovascular System

What You WILL LEARN

After reading this chapter, you will know how to do the following:

- ✔ Differentiate between the various pathologic processes of acute coronary syndrome.
- ✔ Describe the physical manifestations most commonly associated with the various types of acute coronary syndromes.
- ✔ Compare and contrast the various types of acute coronary syndromes.
- ✔ Establish a prioritized plan of care for patients with acute coronary syndrome.
- ✔ Discuss the complications of acute coronary syndrome.
- ✔ Explain the physiologic changes associated with heart failure.
- ✔ Identify risk factors that predispose patients to the development of heart failure.
- ✔ Compare and contrast the clinical manifestations for right- and left-sided heart failure.
- ✔ Identify appropriate nursing interventions for caring for a patient with heart failure.
- ✔ Describe prevention approaches that can be instituted in the critical care environment.
- ✔ Discuss relevant patient education topics.

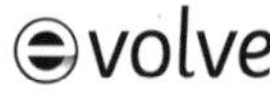

See http://evolve.elsevier.com/Schumacher/criticalcare for additional NCLEX® review questions.

V ... ndrome?

... ed to the cascade of
... nia with or without
... inclusion of all the
... port to the myocar-
... farction (NSTEMI),
... (Q wave). The classic
... sternal (retrosternal)
... ate to the shoulders,
... s pressure, heaviness,
... usea, diaphoresis, and

... I

... when the heart muscle is
... However, in the case of
... f an acute plaque rupture
... n delivery to the point of
irreversible ... rivation leads to structural
and functional changes within the affected area of myocardial tissue. As with acute coronary syndrome, CAD is the most common cause of AMI. With these basic similarities in mind, many components of the AMI disease process and treatment either overlap to some degree or further develop along the continuum of cardiovascular diseases.

With continued advances in medical research and pharmacologic therapies, the nurse has incredible potential for playing a crucial role in not only improving AMI survival rates but also preserving the highest level of long-term functionality in these patients. Therefore, it is essential that all nurses be able to identify quickly the signs and symptoms of AMI and then implement evidence-based interventions known to increase patients' survival rates and quality of life.

What You NEED TO KNOW

Most often, atherosclerosis (CAD) is the underlying cause of AMI, although in rare cases AMI has been attributed to direct trauma or electrocution. However, it is not clear whether some degree of undiagnosed atherosclerosis actually existed in these cases. Nonetheless, when AMI occurs because of CAD, the offending incident is usually a thromboembolic occlusion of one or more coronary vessels.

In the presence of atherosclerotic plaques, particularly during the more advanced stages, myocardial blood supply is already compromised. In these instances in which myocardial reserve is extremely limited, any event that increases the workload or further impairs the blood supply to the heart places the individual at increased risk for suffering ischemic cardiac changes. The situation is one of simple supply and demand: An oxygen deficit results when there is demand that outweighs the supply, which results in myocardial ischemia and possibly even infarction. Precipitating factors that can cause an imbalance in supply and demand include:

- Physical exertion
- Emotional stress
- Temperature extremes
- Digestion of a heavy meal
- Valsalva maneuver
- Sexual excitation
- Pathophysiologic characteristics

As previously discussed, when an individual has CAD, the danger of plaque rupture is present at any time. This event can lead to two disastrous consequences. Upon rupture, the embolic plaque travels into the coronary vasculature and obstructs flow. Alternatively, even if the plaque does not become an embolus, the irregular surface of the damaged endothelium causes platelet aggregation and fibrin deposits, which lead to thrombus formation and result in the partial or total occlusion of the artery. The area of myocardium served by this coronary artery branch is then subjected to a lack of perfusion.

The lack of oxygen available for oxidative phosphorylation to take place results in cellular anaerobic metabolism. Lactic acid, a deleterious by-product of anaerobic metabolism, accumulates rapidly within the myocardium and inhibits normal enzyme physiologic activity. In the presence of lactic acid, enzymes, which are essential for intracellular function, cease to work. In addition, the necessary reserves of adenosine triphosphate (ATP) are exhausted within minutes and the myocardium is unable to sustain anaerobic activity. Without ATP, the transmembrane pump fails to work, resulting in free movement of ions across the plasma membrane. The most crucial effect of this ionic movement is the change in membrane potential as sodium moves into the cell and potassium moves out. This change ultimately inhibits the conduction of electrical impulses and thus myocardium contractility. Additionally, because water follows sodium into the cell, swelling occurs.

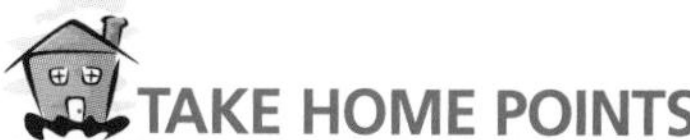

TAKE HOME POINTS

The cardiac output (CO) and peripheral vascular resistance directly affects BP. If a patient's BP decreases, then either the flow CO or the systemic vascular resistance (SVR) has changed.

Cardiac cells can withstand ischemic conditions for approximately 20 minutes before irreversible cellular death begins. If these ischemic changes are not reversed, water continues to move into the cytoplasm, eventually causing structural and functional changes, including lysosomal and mitochondrial swelling. The eventual rupture in these membranes leads to the autodigestion of cellular contents by the hydrolytic lysosomal enzymes as well as disruption of organelles and genetic material. Cardiac contractility and output are negatively impacted as the affected area of the myocardium loses the ability to meet the metabolic requirements of the body.

TAKE HOME POINTS

- Initially, when blood flow to the myocardium is prevented, ischemia ensues in the area distal to the obstruction. If blood flow is not soon restored, the ischemia progresses to infarction.
- Infarction results from sustained ischemia and is irreversible, causing cellular death and necrosis.

Cellular necrosis causes the release of endogenous catecholamines and activates the body's inflammatory process. The increase in circulating epinephrine and norepinephrine levels stimulates glycogenolysis and lipolysis, which causes a surge in plasma concentrations of glucose and free fatty acids. In an attempt to heal the injured cells, the inflammatory process initiates the release of leukocytes, which infiltrate the area. These neutrophils and macrophages begin the process of phagocytosis to degrade and remove the necrotic tissue. When this process is completed, a collagen matrix is laid down, which eventually forms scar tissue. Although the scar tissue is strong, it is unable to contract and relax like healthy cardiac muscle, which can lead to ventricular dysfunction or pump failure.

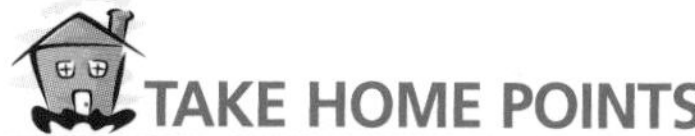

TAKE HOME POINTS

For a period after AMI, a pseudodiabetic state frequently develops because of glycogenolysis.

Determining the Severity of Acute Myocardial Infarction

The degree of altered function depends on the specific area of the heart involved, the presence of collateral circulation, and the size and the duration of the infarction. When describing infarctions in terms of the location of occurrence, the following terms are used: anterior, inferior, lateral, or posterior wall. Common combinations of areas are the anterolateral or anteroseptal MI. The location and area of the infarction correlate with the

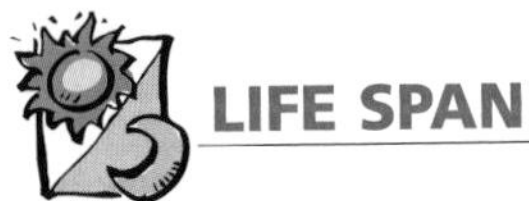

LIFE SPAN

The younger person who has a severe MI and has not had sufficient time to develop preestablished collateral circulation is often more likely to have more serious impairment than an older person with the same degree of occlusion.

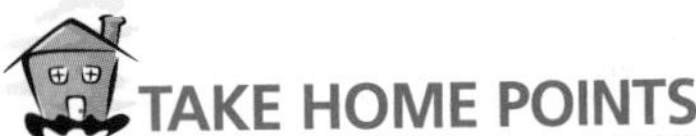

TAKE HOME POINTS

A transmural infarction impairs contractility to a greater extent than does a subendocardial infarction.

Myocardial cell death begins after 20 minutes of ischemia; the damage is not complete and irreversible until after 3 to 4 hours.

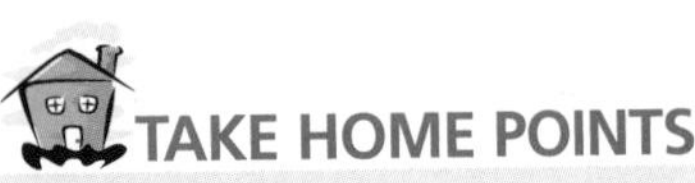

TAKE HOME POINTS

Cells in the ischemic area are salvageable if reperfusion therapies and inotropic support is promptly instituted.

part of the coronary circulation involved. For example, inferior wall infarctions are usually the result of right coronary artery lesions. Left circumflex artery lesions usually cause posterior or inferior AMIs. Lesions in the left anterior descending artery usually cause anterior wall infarctions. (See Color Plate 4 of coronary arteries and localization of AMI.)

The degree of preestablished collateral circulation also determines the severity of infarction. In an individual with a history of heart disease, adequate collateral circulation channels may have been established that provide the area surrounding the infarction site with sufficient blood supply.

Another AMI descriptor refers to the depth or extent of muscle affected. A transmural infarction occurs when the entire thickness of the myocardium in a region is involved, and a subendocardial infarction (nontransmural) exists when the damage has not penetrated through the entire thickness of the ventricular wall, usually only the inner ⅓ to ½.

During the infarction process, so-called *zones* develop. The central core is the *zone of infarction and necrosis.* The tissue immediately beyond the central core is the *zone of hypoxic injury.* The outermost region is the *zone of ischemia.* The amount of tissue included in each area depends on the duration or lack of impaired perfusion. As the area of infarction grows, the degree of resulting functional impairment also increases.

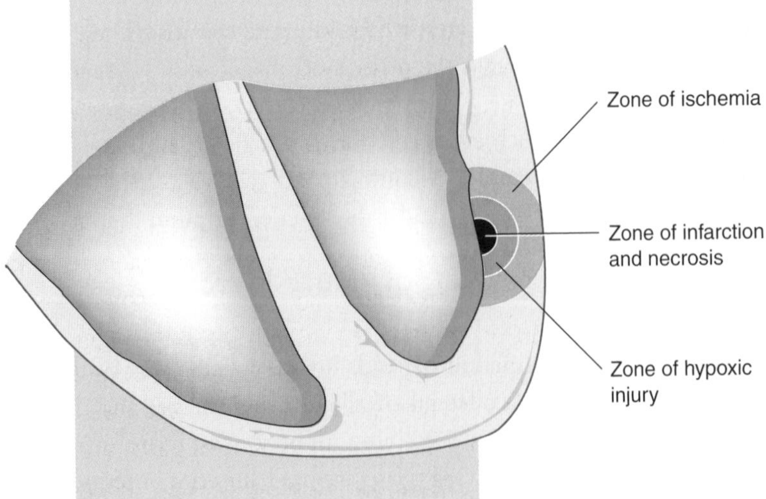

Myocardial infarction (MI) zones. *(From Phipps WJ et al:* Medical-surgical nursing: health and illness perspectives, *ed 7, St Louis, 2003, Mosby)*

Clinical Manifestations of Acute Myocardial Infarction

The hallmark of AMI is severe, unrelenting chest pain. As with angina, the pain is typically described as crushing, pressure-filled, tight, constricting, or squeezing. The most common location of the pain is substernal, with radiation to the neck, jaw, or left arm. Less frequently, pain is reported in the shoulders, back, or right arm. In addition, a positive Levine's sign (one or two fists clenched over the chest area when the patient is asked to localize the pain) can contribute to the diagnosis.

The major difference in the clinical presentation of AMI compared with that of angina is the onset, severity, and duration. Chest pain associated with AMI usually has an abrupt onset and can occur during activity, rest, or even sleep. The pain described during AMI is typically more severe than anginal pain, lasting at least 20 to 30 minutes, and it is not relieved with either rest or nitroglycerin. However, not all patients will experience the same clinical presentation.

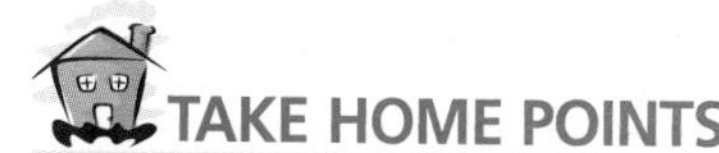

Chest pain from an AMI is unrelieved with rest.

Some patients who experience cardiac ischemia or infarction can have an atypical clinical presentation, particularly women, individuals with diabetes, and older adults. In these populations, cardiac pain can go unrecognized because of diminished or altered pain perception; up to 25% of all patients may experience what is known as a *silent infarction*. Usually, individuals experiencing a silent infarction report one or more of the *associated clinical manifestations*.

Some patients report vague feelings of discomfort or pain that comes and goes, and some attribute their pain to indigestion.

During AMI, associated clinical manifestations can range from vague sensations of "just not feeling well" to the loss of consciousness or cardiac arrest. Often the skin is cold and diaphoretic with a pale or ashen appearance, which occurs because of peripheral vasoconstriction as the body shunts blood to the vital core. The initial surge of catecholamines can contribute to a variety of signs and symptoms such as tachycardia, hypertension, anxiety, palpitations, apprehension, and feelings of impending doom. Stimulation of the medulla is mediated via vasovagal reflexes and can result in nausea and vomiting. Fever may be present secondary to the activation of the inflammatory process. As the infarction progresses and the heart's pumping ability becomes impaired, cardiac output drops. Symptoms associated with decreased cardiac output include hypotension, restlessness, dyspnea, jugular vein distention, oliguria, and confusion. On auscultation, a murmur, S3, S4, or splitting of heart sounds might be heard, which suggests ventricular dysfunction and disruption of normal valvular function. Additional findings may also include a

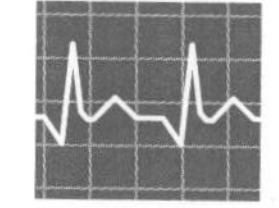

Clinical signs/symptoms of MI can be different between men and women.

newly developed right or left bundle branch on the ECG tracing as well as a pronounced Q-wave and ST-segment elevation.

Complications of Acute Myocardial Infarction

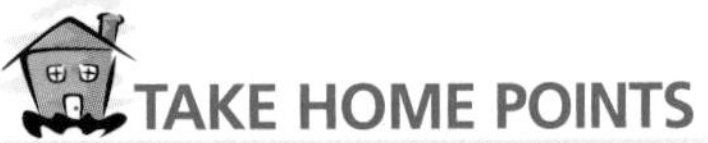

TAKE HOME POINTS

The conduction disturbances (arrhythmias) may be transient or chronic, and their seriousness depends on the hemodynamic consequences.

AMI can result in an array of cardiac functional impairments that can range from mild to severe depending on the factors previously discussed. Physiologic changes can include reduced contractility with abnormal wall motion, decreased stroke volume, altered left ventricular compliance, decreased ejection fraction, increased left ventricular end-diastolic pressure, and sinoatrial node malfunction. These impairments can lead to a variety of clinical complications such as:

- Arrhythmias (affect 90% of patients)
  - First-degree AV block
  - Second-degree AV block
  - Third-degree AV block
  - Atrial fibrillation
  - Ventricular tachycardia
  - Ventricular fibrillation
- Pericarditis
- Cardiac tamponade
- Papillary muscle rupture
- Chordae tendineae cordis rupture
- Myocardial wall rupture
- Pulmonary embolus
- Cerebrovascular accident
- Heart failure
- Pulmonary edema
- Cardiogenic shock
- Cardiac arrest
- Death

What You DO

A rapid, yet thorough and focused, health history and physical assessment are instrumental in the diagnosis of AMI. The goal of the health history is to determine the presence of CAD risk factors, angina, or previous infarctions. As with angina, the physical assessment primarily focuses on the current episode of chest pain, general appearance, determination of frequent vital signs, and continuous monitoring of cardiac rhythm and pulse, as well as an ongoing evaluation of mental status, heart, lungs, abdomen, urine output, and extremities. This assessment is helpful in gauging the extent of the infarction and in guiding appropriate therapies.

In addition to the history and physical examination, a 12-lead ECG and serial cardiac enzyme studies are the current gold standard for the diagnosis of AMI. Other clinical findings that are not solely diagnostic but will help contribute to the clinical picture of AMI include fever, hyperglycemia, hyperlipidemia, elevated sedimentation rate, and leukocytosis. Additionally, a chest x-ray film may be examined for cardiac enlargement, cardiac calcifications, and pulmonary congestion. Nuclear imaging is an extremely sensitive, although invasive, diagnostic study that is commonly used to establish a diagnosis of AMI when other data are inconclusive.

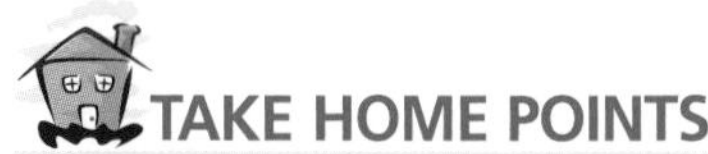

A focused history and physical assist in collecting findings for the diagnosis of AMI and the exclusion of other causes of chest pain.

Electrocardiographic Tracings

The 12-lead ECG is capable of diagnosing AMI in 80% of patients, making it an indispensable, noninvasive, and cost-effective tool. Because of the pathophysiologic manifestations previously described, the membrane potential is altered in the infarcted area of the myocardium, making it unable to depolarize and repolarize. Thus, conduction abnormalities can usually be detected. Whereas routine cardiac monitors look only at the conduction system from one angle, the 12-lead ECG allows the clinician 12 views from many perspectives on the body surface, making it far superior in diagnosing AMI. Because each of the 12 leads correlates with a specific region of the myocardium, the exact location of the infarction can be determined (see Color Plate 4). Conduction abnormalities represented in the leads adjacent to the infarcted area are called *indicative changes.* Conversely, abnormalities seen in the leads opposite the infarcted area are called *reciprocal changes,* and these are the inverse of those observed in the indicative leads.

Typically, an evolving AMI will show ST segment elevation on an ECG, which indicates acute, evolving myocardial necrosis. To confirm a diagnosis of AMI, these elevations must be greater than 1 mm and be observed in two or more contiguous leads. As AMI evolves, the development of a Q wave may be observed, which signifies further electrical abnormalities. The emergence of Q waves may indicate worsening ischemia and necrosis. During the healing process, the ST segment gradually returns to normal; however, Q waves remain unchanged.

It is recommended that serial ECGs be performed every 30 minutes for 2 hours for those patients at high risk for AMI.

Electrocardiograph Changes Localizing a Myocardial Infarction

Location of MI	Indicative Changes*	Reciprocal Changes†	Affected Coronary Artery
Lateral	I, aVL, V_5, V_6	V_1-V_3	Left coronary artery—circumflex branch
Inferior	II, III, aVF	I, aVL	Right coronary artery—posterior descending branch
Septum	V_1, V_2	None	Left coronary artery—left anterior descending artery, septal branch
Anterior	V_3, V_4	II, III, aVF	Left coronary artery—left anterior descending artery, diagonal branch
Posterior	Not visualized	V_1, V_2, V_3, V_4	Right coronary artery or left circumflex artery
Right ventricle	V_1-R-V_6R		Right coronary artery—proximal branches

*Leads facing affected areas.
†Leads opposite affected areas.
Aehlert B: *ECGs made easy*, ed 2, St Louis, 2002, Mosby.

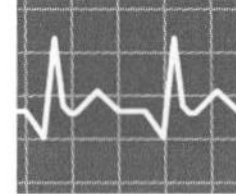

ST-segment monitoring should be performed on all patients at risk for AMI.

The diagnosis of AMI solely with the use of ECG is complicated by the fact that not all patients demonstrate ST elevations. In fact, persistent ST depression and T-wave inversion, with or without Q waves, indicate some subendothelial infarctions. In addition, left bundle branch block (LBBB), a common arrhythmia seen during AMI, may obscure the detection of ST-segment elevations. Furthermore, because the ECG represents the cardiac conduction system, which is a dynamic process subject to change over time, one single ECG is not sufficient to confirm or exclude a diagnosis of AMI.

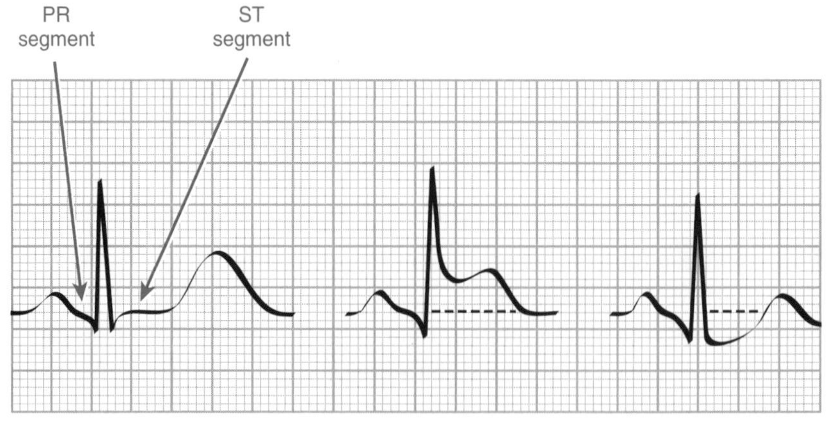

ECG, 12-lead changes in acute myocardial infarction (AMI). *(From Aehlert B:* ECGs made easy, *ed 2, St Louis, 2002, Mosby.)*

Anteroseptal Acute Myocardial Infarction

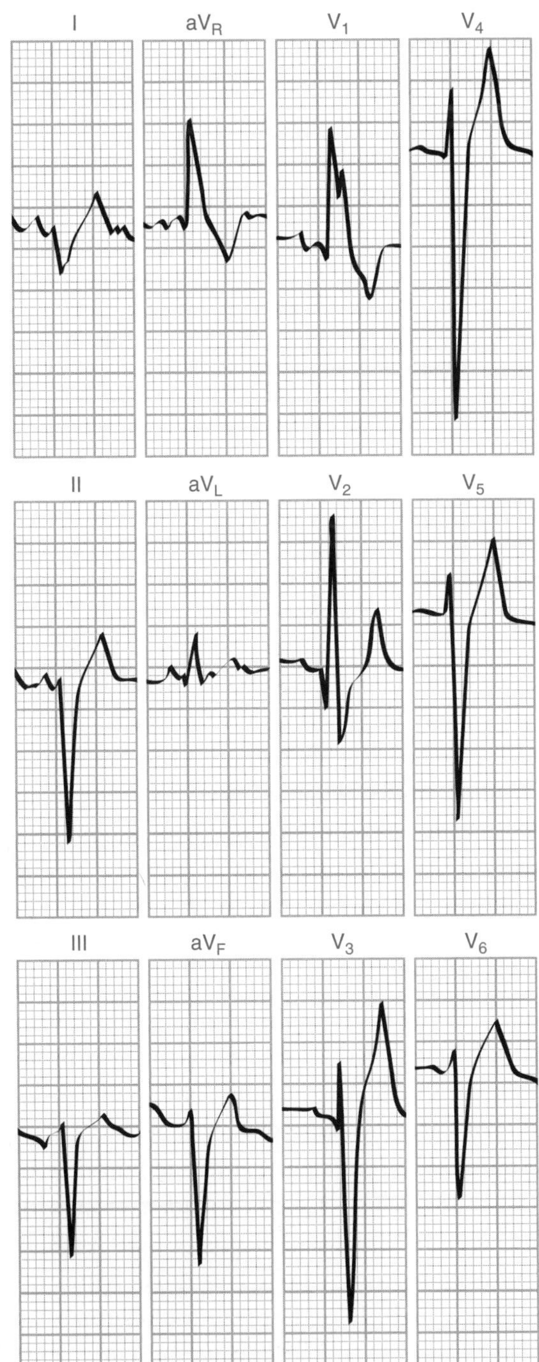

Q wave in leads V_1 to V_3 along with a broad R wave

(From Conover M: Understanding electrocardiography, *ed 8, St Louis, 2003, Mosby.)*

Cardiac Enzymes

During the infarction process, cell membranes rupture, allowing intracellular enzymes to spill out into the bloodstream. A blood sample drawn at certain times during or after AMI can be sent to the laboratory where enzymes can be measured and interpreted to determine the presence of an infarction. The problem is that most of these enzymes are not found exclusively in cardiac tissue. Therefore, injury to many tissues in the body causes an elevation in some of the markers routinely measured during AMI diagnosis.

Cardiac Enzyme Laboratory Findings

Enzyme	Earliest Rise (hr)	Peak (hr)	Return to Baseline
CK	2 to 6	18 to 36	3 to 6 days
CK-MB	4 to 8	15 to 24	3 to 4 days
Myoglobin	0.5 to 1	6 to 9	12 hours
Troponin I & T	1 to 6	7 to 24	10 to 14 days

CK, Creatine kinase; *MB*, cardiac muscle marker.

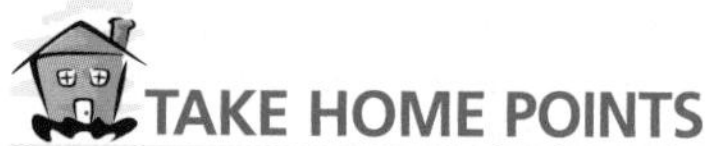

TAKE HOME POINTS

Troponin I is a protein found only in myocardial cells. It is a quick, rapid test that, when elevated, indicates AMI.

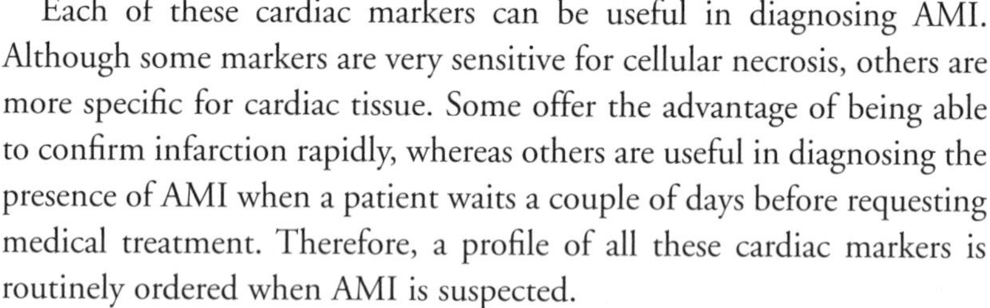

Each of these cardiac markers can be useful in diagnosing AMI. Although some markers are very sensitive for cellular necrosis, others are more specific for cardiac tissue. Some offer the advantage of being able to confirm infarction rapidly, whereas others are useful in diagnosing the presence of AMI when a patient waits a couple of days before requesting medical treatment. Therefore, a profile of all these cardiac markers is routinely ordered when AMI is suspected.

Medical Management

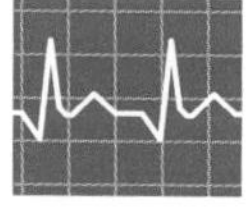

Amiodarone treats ventricular and supraventricular arrhythmias, particularly atrial fibrillation.

When any patient complains of chest pain suggestive of AMI, certain protocols should be instituted while the diagnosis is being made. The physical assessment should be ongoing and must include frequent monitoring of vital signs and pulse oximetry. Serial 12-lead ECGs with subsequent continuous ST-segment cardiac monitoring is imperative. Laboratory tests must include a cardiac marker profile and possibly a complete blood count (CBC), basic chemistry, lipid levels, liver function studies, and coagulation panel (PT/PTT or INR). Supplemental oxygen and IV access are essential. In addition to the pharmacologic therapies (fibrinolytics, antiplatelets, anticoagulants, nitrates, morphine, and beta-blockers), it may also be necessary to begin an amiodarone infusion if life-threatening dysrhythmias occur.

FIRST-LINE AND INITIAL TREATMENT FOR AMI

- Provide oxygen.
- Obtain a 12-lead ECG within 10 minutes of arrival.
- Monitor vital signs and pulse oximetry.
- Order laboratory tests.
- Monitor continuous cardiac rhythm with ST-segment monitoring.
- Conduct history and physical examination.
- Administer medications.

The patient will be admitted to the CCU where invasive lines such as an arterial line and a pulmonary artery (PA) catheter may be placed to provide further data to monitor ventricular function and guide the therapeutic regimen. In the event of severe left ventricular dysfunction, an intra-aortic balloon pump (IABP) may be used to assist ventricular ejection and promote coronary artery perfusion. Last, revascularization procedures such as emergency percutaneous coronary intervention with stent deployment or CABG should be anticipated if thrombolytics are either contraindicated or unsuccessful.

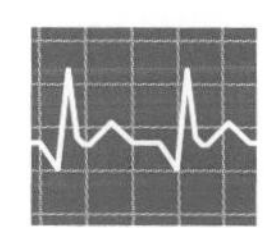

Medications used in AMI care: Nitrates = vasodilator decreases preload. Betablocker = beta-adrenergic antagonists. Morphine = relieves pain of MI and dyspnea of acute left ventricular failure. Decreases preload. Clopidogrel (Plavix) = prolongs bleeding time, reduction of restenosis post stent placement.

Pharmacologic Interventions

The American Heart Association (AHA) (2003) reports that more than 85% of all AMIs are due to thrombus formation. Therefore, in today's health care arena, thrombolytic and anticoagulant therapies are standards of practice in the treatment of AMI. Other agents frequently used in the management of AMI include nitrates, beta-adrenergic blockers, morphine sulfate, and antiplatelets such as aspirin, clopidogrel (Plavix), and GIIb/IIIa inhibitors such as abciximab (ReoPro), eptifibatide (Integrilin), or tirofiban (Aggrastat).

Thrombolytic Therapy

The survival rate for patients with AMI who receive thrombolytic reperfusion therapy is estimated to be 95%. Prompt and complete revascularization reduces infarction size, preserves left ventricular function, reduces morbidity, and prolongs survival. Thus, the treatment goals are to institute thrombolytic therapy as quickly as possible to halt the infarction process, salvage the greatest amount of myocardial muscle, and prevent any subsequent infarctions.

An adverse bleeding event is the major complication of thrombolytics, but allergic reaction is also possible because fibrinolytic agents are derived from bacterial proteins.

Thrombolytics, such as streptokinase, tissue plasminogen activator (t-PA), reteplase (r-PA), alteplase (Activase), and tenecteplase (TNK-tPA) are administered with the intention of dissolving the clots that occlude coronary arteries, thus promoting vasodilation and restoring myocardial blood flow. However, because thrombolytics produce lysis of the pathologic clot, they may also lyse homeostatic clots, such as in those in the cerebrovasculature, gastrointestinal tract, or operative site. Therefore, patient selection is important because individuals receiving thrombolytic therapy may have a minor or major bleeding episode as a consequence of the therapy.

To be maximally beneficial, thrombolytic treatment should be instituted within 12 hours of symptom onset and ECG changes, although current preference is 6 hours. Beyond 12 hours, few patients will benefit, and no clear evidence exists that confirms whether the benefits outweigh the risk of hemorrhage. All patients with a history and physical examination suggestive of AMI in conjunction with substantiating ECG changes (either ST segment elevation or new RBBB or LBBB), regardless of age, sex, or race, should be considered for thrombolytic therapy, as long as no absolute or relative contraindications exist. Successful reperfusion therapy should result in an abrupt cessation of chest pain, a rapid return of the ST elevation to normal, reperfusion arrhythmias or conduction abnormalities, and improved left ventricular function.

Thrombolytic Contraindications

Absolute	Relative
Aortic dissection	Uncontrolled hypertension (> 180/110 mm Hg)
Previous cerebral hemorrhage	Current use of anticoagulants
Known history of AVM or cerebral aneurysm	Known bleeding diathesis
Active internal bleeding (excludes menstruation)	Traumatic head injury (in the past 4 weeks)
Thromboembolic stroke (in past 6 months)	Major surgery (in past 3 weeks)
Known intracranial neoplasm	Internal bleeding (in past 6 months)
	Pregnancy
	Active peptic ulcer disease

AVM, Arteriovenous malformation.

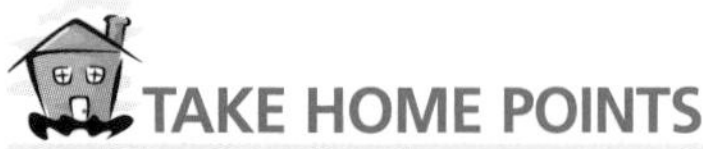

Is patient allergic to MSO4 (morphine)? Don't give MSO4, but instead, administer titrite nitro if it is a true allergen. Otherwise, premedicate with Benadryl or steroids.

Anticoagulant Therapy

Anticoagulant therapy is commonly used in the patient with AMI for three prophylactic reasons. First, after or concurrent with thrombolytic therapy, unfractionated heparin (UFH) or low–molecular-weight heparin (LMWH) is frequently administered to prevent reocclusion of the reperfused artery; second, to prevent pulmonary embolism, a common cause of death as debris or clots break free from the infarcted endocardium; third, because AMI routinely results in arrhythmias (as does atrial or ventricular fibrillation, which causes blood to pool in the chambers of the heart), UFH or LMWH can decrease the likelihood for subsequent clot formation. The mechanism by which these drugs work is as follows: UFH or LMWH in low doses prevents the conversion of prothrombin to thrombin; in high doses, they neutralize thrombin, which prevents the conversion of fibrin to fibrinogen and, consequently, prevents new clot formation.

TAKE HOME POINTS

Anticoagulants, like heparin, prevent thrombus formation and the extension of existing thrombi; they do not lyse (dissolve) existing thrombi.

Nursing Management

The nurse's primary responsibility during an evolving AMI is to ensure that life-saving therapies are instituted as quickly and safely as possible to limit the severity of the infarction and the functional impairment it causes. Long-term nursing responsibilities primarily focus on helping the patient return to a functional, high-quality life with prevention of future AMI being a primary goal.

Acute Nursing Interventions

During a suspected or evolving AMI, the nurse must perform a rapid and focused physical assessment and health history. Frequent monitoring of vital signs and continuous cardiac monitoring are essential parts of the nurse's ongoing assessment. A critical nursing function is the prompt institution of prescribed medical and pharmacologic therapies, particularly the expeditious administration of thrombolytic agents or preparation for revascularization by percutaneous intervention or coronary artery bypass grafting.

If thrombolytic agents are prescribed, the nurse must frequently assess for signs and symptoms of internal hemorrhage like changes in mental status or level of consciousness, hematuria, hemoptysis, and gastrointestinal pain or bleeding. Although minor bleeding (e.g., superficial bleeding from IV sites) is to be expected, any sign of major bleeding should be emergently communicated with the physician.

The administration of thrombolytic agents may cause reperfusion arrhythmias.

During the acute phase, all nursing actions should be aimed at reducing myocardial oxygen demand and increasing supply. Therefore, the delivery of oxygen must be ensured via nasal cannula or mask unless otherwise contraindicated. Continuous monitoring of pulse oximetry is also indicated. The nurse must frequently assess for pain and anxiety and, if present, promptly treat with prescribed agents. A quiet, calm, nonstimulating environment can greatly help reduce stress and anxiety. Activity initially is assisted while monitoring the patient's cardiac

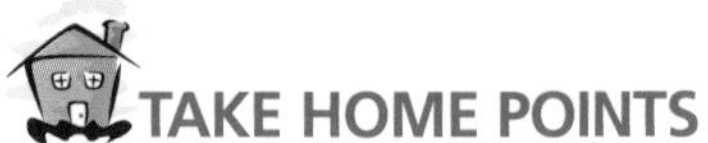

TAKE HOME POINTS

As with all nursing interventions, continuous evaluation of effectiveness is essential to modify therapies appropriately.

response to increased workload. Activity is then incrementally increased to allow the patient to resume a more normal activity pattern before discharge, with the recommendation for participation in a structured cardiac rehabilitation program with monitored exercise. Accurate measurements of intake and output must be maintained, particularly urine output because this is a reliable indicator of cardiac output and systemic perfusion. A stool softener should be prescribed to prevent straining and possible vasovagal stimulation, which can cause precipitous bradycardia. Emotional support is important. Therefore, the nurse's demeanor should be calming and reassuring, although not misleading. In addition, sufficient and appropriate explanations of all medical therapies should be provided.

Long-Term Nursing Management

The prevention of subsequent coronary events and the maintenance of physical functioning are important aspects of preventive care in patients with AMI. Therefore, comprehensive and extensive counseling is essential not only for the patient but also for the family. Education regarding prevention of recurrence primarily focuses on risk reduction. However, it is also vital to teach the patient and family the signs and symptoms of myocardial ischemia and the appropriate responsive actions. In addition, the patient must understand the importance of adhering to whichever pharmacologic regimen is prescribed, including specifics of dose, how and when to administer the medication, drug side effects, and drug interactions.

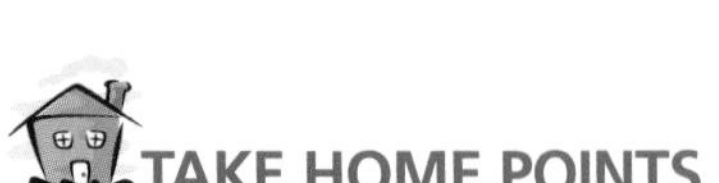

TAKE HOME POINTS

It is important to determine whether the patient can financially afford the prescribed medications.

The patient cannot alter unmodifiable risk factors. Therefore, all efforts must be directed toward identifying and altering modifiable risk factors. Although numerous modifiable risk factors exist for CAD, education should be tailored to each patient's particular risk factors.

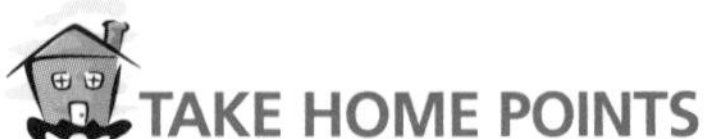

TAKE HOME POINTS

Sodium intake should be <2 grams per day to prevent edema. Discuss avoidance of frozen foods and prepared canned foods.

Effective management of hypertension requires frequent blood pressure monitoring, adherence to appropriate drug therapy, and nutritional counseling regarding a low-sodium diet. In addition, a prescribed exercise program helps control blood pressure levels and promote cardiac rehabilitation in general. Smoking cessation is another focus because cessation has been shown to reduce mortality and reinfarction rates by 50% within 1 year. Interventions in this area include nicotine supplements with subsequent weaning; participation in a support group; relaxation training; instruction on behavioral skills for coping with high-stress situations; and maintenance of long-term, periodic telephone contact with counselors. Psychosocial interventions should be directed at identifying and alleviating sources of anxiety and depression, including specific stress management therapies. Patients may need to consider a change in occupation to address this particular risk factor. Overall, MI survivors need to be taught how to individualize the necessary changes in lifestyle and medical treatment to reduce the progression of coronary disease and prevent any recurrence of coronary events.

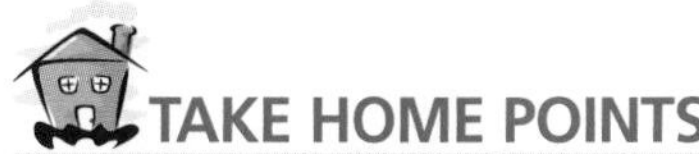

TAKE HOME POINTS

- Promotion of cardiac wellness should be a fundamental goal of all nurses.
- Prevention is better than cure, and healthy lifestyle changes that are instituted early in life are not only easier but also can ultimately lead to a longer, more productive and fulfilling life.

Do You UNDERSTAND?

DIRECTIONS: Fill in the blanks to complete each of the following statements.

1. AMI results from ________________ ischemia and may cause ________________ cellular death and necrosis.
2. In terms of myocardial oxygen, a ________________ that outweighs the ________________ will result in myocardial ischemia and possibly infarction.
3. Potential precipitating factors of AMI include the following:
   a. ________________
   b. ________________
   c. ________________
   d. ________________
   e. ________________
   f. ________________
   g. ________________
4. Cardiac cells can withstand ischemic conditions for approximately ________________ minutes before irreversible cellular death begins.
5. After AMI, the degree of altered cardiac function depends on the following:
   a. ________________
   b. ________________
   c. ________________
   d. ________________

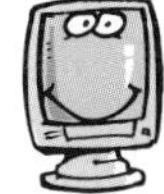

www.americanheart.org

Answers: 1. sustained, irreversible; 2. demand, supply; 3. a. physical exertion; b. emotional stress; c. weather extremes; d. digestion of a heavy meal; e. Valsalva maneuver; f. hot baths or showers; g. sexual excitation; 4. 20; 5. a. the specific area of the heart involved; b. the presence of collateral circulation; c. the size of the infarct; d. the duration of the infarct.

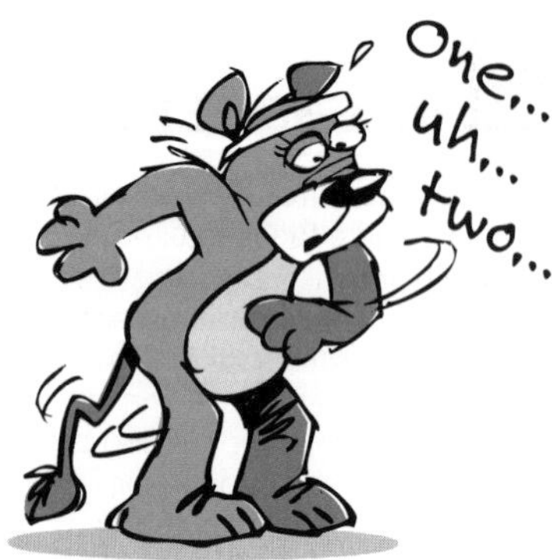

Exercise intolerance is a sign of heart failure.

What IS Heart Failure?

"**Heart failure**" sounds as if the heart will quit working at any moment. What heart failure actually means is that the heart muscle is weakened. The pumping chambers (ventricles) cannot pump forcefully enough to send blood out to meet the metabolic needs of the body. The inadequate tissue perfusion causes fatigue and poor exercise tolerance. Blood backs up from the left ventricle into the veins of the lungs, causing shortness of breath and lung crackles. Blood backs up from the right ventricle into the veins of the systemic circulation, causing edema as a result of fluid retention and volume overload. Not all patients have all of these symptoms. Some patients have no fluid retention but have exercise intolerance. Some complain of edema but experience few symptoms of dyspnea or fatigue. Because not all patients have volume overload, the term *heart failure* is now preferred over the more common term "congestive heart failure."

What You NEED TO KNOW

The most common causes of heart failure are:

- Coronary artery disease. Sluggish blood flow due to narrowed arteries can decrease the pumping ability of the heart.
- Previous heart attack (MI). Prolonged ischemia to the myocardium can cause muscle injury and cell death, which weakens the heart muscle.
- Hypertension. Long-standing high blood pressure causes the heart to work extra hard to overcome the resistance and can, over time, weaken the muscle.
- Cardiomyopathy. A generalized degeneration and enlargement of the heart muscle linked to heredity, excessive alcohol intake, infections, pregnancy, drug toxicity including chemotherapy, or other unknown cause (idiopathic).
- Valvular heart disease. A damaged heart valve forces the heart to work harder to keep the blood flowing in the right direction. Heart valves may be damaged by rheumatic fever, congenital defect, calcification build-up, or infective endocarditis.

Other, less common causes of heart failure include anemia, hyperthyroidism, dysrhythmias, and myocarditis.

Systolic Heart Failure

Systolic heart failure is an impairment in the ability of the heart to contract and empty. It is defined as an *ejection fraction* (EF) of less than 40%. EF is the percentage of blood ejected with each contraction. Normal EF is 55% to 75%. The heart enlarges in systolic heart failure in an attempt to pump more blood. Neurohormonal influences cause the kidneys to hold on to sodium and water and cause the blood vessels to constrict. The body's attempts to compensate for the lack of blood supply actually make the problem worse. Pharmacologic treatment is aimed at counteracting the body's own compensatory mechanisms.

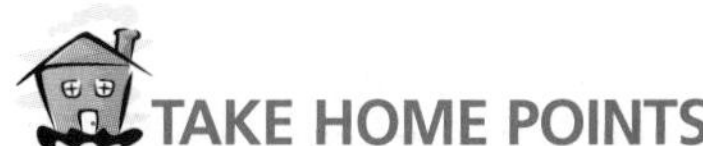

TAKE HOME POINTS

The term *heart failure* is preferred over the older term, "congestive heart failure," because not all patients have pulmonary or systemic congestion.

Diastolic Heart Failure

Diastolic heart failure is an impairment of the heart's ability to relax. The myocardial wall becomes stiff and thickened, impairing the heart's ability to fill. EF is not decreased in diastolic heart failure. It is sometimes called heart failure with "preserved systolic function." Although the ventricle enlarges, it does so concentrically as it thickens more on the inside; consequently, the overall heart size remains normal. The inward thickening decreases the chamber size, resulting in less blood flow into the pulmonary and systemic circulation.

The same symptoms of pulmonary congestion can occur in systolic and diastolic heart failure. Some patients have components of both systolic and diastolic heart failure. Although most studies have been conducted in systolic heart failure patients, it is now being discovered that the prevalence of diastolic heart failure is greater than was once believed. Because there are no specific guidelines published for the treatment of diastolic heart failure, the emphasis of this chapter is on systolic heart failure. A thorough discussion of diastolic heart failure is beyond the scope of this text.

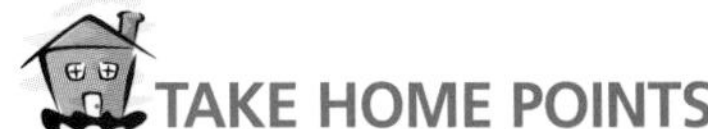

TAKE HOME POINTS

- Systolic heart failure: EF less than 40%.
- Diastolic heart failure: When the mitral valve opens, the left ventricle cannot relax to let blood in. Left ventricular (LV) and left atrial (LA) pressures increase, which back up into the pulmonary circulation. EF is normal.
- Systolic and diastolic heart failure can both present with symptoms of fluid overload.

Common Causes of Systolic and Diastolic Heart Failure

Systolic	Diastolic
Coronary artery disease, MI	Restrictive cardiomyopathy
Idiopathic dilated cardiomyopathy	Hypertrophic cardiomyopathy
Hypertension	Aortic stenosis
Valvular disease (MR)	Hypertension/ischemia

MI, Myocardial infarction; *MR*, mitral regurgitation.

Chronic Versus Acute Heart Failure

Most heart failure is chronic. *Chronic heart failure* is a gradual, progressive deterioration of left ventricular function. Unless the chronic heart failure is due to a mechanical cause such as coronary artery obstruction or an

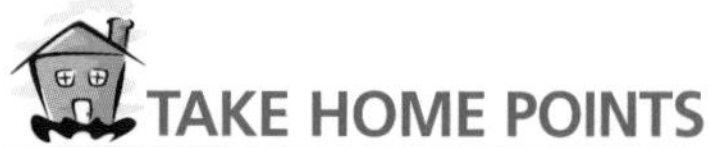

Chronic use of NSAIDs can cause heart failure.

abnormal heart valve, it cannot be cured but only managed through medications and lifestyle changes. A diagnosis of chronic heart failure is made only after treatable causes have been ruled out. The problem is that once an initial insult has occurred to initiate heart failure, the body's compensatory mechanisms become maladaptive and aggravate the situation. Symptoms of volume overload and decreased cardiac output may initially be mild (decreased exercise tolerance) but gradually progress in severity to symptoms of fatigue and dyspnea, even dyspnea at rest. The immediate goal of treatment is to decrease the workload of the heart by preventing volume overload (preload) and decreasing resistance to pumping (afterload). As heart failure progresses and the heart enlarges, a vicious cycle begins, which can lead to permanent cellular changes and a change in the shape of the heart. (Think of it loosely as changing from a football shape into a basketball shape.) This change is called *remodeling.*

Acute heart failure can result from a new-onset cardiac event (e.g., MI, dysrhythmias, valve rupture, tamponade). More often, acute heart failure is a complication of chronic heart failure. A patient with chronic heart failure who was previously stable on medications but comes to the emergency department with extreme SOB (decompensation) is in acute heart failure. For some reason (see the following box), the patient's oral dose of diuretic fails to control congestive symptoms.

Reasons for Heart Failure Exacerbations

- Noncompliance with drug or diet regimens (increased salt and fluid intake)
- Increased alcohol intake
- Impaired drug absorption
- Renal insufficiency
- Underlying disease progression (MI, valvular disease)
- Anemia
- Fever (2° sudden increase in metabolic demand)
- Increased exercise or emotional upset
- Increased use of nonsteroidal antiinflammatory drugs (can cause sodium retention and peripheral vasoconstriction)

Left Versus Right Heart Failure

Heart failure is a disease of the ventricles of the heart. Although the ventricles may fail independently of one another, left ventricular failure usually occurs first, which causes blood to back up into the pulmonary circulation. This action causes pulmonary hypertension, which leads to right ventricular failure over time. In most chronic advanced heart failure, patients exhibit symptoms of both left and right ventricular failure. Consequently, patients with chronic heart failure have combined symptoms of left and right heart failure. (See Color Plate 5 for diagram showing blood flow through the heart.)

Signs and Symptoms of Volume Overload

	Left Heart Failure (Pulmonary Congestion)	Right Heart Failure (Systemic Congestion)
Symptoms	Dyspnea* Paroxysmal nocturnal dyspnea* Orthopnea* Fatigue* Dry cough, worse at night Nocturia	Peripheral pitting edema* Weight gain Ascites Liver engorgement or discomfort Anorexia, nausea Abdominal bloating Nocturia
Signs	Cardiomegaly Tachypnea Tachycardia Third heart sound* (listen in left lateral decubitus position) Crackles bilaterally*	Hepatosplenomegaly Jugular venous distention* Positive HJ reflux Elevated CVP

*Classic sign or symptom.
HJ, Hepatojugular; *CVP*, central venous pressure.

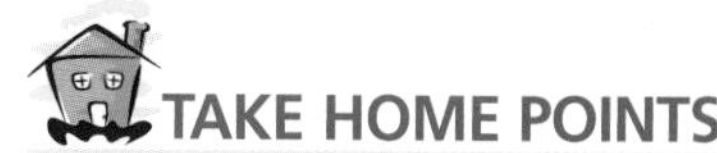

Paroxysmal nocturnal dyspnea (PND) is the sudden onset and severe SOB that wakes a person up out of a sound sleep. The cause is extra interstitial fluid in legs that reenters general circulation, producing hypervolemias and hence more fluid into interstitial lung spaces causing SOB.

What You DO

Diagnosis

Heart failure is largely a clinical diagnosis, which is not based on a single diagnostic or laboratory test but primarily on a careful history and physical examination. Diagnostic tests such as echocardiogram, chest x-ray studies, and radionuclide ventriculography are confirmatory rather than diagnostic in nature.

The signs and symptoms of heart failure (e.g., SOB, fatigue) are often difficult to identify because they are frequently confused with other disorders or attributed to aging, obesity, or lack of conditioning. Exercise intolerance can occur so gradually that patients may adapt their lifestyles to minimize symptoms and thus fail to report them.

Diagnostic tests may include:

- **Echocardiogram.** Two-dimensional echocardiography with Doppler flow is the gold standard of diagnostic tests. It can determine ventricular wall size and motion, and can differentiate systolic from diastolic dysfunction. Findings in systolic heart failure include a dilated left ventricle and decreased EF (<40%). An echocardiogram can evaluate valvular status as a mechanical cause of heart failure.

- **Chest x-ray studies.** The chest x-ray may be used to rule out other causes of SOB such as chronic obstructive pulmonary disorder (COPD) or pneumonia. When the patient is first examined, a chest x-ray film will show an enlarged heart and prominent pulmonary vasculature. Early cardiomegaly in symptomatic patients is highly suggestive but not diagnostic of heart failure.
- **ECG.** A 12-lead ECG may show a prior MI, ventricular enlargement, or the presence of dysrhythmias.
- **Radionuclide ventriculography.** Radionuclide ventriculography gives an accurate measurement of global and regional function by measuring the amount of blood pumped out but is unable to assess valvular abnormalities or cardiac hypertrophy directly.
- **Brain natriuretic peptide (BNP) measurement.** BNP is a hormone that is released into the bloodstream by the failing ventricle in an attempt to help out by its natural vasodilatory and diuretic responses. The BNP blood level can help differentiate whether shortness of breath is due to heart failure or a primary pulmonary problem. An elevated level is an indication of heart failure.
- **Treadmill stress test and cardiac catheterization.** A treadmill stress test or cardiac catheterization (or both) may be performed to rule out CAD as a treatable cause of heart failure.

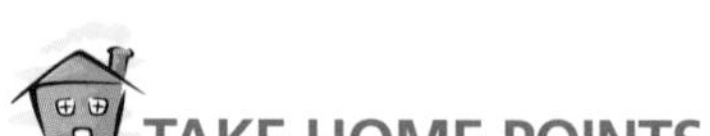

Heart failure is classified in two ways: (1) by functional classification or severity of symptoms using the NYHA Functional Classification System and (2) by level of treatment and prevention using the AHA/ACC Staging System.

NYHA Functional Classification System

CLASS I: Ordinary physical activity causes no symptoms of HF.
CLASS II: Ordinary physical activity causes HF symptoms.
CLASS III: Less than ordinary physical activity causes HF symptoms.
CLASS IV: HF symptoms at rest.

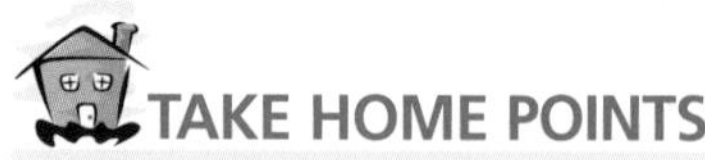

Acute pulmonary edema occurs when the pressure in the pulmonary vessels becomes so great that fluid floods the alveoli and decreases the availability for air exchange.

AHA/ACC Staging System

STAGE A: Patients at high risk for developing HF (prevention-based)
STAGE B: Patients with cardiac structural abnormalities or remodeling who have not developed HF symptoms
STAGE C: Patients with current or prior symptoms of HF
STAGE D: Patients with known HF and presence of advanced symptoms even with appropriate medical care

Treatment

If the underlying cause of heart failure is mechanical (i.e., a valvular problem or an occluded coronary artery), surgery and/or coronary revascularization should be considered to correct the cause. However, in the majority of cases, the mainstay of treatment is pharmacologic therapy.

Avoid licorice as large amounts cause hypokalemia and sodium retention.

Acute Heart Failure

Inpatient Treatment

During acute exacerbations, hospitalization may be necessary. If the clinical signs are mild to moderate, patients may be treated with IV diuretics until stabilized and then discharged. However, if there are symptoms of acute pulmonary edema or shock or complications such as ventricular dysrhythmias, admission to the coronary care unit is indicated. This situation requires emergency treatment with oxygen and medications. Mechanical ventilation, a PA catheter, or an IABP may be needed, depending on the severity.

FIRST-LINE AND INITIAL TREATMENT FOR ACUTE HEART FAILURE

- Provide oxygen; possible endotracheal intubation.
- Administer intravenous medications.

Medications

Loop diuretics such as furosemide (Lasix), bumetanide (Bumex), ethacrynic acid (Edecrin), or torsemide (Demadex) are intravenously administered to decrease preload. Venous vasodilators such as nitroglycerin may also be given to decrease preload. Morphine sulfate not only decreases anxiety, but it also helps decrease preload by venous vasodilation. Nesiritide (Natrecor) is a newer class of IV drug that is effective in acute exacerbations of heart failure that are refractory to diuretics. It decreases both afterload and preload. Positive inotropic drugs such as milrinone (Primacor) and dobutamine (Dobutrex) or intropin (Dopamine) are used to increase contractility in acute heart failure.

If the patient has been taking beta-blockers at home and comes to the emergency department with acute distress with a need for increased contractility, Primacor is the drug of choice. Intropin (Dopamine) will not work if the receptor sites have been blocked.

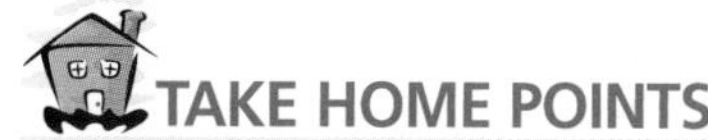

Beta-blockers: Carvedilol (Coreg), Metoprolol-SR (Lopressor, Toprol XL), Bisoprolol (Zebeta), Atenolol (Ternormin), Propranolol (Inderal)

Chronic Heart Failure

Outpatient Treatment

Chronic heart failure is usually managed on an outpatient basis. In the past, emphasis was placed on the treatment of symptoms only—digitalis to strengthen the heart and diuretics to unload the extra fluid to decrease

SOB. Currently, more emphasis is placed not only on stabilizing the patient but also on stabilizing the disease, breaking the vicious cycle of compensation and preventing the permanent changes of remodeling. This treatment regimen should ultimately lead to an increase in the quality of life and a decrease in hospital readmissions. Treatment of the patient, as well as the disease, is accomplished primarily with medications. Patients are expected to become educated about their disease and to be compliant with their medication regimen, daily weights, sodium restriction, and rest/activity habits.

TAKE HOME POINTS

- A positive inotropic drug increases the force of the heart's contraction, and a negative inotropic drug decreases the force of the heart's contraction.
- IV medications may be switched to those taken orally when the patient transfers out of the coronary care unit, has been hemodynamically stable for 24 hours, and exhibits no remaining symptoms when at rest.
- Patient still exhibits chronic heart failure even though his or her acute episode has been treated.

Regular follow-up physical examinations should include evaluation of fluid status. At each visit, the health care provider should record the patient's body weight, BP both sitting and standing, measurement of degree of jugular venous distention (JVD) and its response to abdominal pressure, the presence and severity of organ congestion (pulmonary crackles and/or hepatomegaly), and the magnitude of peripheral edema in the legs, abdomen, or presacral area. Medications are reviewed at each visit and regulated as needed to minimize symptoms. With the proper treatment regimen, patients with heart failure are living longer, better quality lives.

The long-term goal of treatment in chronic heart failure is to break the cycle of hypertrophy and remodeling by suppressing the compensatory mechanisms. How is this done? The harmful effects of the sympathetic nervous system (SNS), renin-angiotensin-aldosterone, and decreased myocardial contractility need to be suppressed by angiotensin-converting enzyme (ACE) inhibitors, angiotensin II–receptor blockers (ARB-II), and beta-blockers.

The short-term goal of chronic heart failure treatment is to treat the patient's symptoms. Systolic heart failure is treated with vasodilators to decrease afterload, diuretics to decrease preload, and positive inotropes to increase contractility.

Medications (Chronic Heart Failure)

ACE inhibitors help decrease preload by preventing sodium and water reabsorption. They indirectly vasodilate and decrease afterload by interfering with the conversion of angiotensin-1 (AT-1) to angiotensin-2 (AT-2). This interference breaks the cycle and prevents the release of aldosterone. No vasoconstriction and no reabsorption of sodium and water occur.

- An ACE inhibitor is the "number one" drug prescribed for all patients with heart failure.

- Some patients cannot take ACE inhibitors because of cough, renal insufficiency, allergy, or angioneurotic edema. If contraindicated due to cough, an angiotensin-receptor blocker (ARB) should be substituted.
- Patients intolerant to ACE inhibitors due to hyperkalemia or renal insufficiency are likely to experience the same side effects with ARBs. In these cases, a combination of hydralazine and isosorbide dinitrate should be considered.
- Side effects of ACE inhibitors may include hypotension and lightheadedness.

Beta-blockers are also now considered the standard of care in the treatment of heart failure because they have been shown to reduce mortality. Beta-blockers block the effects of the SNS so that the compensatory tachycardia, hypertension, and vasoconstriction cannot occur and therefore the workload of the heart decreases and hypertrophy and remodeling cannot occur.

- Some beta-blockers are more effective and safer than others for certain conditions. At present, **only** carvedilol (Coreg), sustained-release metoprolol (Toprol XL), and bisoprolol (Zebeta) are approved by the Food and Drug Administration (FDA) for the treatment of heart failure because they have been proven to reduce mortality.
- Doses of beta-blockers must be gradually increased as tolerated. It may take days or weeks before improvement is observed.
- A major side effect of beta-blockers, especially during up-titration, is fatigue.
- Beta-blockers are relatively contraindicated in patients with asthma, COPD, or conduction disorders. (A slowly titrated test dose may be used initially.)

Diuretics are prescribed to prevent and treat the symptoms of fluid overload in patients with chronic heart failure. Loop diuretics are normally used as in acute heart failure, but they are administered by mouth rather than IV routes. Side effects of diuretics include hypotension, dizziness, nocturia, and hypokalemia. If two daily doses are needed, the second dose should be administered no later than 4:00 PM because of the increased potential for nocturia. Potassium supplements are given to prevent hypokalemia, unless the patient is on a potassium-sparing diuretic or an aldosterone antagonist. In these patients, monitoring of serum creatinine and serum potassium is recommended.

The major medication prescribed historically to increase contractility in chronic heart failure is *digoxin* (Lanoxin). Lanoxin is inexpensive and very effective in decreasing symptoms. It may also be prescribed to control the

ACE inhibitors and beta-blockers are not prescribed for acute heart failure.

TAKE HOME POINTS

In heart failure, it is **BAD** to have an increased heart rate, increased BP, increased volume, and vasoconstriction. Any medication that counteracts these effects is **GOOD**.

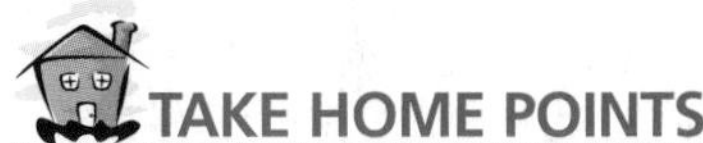

Foods high in potassium include bananas, green vegetables, potato skins, and salt substitutes.

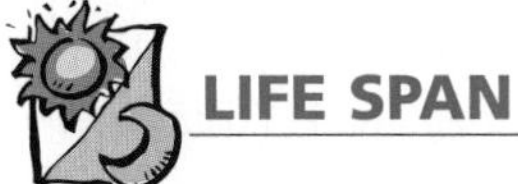

Risk of hyperkalemia increases in elderly on potassium supplements due to decreased kidney function and/or increased potassium food intake.

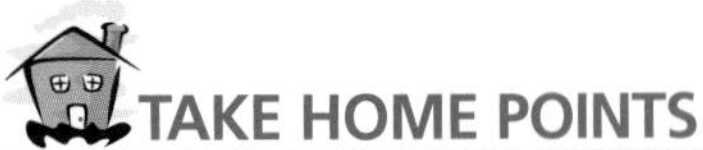

TAKE HOME POINTS

The *long-term treatment goal* of chronic heart failure is to treat the *disease*. The *short-term treatment goal* of chronic heart failure is to treat the *patient*.

ventricular rate in atrial fibrillation. Signs of toxicity include nausea, blurred vision, and dysrhythmias. A "fine line" exists between therapeutic digoxin (Lanoxin) doses and toxicity, especially in patients with renal insufficiency, so routine serum monitoring is recommended.

Other drugs that can be useful in heart failure include antiarrhythmics such as amiodarone. Amiodarone can be prescribed to decrease the recurrence of atrial arrhythmias and to decrease the incidence of implantable cardiodefibrillator (ICD) discharge in ventricular dysrhythmias.

The addition of isosorbide dinitrate and hydralazine to the aforementioned standard regimen is reasonable for patients with persistent symptoms and can be especially effective in blacks with NYHA functional class III or IV heart failure.

Infusions of positive inotropic agents such as milrinone, dobutamine, and nesiritide have been used in an outpatient setting to provide symptom relief in patients who are unresponsive to the standard medical regimen. The *ACC/AHA 2005 Guidelines for the Diagnosis and Management of Heart Failure* recommend only short-term use of these infusions in patients awaiting heart transplantation or palliatively in end-stage heart failure.

TAKE HOME POINTS

- ACE inhibitors are preventive in nature and therefore not given in acute heart failure.
- An aldosterone blocker such as spironolactone (Aldactone) may also be given along with ACE inhibitors for a more sustained effect in chronic heart failure.
- Beta-blockers are effective at blocking the excessive exercise-induced tachycardia that can limit the patient's activities.
- Beta-blockers vasodilate and decrease resistance to flow.
- Beta-blockers are not given in acute exacerbations of heart failure.

Medications Used to Treat Acute and Chronic Heart Failure

Drug Name (Brand)	Drug Name (Generic)	Purpose	Used to Treat AHF	Used to Treat CHF
Loop Diuretics				
Lasix	furosemide	Decrease preload. Used to prevent	Yes (IV)	Yes
Bumex	bumetanide	symptoms of volume overload.	Yes (IV)	Yes
Demadex	torsemide		Yes (IV)	Yes
Edecrin	ethacrynic acid		Yes (IV)	Yes
Angiotensin Converting Enzyme (ACE) Inhibitors				
Capoten	captopril	Prevent conversion of AT-1 to AT-2.	No	Yes
Vasotec	enalapril	Decrease fluid retention.	No	Yes
Monopril	fosinopril	Decrease afterload by vasodilation.	No	Yes
Zestril	lisinopril	Prevent remodeling.	No	Yes
Altace	ramipril		No	Yes
Aceon	trandolapril		No	Yes
AT-2 Receptor Blockers (ARBs)				
Use when AT-1 is contraindicated due to cough (NOT in renal insufficiency)				
Atacand	candesartan	Block AT-2.	No	Yes
Avapro	irbesartan	Decrease fluid retention.	No	Yes
Cozaar	losartan	Decrease afterload by vasodilation.	No	Yes
Diovan	valsartan	Prevent remodeling.	No	Yes

TAKE HOME POINTS

- Most medications used in acute heart failure are given via IV routes.
- Medications used in patients with chronic heart failure are all administered orally.

Medications Used to Treat Acute and Chronic Heart Failure—cont'd

Drug Name (Brand)	Drug Name (Generic)	Purpose	Used to Treat AHF	Used to Treat CHF
Beta-Blockers				
Coreg Toprol XL Zebeta	carvedilol metoprolol succinate bisoprolol	Block sympathetic response. Prevent excessive increases in HR and BP. Vasodilate to improve symptoms and clinical status. Prevent remodeling. Decrease mortality.	No No No	Yes Yes Yes
Aldosterone Antagonists				
Aldactone Inspra	spironolactone eplerenone	Block aldosterone to elicit a diuretic effect.	No No	Yes Yes
Other				
Natrecor	nesiritide	Naturally occurring hormone that counteracts the compensatory responses to heart failure so decreases preload, afterload.	Yes	No
Lanoxin	digoxin (cardiac glycoside) dobutamine	Increases cardiac contractility.	No	Yes
Dobutrex	milrinone	Increases cardiac contractility.	Yes	No
Primacor	(phosphodiesterase inhibitor)	Increases cardiac contractility.	Yes	No
Nitrobid	nitroglycerin	Decreases preload by dilating venous capacitance vessels.	Yes	No
Duramorph	morphine sulfate	Decreases preload by dilating venous capacitance vessels	Yes	No

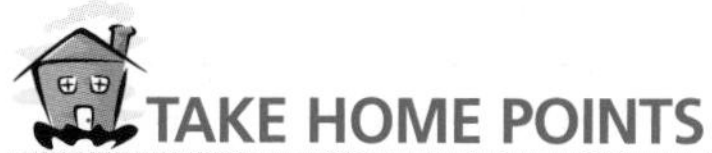

Foods usually high in sodium include frozen entrees, canned foods, and processed meals (i.e., lunch meats).

Nonpharmacologic Treatment

In addition to treating with medication, patients also are advised to do the following:

- Stop smoking. Smoking damages the blood vessels, makes the heart beat faster, and decreases the amount of oxygen in the blood.
- Control BP levels to decrease the workload of the heart.
- Limit sodium intake. Excess sodium contributes to water retention, which makes the heart work harder. The usual recommendation is limited to 2 g/day. Fluids may also be restricted in patients with fluid overload.
- Learn to read medication, food, and herbal labels for sodium content.
- Lose weight, if necessary.
- Limit use of alcohol. Alcohol can weaken the heart muscle or increase the risk of dysrhythmias.

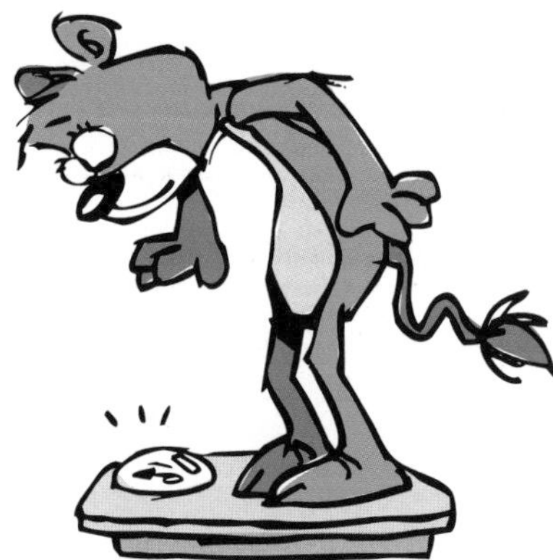

Assessment of change in weight is important in patients with heart failure.

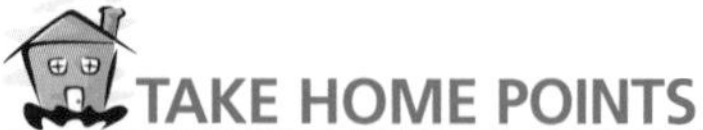

TAKE HOME POINTS

- Diastolic heart failure is treated differently than systolic heart failure. Calcium channel blockers are used in diastolic heart failure to help relax the work of the left ventricle.
- Vasodilators are used to treat systolic heart failure.

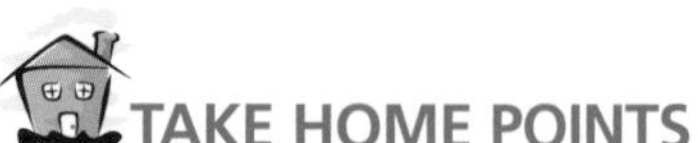

TAKE HOME POINTS

Weighing daily is the best indicator of fluid losses or gains in the patient with heart failure. Significant weight changes can indicate problems before symptoms occur. Approximately 10 pounds of extra fluid must accumulate before symptoms of increased volume develop.

A weight change of more than 3 pounds per day is a result of fluid gains or losses rather than fat gains or losses.

- Get plenty of rest, at least 8 hours daily.
- Minimize stress and find ways to manage stress effectively.
- Weigh daily to maintain fluid volume status; notify physician if weight gain is greater than 3 pounds per day or 5 pounds per week.
- Avoid NSAIDs. They can increase sodium and water retention.
- Improve physical conditioning with moderate exercise to prevent deconditioning; avoid isometric exercises such as push-ups and weightlifting.
- Report worsening of symptoms or new symptoms such as hypotension or dizziness that might be drug-related developments.

Other treatment options include the following:

Cardiac Resynchronization Therapy. Also called a biventricular pacemaker, pacer leads are inserted into the left and right ventricles and the coronary sinus to resynchronize the contractility of the ventricles. This treatment is indicated for severe heart failure and useful only in patients with asynchrony of the ventricles (i.e., bundle branch block). Cardiac resynchronization therapy allows the ventricles to regain synchrony in pumping, which is lost in bundle branch block. Indications include a QRS greater than or equal to 130 msec. The use of a regular pacemaker is not an appropriate treatment for heart failure because the problem lies with the mechanical system (contractility), not the electrical system.

Heart Transplantation. Several centers perform heart transplants on appropriate patients. Heart transplantation is a drastic step, and the entire patient profile must be carefully considered. Heart failure must be end-stage, with refractory cardiogenic shock or dependence on IV inotropic support to maintain adequate organ perfusion. The other organs must be healthy. Low LV ejection fraction alone is an insufficient indication for transplantation. Other considerations include the stress of surgery, side effects of antirejection immunosuppressive drugs, availability of compatible donor organs, and the cost of and need for continuous follow-up.

Left Ventricular Assist Device (LVAD) or Mechanical Heart Pump. An LVAD is a mechanical device that is implanted into the abdomen and attached to the weakened heart to help it pump. It may be used as an alternative to transplant or may help a failing heart until a donor heart becomes available. Indications include patients with refractory end-stage heart failure who have an estimated mortality rate of greater than 50% within 1 year with medical therapy alone. Age considerations and co-morbidity do not restrict its use as significantly as that for heart transplantation.

COMPLICATIONS

Heart failure can result in an array of cardiac impairments such as:

- Mitral regurgitation from the dilated ventricle stretching the mitral valve leaflets.
- Atrial fibrillation from increased LA pressures and stretching caused from backflow of blood.
- Thrombi from stagnant blood flow as a result of incomplete emptying in a dilated, inefficient heart or because of atrial fibrillation.
- Ventricular dysrhythmias from ischemia, cardiomegaly, or electrolyte imbalances. Antidysrhythmic medications and an ICD may be needed to prevent sudden cardiac death from life-threatening dysrhythmias.

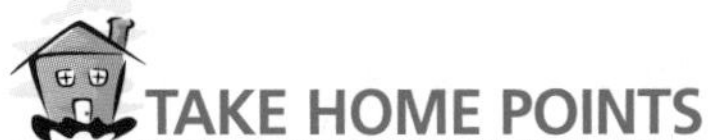

What is new in the treatment of heart failure? Scientists have recently begun transplanting skeletal muscle cells (myoblasts) into dead heart muscle or scar tissue in an attempt to regenerate new muscle. Results are promising.

Do You UNDERSTAND?

DIRECTIONS: **Select the best answer to complete the following statements. Place the corresponding letters in the spaces provided.**

______1. Which condition best describes heart failure?
  a. The heart stops beating.
  b. The heart cannot beat strongly enough to meet the needs of the body.

______2. Which of the following are the patient's responsibilities?
  a. Compliance with prescribed medications
  b. Monthly weighings and reporting any sudden headache
  c. Compliance with weekly uses of cathartics
  d. Performing aerobic and strength exercises within 1 week of AMI

______3. Heart failure is one of the most common causes of recurrent readmissions to hospitals, some of which may be avoided. What nursing action will decrease the readmission rate?
  a. Allow the patient to stay an extra 2 days in the hospital before discharging.
  b. Double the diuretic dose on discharge.
  c. Ask the patient to move physically closer to his or her primary care provider.
  d. Provide adequate patient education information on discharge and follow up on the patient within 7 days of discharge from the hospital.

_____4. A patient can have chronic and acute heart failure at the same time.
a. True
b. False

DIRECTIONS: Provide a short answer to the following question.

5. Which diagnostic test is the gold standard for diagnosing systolic heart failure?

____

DIRECTIONS: Circle the word in each group that accurately describes the goals in the treatment of systolic heart failure.

6. Preload: *increase* or *decrease*
7. Afterload: *increase* or *decrease*
8. Contractility: *increase* or *decrease*
9. Heart rate and BP: *increase* or *decrease*
10. *Vasodilation* or *vasoconstriction*

DIRECTIONS: Match the following drug names in Column A with the actions used to treat heart failure in Column B.

Column A

_____ 11. Increases the pumping ability of the heart (contractility)

_____12. Prevents the conversion of AT-1 to AT-2, thereby reducing afterload by dilating peripheral arterioles

_____13. Decreases heart rate and BP (oxygen demand to the heart)

_____14. Decreases preload by its diuretic action

Column B

a. Nesiritide
b. Furosemide
c. Lanoxin
d. ACE inhibitors
e. Beta-blocker
f. Morphine
g. ARB

Column A

_____15. May be substituted for ACE inhibitors if they are contraindicated

_____16. Natural-occurring hormone that counteracts the body's compensatory responses to heart failure

_____17. Dilates venous capacitance beds to decrease preload

Answers: **1. b; 2. a; 3. d; 4. a; 5. echocardiogram; 6. decrease; 7. decrease; 8. increase; 9. decrease; 10. vasodilation; 11. c; 12. d; 13. e; 14. b; 15. g; 16. a; 17. f.**

References

Adams KF, Lindenfield J, et al: 2006 Heart Failure Society of America comprehensive heart failure practice guidelines, *J Card Failure,* 12:e1-e122, 2006.

Albert N: Heart failure with preserved systolic function: giving well-deserved attention to the "other" heart failure, *Critical Care Nursing Quarterly,* 30(4):287-296, 2007.

American Heart Association web site: Retrieved January 6, 2003, from www.americanheart.org.

Antman EM, Braunwald E: ST elevation myocardial infarction: pathology, pathophysiology, and clinical features. In E Braunwald, DP Zipes, P Libby, & R Bownow: *Braunwald's heart disease: a textbook of cardiovascular medicine,* ed 7, Philadelphia, 2005, Saunders.

Bowman MA: *Current concepts in the management of heart failure: maximizing medical therapy.* Presentation at St. Joseph Hospital, Augusta, GA, January 2002.

Cannon CP, Braunwald E: Unstable angina and non-ST elevation myocardial infarction. In E Braunwald, DP Zipes, P Libby, & R Bownow: *Braunwald's heart disease: a textbook of cardiovascular medicine,* ed 7, Philadelphia, 2005, Saunders.

Carroll DL: Acute coronary syndrome: updates. Presented at the AACN National Teaching Institute, Chicago, May 2008.

Fraker TD, et al: 2007 Chronic angina focused update of the ACC/AHA 2002 guidelines for the management of patients with chronic stable angina: a report of the American College of Cardiology/American Heart Association task force on practice guidelines writing group to develop the focused update of the 2002 guidelines for the management of patients with chronic stable angina, *Circulation* 116:2762-2772, 2007.

Gibler WB, et al: Practical implementation of the guidelines for unstable angina/non-ST-segment elevation myocardial infarction in the emergency department: a scientific statement from the American Heart Association on Cardiovascular Nursing, and Quality of Care and Outcomes Research Interdisciplinary Working Group, in collaboration with the Society of Chest Pain Centers, *Circulation* 111:2699-2710, 2005.

Heart Failure Practice Guidelines 2006. Heart Failure Society of America. Retrieved May 23, 2008, from www.HFSAorg.

Hochman JS, Califf RM: Acute myocardial infarction. In Elliott M: *Antman's cardiovascular therapeutics,* Philadelphia, 2002, Saunders 2002, pp 233-280.

Hunt SA, Abraham WT, Chin MH, et al: ACC/AHA guideline update for the diagnosis and management of chronic heart failure in the adult: a report of the American College of Cardiology/American Heart Association Task Force on Practice Guidelines. *J Am Coll Cardiol* 20:46(6)e1-e82, 2005.

Jacobson C: Cardiovascular drugs: why we use what we use. Presented at AACN National Teaching Institute, Chicago, May 2008.

Jacobson D, Marzlin K, Webner C: *Cardiovascular nursing practice: a comprehensive resource manual and study guide for clinical nurses,* Seattle, WA, 2007, Cardiovascular Nursing Education Associates.

Mayo Clinic Health Solutions: Heart failure: living better and longer with a damaged heart. *Mayo Clinic Health Letter,* Rochester, MN, June 2007, Mayo Foundation for Medical Education and Research.

Monroe S, Pepine CJ: Management of unstable angina. In Elliott M: *Antman's cardiovascular therapeutics,* Philadelphia, 2002, Saunders, pp 205-228.

Pearson TA, et al: AHA Guidelines for primary prevention of cardiovascular disease and stroke: 2002 update: consensus panel guide to comprehensive risk reduction for adult patients without coronary or other atherosclerotic vascular diseases, *Circulation* 106:388-391, 2002.

Webner CL, Marzlin KM: From door to discharge: acute care strategies in acute coronary syndrome. Presented at AACN National Teaching Institute, Chicago, May 2008.

NCLEX® Review

1. The most common complication after an AMI is:
   1 Cardiogenic shock.
   2 Dysrhythmias.
   3 Congestive heart failure.
   4 Myocardial wall rupture.

2. An AMI causes conduction abnormalities because the:
   1 Myocardial cells are forced to engage in aerobic metabolism.
   2 Myocardial cells are overexcited.
   3 Myocardial membrane potential is altered.
   4 Myocardial cells contain too much potassium.

3. A patient complains of unrelenting, crushing chest pain, nausea, dyspnea, and is cold and clammy. The nurse suspects the patient is having an AMI and expects to see which of the following changes on the ECG?
   1 T-wave depression.
   2 ST-segment elevation.
   3 T-wave inversion.
   4 P-wave inversion.

4. The nurse notices ECG changes in leads II, III, and aVF that are strongly suggestive of an AMI. What area of the myocardium is affected?
   1 Inferior.
   2 Anterior.
   3 Posterior.
   4 Lateral.

5. Which of the following cardiac markers is very effective in determining an AMI because it is sensitive, specific, begins rising within 1 to 6 hours, and remains elevated for 10 to 14 days?
   1 Myoglobin.
   2 Creatinine kinase (CK).
   3 Lactic dehydrogenase (LDH).
   4 Troponin I.

6. LR is a 60-year-old man with a 6-week history of generalized malaise, an incessant cough, worse at night. He has a positive medical history for gouty arthritis. A chest x-ray study shows generalized cardiomegaly. Upon questioning, he reports a recent weight gain of about 10 pounds. The patient is referred to a cardiologist, who orders a two-dimensional echocardiogram with Doppler flow. Which of the following findings would support a diagnosis of systolic heart failure?
   1 A reduction in pumping power of the left ventricle to the point where the left ventricular (LV) ejection fraction (EF) is less than 40%
   2 An inability of the ventricle to relax during filling
   3 An increase in left atrial pressure due to mitral regurgitation
   4 Increase in ventricular filling pressure with normal EF.

7. LR's ejection fraction is 30%. Considering his history, which of the following is the most likely cause?
   1 Long-standing hypertension.
   2 Recent myocardial infarction.
   3 Congenital valvular defect.
   4 Viral cardiomyopathy.

8. LR's physical examination includes subtle findings of peripheral edema and positive jugular venous distention. These are symptoms of:
   1 Left-sided heart failure directly.
   2 Right-sided heart failure secondary to left-sided heart failure.
   3 Right-sided heart failure secondary to primary lung disease.
   4 Acute pulmonary edema.

9. In addition to medication compliance, which of the following instructions should the nurse give to LR?
   1 Limit sodium intake to 4 g/day.
   2 Weigh daily and report a weight gain of 3 to 5 pounds/day.
   3 Avoid all exercise to rest the heart.
   4 Take diuretic at bedtime.
10. Several months after his diagnosis, LR develops a sudden onset of shortness of breath with severe orthopnea. He is rushed to the ED. Vital signs include HR of 150/min, RR of 32/min, BP of 170/110, and SpO_2 of 85%. BNP is 1500 pg/mL. Chest x-ray shows bilateral infiltrates. EF by echocardiogram is 20%. He requires IV diuretics, supplemental oxygen, and narrowly escapes endotracheal intubation. His wife states that he has been taking large doses of ibuprofen for a flare-up of his gouty arthritis. What is the most likely cause of this flash pulmonary edema?
   1 He most likely missed a dose of his diuretic.
   2 He most likely ate too much salt that day.
   3 He most likely has pneumonia, unrelated to his heart failure.
   4 The ibuprofen has caused fluid retention and is contraindicated in heart failure.

NCLEX® Review Answers

1.2 Dysrhythmia is the most common complication after an AMI. Cardiogenic shock is not common, and rupture of the myocardial wall is a rare occurrence. Congestive heart failure is not a complication but a co-morbid disease.

2.3 Alteration in the membrane potential leads to electrical conduction abnormalities. Aerobic metabolism results from lack of oxygen. AMI is not overexcitation. Heart cells do not contain excess potassium that results in dysrhythmias.

3.2 ST elevation in an ECG is classic for AMI. The other three are not observed in an AMI.

4.1 Leads II, III, and aVF are associated with the inferior aspect of the heart.

5.4 Troponin I is a specific cardiac marker for diagnosing AMI, as is Tropinin T. Myoglobin is often the cause of a urinary dysfunction. CK is a nonspecific test with multiple causes for increased values. LDH is an enzyme that is found in all body tissues.

6.1 Systolic dysfunction occurs during systole when the heart is pumping or emptying. Normal EF is 55% to 75% and systolic heart failure is EF less than 40%. The inability of the ventricle to relax during filling and an increase in ventricular filling pressure both define diastolic heart failure along with a normal EF. An increase in LA pressure can be due to mitral regurgitation but is not the cause of systolic heart failure.

7.4 Although hypertension, recent MI, and valvular defects are causes of systolic heart failure, none are present in LR's history. Viral cardiomyopathy is the most likely cause historically.

8.2 Symptoms of left-sided failure include pulmonary congestive symptoms such as shortness of breath. Symptoms of right-sided failure include systemic congestion symptoms such as ascites, peripheral edema, and jugular venous distention. Chronic right-sided failure is most commonly caused by chronic left-sided failure. Left-sided heart failure causes fluid to back up into the lungs, which causes pulmonary resistance to blood that is trying to exit the right ventricle. Blood backs up into the right atrium and further backward into the systemic circulation, causing symptoms of right-sided heart failure. The patient has no evidence of primary pulmonary disease. Acute pulmonary edema would present with primary symptom of severe dyspnea.

9.2 Daily weights can detect fluid excesses before symptoms appear. Sodium intake should not exceed 2 g/day. Mild-moderate aerobic exercise (nonisometric) is encouraged in heart failure patients. Diuretics should not be given after 4 to 5 PM to prevent nocturia.

10.4 The patient now has acute heart failure superimposed on his chronic heart failure. Although missing a dose of diuretic and increasing the sodium intake could precipitate an acute onset of pulmonary edema, the most likely cause is the excess fluid retention caused by the high doses of ibuprofen. Elevated BNP level supports the diagnosis of heart failure, not pneumonia.

Chapter 5 Respiratory System

What You WILL LEARN

After reading this chapter, you will know how to do the following:

- ✔ Discuss reasons for initiating mechanical ventilation.
- ✔ Describes modes of invasive ventilation.
- ✔ Identify appropriate nursing interventions for caring for a patient who is mechanically ventilated.
- ✔ Discuss complications of mechanical ventilation.
- ✔ Describe the pathophysiology of pulmonary embolus and acute respiratory distress syndrome.
- ✔ Identify risk factors that predispose patients to the development of a pulmonary embolus and acute respiratory distress syndrome.
- ✔ Explain the nursing management for the care of a patient with a pulmonary embolus.
- ✔ Discuss the plan of care for a patient with acute respiratory distress.
- ✔ Discuss relevant patient education topics.

evolve

See http://evolve.elsevier.com/Schumacher/criticalcare for additional NCLEX® review questions.

What IS Mechanical Ventilation?

Mechanical ventilation is a form of assisted ventilation that takes over all or part of the work performed by the respiratory muscles and organs. It is initiated when the patient's ability to oxygenate and exchange carbon dioxide (CO_2) is impaired. Mechanical ventilation may be indicated for the following reasons:

- Hypoxemia
- Respiratory failure
- Atelectasis
- Aspiration
- Airway burns
- Pulmonary edema
- Pulmonary embolism (PE)
- Respiratory muscle fatigue
- Loss of spinal innervation
- Acute respiratory distress syndrome (ARDS)
- Oversedation/overdose
- To reduce intracranial pressure
- To stabilize the chest wall

The main goal of mechanical ventilation is to support gas exchange until the disease process or condition is resolved.

TAKE HOME POINTS

- Before mechanically ventilating a patient, other oxygen delivery devices such as a nasal cannula or facemask may be used. A nasal cannula delivers low-flow oxygen (1 to 6 L/min) through prongs inserted into the nose; a facemask, which covers the nose and mouth, delivers higher concentrations of oxygen (40% to 60%).
- A non-rebreather mask will deliver an FiO_2 concentration of 100% but is used only as bridge therapy until intubation and ventilation can be performed.

What You NEED TO KNOW

Positive-Pressure Ventilation

Positive-pressure ventilation (PPV) is the most common form of mechanical ventilation used in the acute care setting. This form of ventilation forces oxygen into the lungs with each breath through an endotracheal or tracheostomy tube. Volume- and pressure-cycled types are the most frequently used modes of PPV in the critical care setting. *Volume-cycled modes* deliver a breath until a preset tidal volume is reached with each breath. *Pressure-cycled modes* deliver a breath until a preset pressure is achieved within the airway. Advances in microprocessor ventilators allow for combinations of ventilation modes, which can be confusing for the novice critical care nurse.

For patients with chronic lung disease who retain $PaCO_2$ (i.e., chronic obstructive pulmonary disease [COPD]), high levels of oxygen must be delivered cautiously because too much oxygen can cause them to lose their drive to breathe. Therefore, low-flow oxygen devices are usually tried first. Although the care team may accept slightly lower SpO_2 levels in these patients, this decision would be made on an individual basis.

Modes of Ventilation

A variety of ventilation modes are available to ventilate and oxygenate the patient; selection is based on the goals of therapy. Essentially, these modes are ways in which ventilation is triggered, allowing the patient partial or complete control over their breathing. Factors that influence the selection of the primary ventilation mode include the underlying pulmonary status (i.e., ease or difficulty of ventilation), oxygenation, and ability of the patient to breathe spontaneously.

TAKE HOME POINTS

- The most common type of mechanical ventilation is positive pressure.
- The two nursing interventions to prevent ventilator-associated pneumonia (VAP) are to elevate the head of the bed 30 to 45 degrees unless contraindicated and to advocate for the patient to have a silver-coated endotracheal tube.

TAKE HOME POINTS

- ACV delivers a preset tidal volume each time the ventilator breathes or the patient takes a spontaneous breath.
- SIMV delivers a preset tidal volume with each ventilator breath, and the patient receives a variable tidal volume initiated by each spontaneous breath.

To ensure adequate tidal volume with PCV, sedation and muscle paralysis by neuromuscular blockage (NMB) may be required.

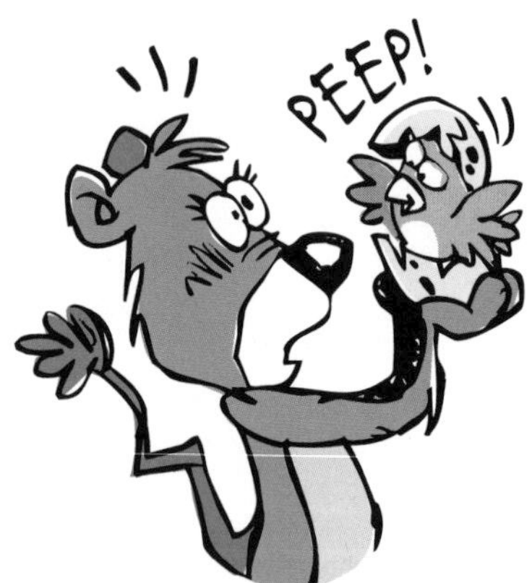

Positive End-Expiratory Pressure

Assist-control ventilation (ACV) delivers a preset volume at a preset rate and whenever the patient initiates a breath. If the patient does not initiate a breath within a preset time, the ventilator will deliver a breath. This mode is used in patients with weak respiratory muscles or those who cannot achieve an adequate tidal volume on their own. One disadvantage is that all breaths, whether initiated by the ventilator or spontaneously, result in delivery of a full tidal volume. Full tidal volumes at respiratory rates higher than the set ventilator rate will create higher minute volumes, lowering $PaCO_2$ levels, resulting in respiratory alkalosis. Sedation may be used to limit spontaneous breathing.

Synchronized intermittent mandatory ventilation (SIMV) delivers a preset volume at a preset rate and is synchronized with the patient's effort. This mode allows for spontaneous breathing between ventilated breaths and prevents competition between the patient and the ventilator. When a spontaneous breath occurs, it is at the patient's own rate and tidal volume. SIMV is a common mode for patients who require minimal ventilatory support and is also used when weaning from the ventilator.

Pressure-controlled ventilation (PCV) delivers a positive-pressure breath until a maximum amount of airway pressure is reached, then the inspiratory phase of the breath stops. The maximum inspiratory pressure limit is preset to help minimize ventilator-induced lung injury (VILI). The delivered tidal volume varies, based on airway resistance and lung compliance. Typically, the settings are adjusted to achieve a goal tidal volume designated by the physician. The tidal volume goal is based on the patient's weight and pulmonary status. This mode is most frequently used in patients with poor lung compliance or those requiring more assistance with gas exchange, such as oxygenation.

Pressure-regulated volume control (PRVC) is a type of PCV in which the ventilator makes pressure adjustments to aim for a predetermined tidal volume. Peak airway pressures vary with changes in lung compliance. For example, a patient with worsening lung compliance has decreasing elasticity of the lung tissue, causing peak inspiratory pressures (PIP) to rise. In PRVC mode, the ventilator senses the increase in PIP and reduces the tidal volume until airway pressures are back within normal range. If tidal volumes become lower than the goal, the health care team needs to reassess ventilatory strategies.

Additional Ventilatory Modes

Positive end-expiratory pressure (PEEP) holds positive pressure in the alveoli during expiration. PEEP is frequently used as a supplement to most modes of ventilation. PEEP, which can range from 2 to 24 cm H_2O

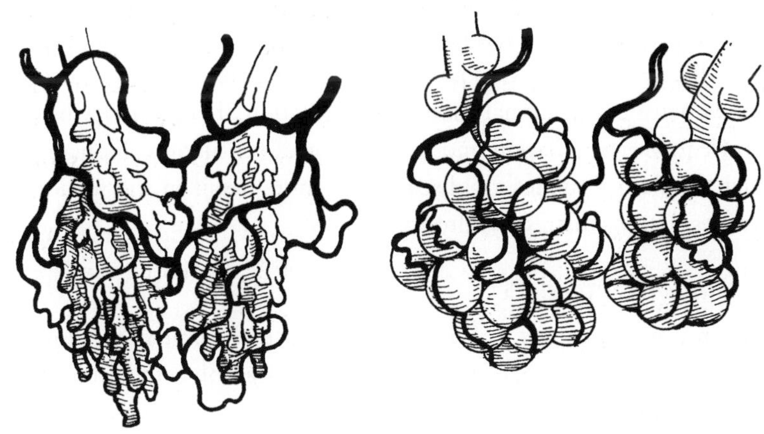

(From Pierce LNB: Guide to mechanical ventilation and intensive respiratory care, *Philadelphia, 1995, WB Saunders.)*

pressure, prevents alveoli from collapsing at end-expiration, improves oxygenation, and increases functional residual capacity (FRC). A negative effect of PEEP greater than 10 cm H_2O is increased intrathoracic pressure, which can cause decreased venous return and cardiac output. With oxygenation being a priority, if hypotension occurs, it may be necessary to increase preload with fluids or use vasopressors to support blood pressure. High levels of PEEP will increase airway pressures, which may lead to such complications as VILI, hypotension, increased intracranial pressure, and alveolar ventilation-perfusion mismatch.

Constant positive airway pressure (CPAP) is similar to PEEP but provides positive pressure during spontaneous breaths. It increases oxygenation by preventing closure of alveoli at end-expiration, thereby maximizing the FRC. CPAP is an independent ventilatory mode and generally ranges from 5 to 10 cm H_2O pressure. It is frequently used to wean patients from the ventilator or as a noninvasive method of ventilation.

Pressure support ventilation (PSV) augments the tidal volume of spontaneous breaths by delivering a preset positive pressure during inspiration. PSV can be added to ventilatory modes such as SIMV or CPAP and is commonly used when weaning patients from the ventilator. PSV settings are typically between 8 and 20 cm H_2O. Higher levels of PSV will assist the patient in obtaining a larger tidal volume. PSV increases patient comfort by decreasing the amount of work required by the patient with each spontaneous breath. More recently, PSV has been used in conjunction with a variety of ventilatory modes when patients are permitted to have spontaneous respiratory effort.

A CPAP of more than 10 cm H_2O pressure may increase intrathoracic pressure to the point that it affects the patient's venous return, decreasing cardiac output and blood pressure. CPAP at this level may also cause the occurence of a pneumothorax.

Nonconventional Ventilation Modes

Other nonconventional ventilation modes have been shown to improve gas exchange in severe respiratory failure when oxygenation does not improve with conventional modes of ventilation. These modes include high-frequency ventilation and extracorporeal ventilation. Nonconventional ventilatory modes are discussed in more detail in the section on acute respiratory distress syndrome (ARDS).

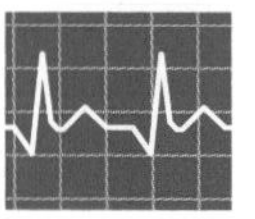

CPAP >10 cm H_2O pressure can cause a pneumothorax.

Ventilator Settings

Ventilator settings must be individualized to each patient to allow for optimal gas exchange. Settings are generally based on arterial blood gas (ABG) measurements. Most acute care institutions have respiratory therapists who set up and manage the ventilator. Nurses should verify the ventilator modes, settings, and alarms at the beginning of each shift, with any ventilator changes, with any worsening of respiratory status, and per institutional policy.

Ventilator Settings, Descriptions, and Ranges

Ventilator Setting	Description	Ranges
Vt	Amount of oxygen delivered to patient with each preset ventilated breath	5-15 mL/kg (average 10 mL/kg)
Respiratory rate	Number of breaths per minute that ventilator is set to deliver	4-20 breaths/min
FiO_2	Percentage of oxygen delivered by ventilator with each breath	21%-100%
I:E Ratio	Duration of inspiratory to expiratory (I:E) time	1:2 (unless IRV is used)
Sensitivity	Determines amount of effort patient must generate before ventilator will give a breath	Too low—patient will have to work harder to obtain a breath Too high—patient's spontaneous respiratory efforts may compete with the ventilator (asynchronous breathing)
Flow rate	Determines how fast Vt will be delivered during inspiration	High—increase airway pressure Low—decrease airway pressure
Pressure limits	Regulates maximum amount of pressure the ventilator will generate to deliver preset Vt	Ventilated breath will stop when pressure limit is reached (in pressure-controlled modes)

Vt, Tidal volume; *FiO_2,* fraction of inspired oxygen; *I:E,* inspiratory to expiratory; *IRV,* inverse-ratio ventilation.

Ventilation Terminology

Terminology	Description	Ranges
Minute volume	Total volume of gas inhaled or exhaled over a 1-minute period. Respiratory rate × tidal volume	5-8 L
Compliance	Elasticity of the lung tissue. Decreased compliance = increased resistance to each breath	
Peak inspiratory pressure (PIP)	Airway pressure at maximum inspiration; also referred to as peak airway pressure.	<30 cm H_2O
Low-pressure alarms	Leak or disconnection in ventilator circuit. Patient is not receiving adequate ventilation. If unable to fix problem immediately, manually ventilate patient with resuscitation bag.	
High-pressure alarms	PIP has exceeded a safe limit, placing patient at risk for VILI.	
Volutrauma	Injury to lung tissue from overdistention of alveoli; a form of VILI.	
Barotrauma	Injury to the lung tissue from too much pressure in the airway; a form of VILI.	
Atelectrauma	VILI from low intraalveolar pressure, causing collapse of the alveoli.	
Rapid shallow breathing index (RSBI)	Quantifiable measure to assess patient's readiness for spontaneous breathing. RSBI = respiratory rate/Vt (Liter)	<105

Mechanical Ventilation Complications

Ventilator-induced lung injury refers to barotrauma, volutrauma, and atelectrauma, conditions that give rise to such complications as pneumothorax, pneumomediastinum, subcutaneous emphysema, and alveolar-capillary membrane damage. Barotrauma occurs secondary to high airway pressures in the alveoli, whereas volutrauma refers to damage caused from overdistention of the alveoli. Atelectrauma is caused by inadequate pressure within the alveolar units, which creates tissue trauma when the alveoli close and reopen.

Hypotension associated with mechanical ventilation occurs because positive-pressure ventilation and PEEP cause an increase in intrathoracic pressure. The increased intrathoracic pressure decreases venous return to the right side of the heart, creating a decrease in preload, which in turn decreases cardiac output.

Peptic ulcers, gastrointestinal (GI) bleeding, inadequate nutrition, and paralytic ileus are some of the more common GI problems associated with mechanical ventilation. Adequate nutrition and the administration of medications to reduce gastric acid help decrease the incidence of these occurrences. Histamine H_2-receptor antagonists (e.g., ranitidine [Zantac],

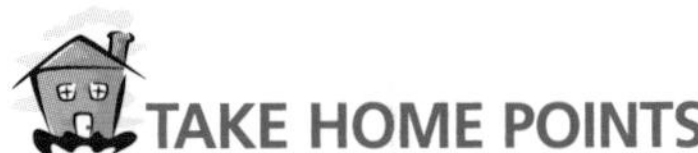

Ventilator setting adjustments are based on arterial oxygen saturation (SaO_2) level and ABG results.

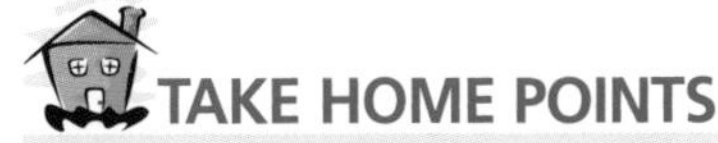

The patient will require a tracheostomy tube if long-term ventilatory management is anticipated. Endotracheal tubes (oral or nasal) are not intended for long-term management and can lead to other problems such as mucosal breakdown, skin ulcerations (lips), sinusitis, and vocal cord paralysis or damage.

cimetadine [Tagamet], or famotidine [Pepcid]) or proton pump inhibitors, (e.g., pantoprazole [Protonix], omeprazole [Prilosec], or esomeprazole [Nexium]) are used to prevent peptic ulcer formation.

Artificial airways bypass many of the body's normal defense mechanisms in the upper respiratory system, such as the cough reflex and ciliary clearance of mucus. Secretions can pool above the cuff of artificial airways and leak into the lower respiratory tract, making suctioning necessary. Within 24 hours the secretions may become contaminated with bacteria, placing the patient at risk for VAP. Effective nursing interventions for VAP prevention include elevating the head of bed 30 to 45 degrees, subglottic suctioning, oral care, and advocating for the use of a silver-coated endotracheal tube. Collaborative interventions that can limit mechanical ventilation days and thus further reduce the risk for VAP include daily sedation vacation, assessment of readiness to wean, deep venous thrombosis (DVT) prophylaxis, and peptic ulcer prophylaxis.

Weaning from Ventilation

Weaning from mechanical ventilation is the gradual withdrawal of ventilatory support, allowing patients to breathe more on their own. The length of the weaning process can vary according to the length of time on the ventilator and the patient's condition. Patients requiring short-term ventilator support (e.g., postoperatively) generally wean more quickly than those who need long-term support (e.g., pneumonia, ARDS). Factors influencing readiness to wean include status of the underlying disease process, nutritional status, cardiovascular status, respiratory status, neuromuscular function, and whether the patient will be able to participate in the weaning process. Assessment of readiness to wean should be performed daily in patients who are considered stable. Readiness to wean should be performed by a quantifiable method, such as rapid shallow breathing index, rather than subjective interpretation by a member of the care team. A spontaneous breathing trial (SBT) is considered necessary before permanent removal of the ventilator. Although different methods may be used for SBT, including T-piece, or CPAP with or without PSV, no difference in efficacy has been demonstrated. During the weaning process patients should be monitored for hemodynamic instability, muscle fatigue, or worsening gas exchange. Oxygenation can be monitored continuously through pulse oximetry, but measures of $PaCO_2$ will require capnography or an ABG. Extubation will depend on the patient's ability to ventilate and protect the airway.

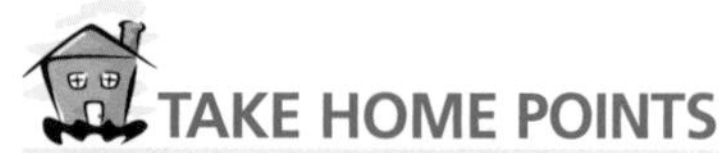

Successful weaning is a team effort among physicians, nurses, respiratory therapy personnel, and patients.

Use of the T-piece (T-tube) for weaning requires that the patient be removed from the ventilator for short periods (SBT) and then placed back on ventilatory support. Supplemental oxygen is administered through the

T-piece while the patient breathes spontaneously. The length of time off the ventilator is gradually extended until ventilatory support is no longer required. When SIMV mode is used for weaning, pressure support is often added to minimize the work of breathing. Ventilatory support is gradually reduced until the patient is able to breathe completely on his or her own. This decrease in ventilatory support includes a reduction in pressure support, often alternating with a decrease in the set respiratory rate. Pressure support augments each spontaneous breath, making the work of breathing easier, allowing the patient to take a larger spontaneous tidal volume. Pressure support continues to be decreased until it reaches a level of 5 to 7 cm H_2O. PEEP, typically used with all ventilatory modes, is converted to CPAP once the patient is able to breathe without a set rate.

CPAP, with or without pressure support, is used for patients who are able to breathe spontaneously for a sustained time. The use of CPAP helps prevent atelectasis during shallow breathing and improves oxygenation by increasing the FRC. Patients on low levels of CPAP (5 cm H_2O) and PSV (5 to 7 cm H_2O) should be assessed for readiness to extubate.

What IS Pulmonary Embolus?

Pulmonary embolus (PE) is a thrombotic (blood clot) or nonthrombotic (fat) emboli that lodges in the pulmonary arterial (PA) system. This blockage obstructs blood flow to the lung tissue supplied by the affected vessel. Venous thromboemboli (VTE) typically originate from the deep veins of the legs, right ventricle (RV) of the heart, or pelvis. Nonthrombotic emboli mainly originate from fat release after skeletal injuries, amniotic fluid, air, and foreign bodies.

What You NEED TO KNOW

Causes

A decrease in blood flow (**venous stasis**), a problem with blood clotting, and some form of injury to the vessel wall are three factors that can lead to the development of venous thrombi. These three factors together are called *Virchow's triad.* The box that follows shows conditions and risk factors that can predispose a patient to or that can precipitate the formation of venous thrombi.

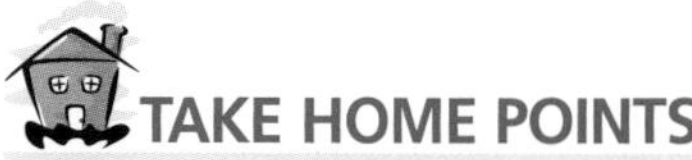

Virchow's triad consists of decreased blood flow (venous stasis), blood-clotting problems, and vessel wall injury.

Venous stasis
Virchow's triad = venous thrombi
Vessel wall injury
Coagulation problems

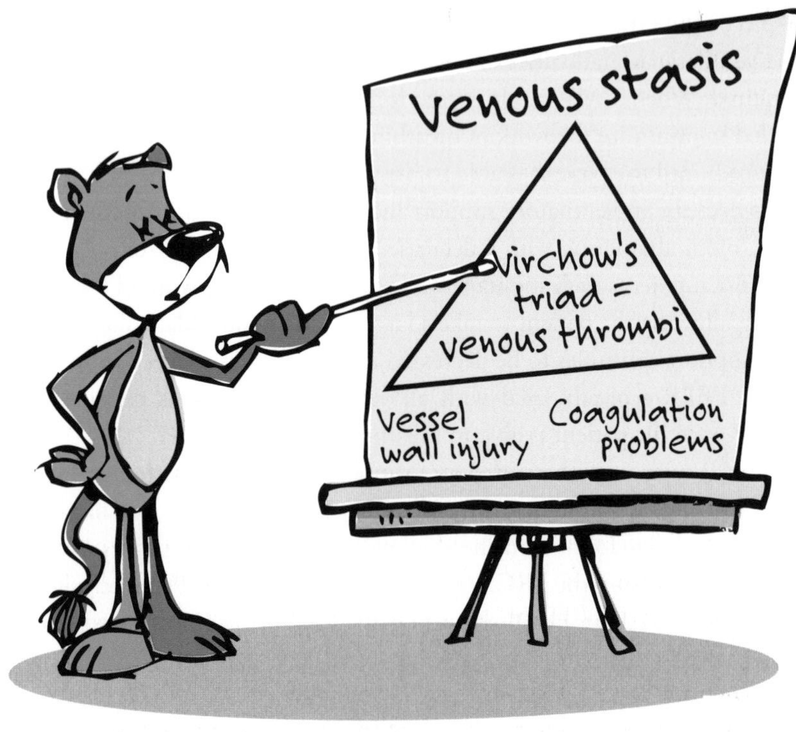

Venous Thrombi: Conditions and Risk Factors

Predisposing Factors to the Development of Venous Thrombi
Atrial fibrillation
Immobility
Infection
Atherosclerosis
Polycythemia
Conditions That Can Precipitate the Formation of Venous Thrombi
Heart failure
Right ventricular heart failure
Cardiomyopathy
Surgery (orthopedic, vascular, abdominal)
Trauma
Pregnancy

Other Risk Factors for Pulmonary Embolism

Immobilization
Obesity
Varicose veins
Long bone fractures
Atrial fibrillation
Venous catheter insertion

Pathophysiologic Changes

When thrombi are formed, break loose, and lodge in the pulmonary vasculature, both respiratory and cardiovascular changes occur. Alveoli distal to the occlusion become ventilated but not perfused. Gas exchange cannot occur, and the level of CO_2 decreases in this area. This decrease causes bronchoconstriction, which shunts blood to ventilated areas of lungs, increases pulmonary resistance, and causes a ventilation-perfusion mismatch. This mismatch causes hypoxia and increases the work of breathing for the patient.

When a PE obstructs more than 50% of the pulmonary vasculature, pulmonary hypertension results. Pulmonary vasoconstriction occurs from the release of mediators at the injury site and from hypoxia. As resistance increases, the workload of the RV of the heart also increases. Failure of the RV eventually occurs, which leads to failure of the left ventricle, decreased cardiac output, decreased blood pressure, and eventually shock.

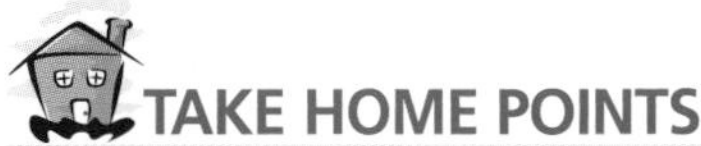

Some patients with hypercoagulable states are prone to the development of thrombi, which can ultimately result in a PE.

Clinical Manifestations of Pulmonary Embolism

Clinical manifestations of PE are often nonspecific, and a thorough history and physical are usually required to help with the diagnosis. The duration and the extent of the embolism often influence the clinical manifestations.

Shortness of breath (SOB) is one of the most common clinical manifestations of PE, although up to 20% of patients have no SOB. SOB can have a sudden onset or occur on exertion. Cough and hemoptysis can be observed in up to one-half of patients diagnosed with PE. Hemoptysis occurs when an area of infarction at or near the periphery of the lung begins to hemorrhage. Tachypnea (respiratory rate $>$ 24 breaths per minute) is a response to the hypoxia that develops from impaired gas exchange.

Chest pain occurs in more than one-half of patients diagnosed with PE. The pain generally comes from an infarction of the pulmonary vessel near the area in which the pleural nerves innervate. The pain is usually worse when taking a deep breath. Tachycardia (heart rate >100 beats per minute) occurs in response to the decrease in oxygenation and impaired gas exchange. Jugular vein distention (JVD) results from pulmonary hypertension and the decreased effectiveness of the RV. Hypotension can be observed in patients with a large PE and is related to the decrease in cardiac output from ventricular dysfunction.

Other clinical manifestations that can occur but are not specific to PE include a statement such as "I just don't feel well," apprehension, palpitations, syncope, rales and crackles, fever, diaphoresis, murmur or gallop, and cyanosis.

Diagnosis

A thorough history and physical examination must be obtained and must include risk factors (see boxes titled "Venous Thrombi: Conditions and Risk Factors" and "Other Risk Factors for Pulmonary Embolism"), recent medical and surgical history, and any physical findings. SOB and chest pain should be described and include time of onset, when it occurs (rest or exertion), location, duration, and position. The Well's Prediction Rule estimates the probability of pulmonary embolism, but clinical judgment should be used, especially with older patients or those with comorbidities.

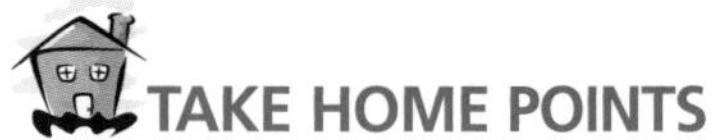

Well's Clinical Prediction Rule states a score of 1 or less, with a normal D-dimer test, makes diagnostic ultrasound unnecessary for DVT. Current research says this rule is beneficial for outpatients but not primary care patients (Oudega et al., 2005).

Common initial diagnostic tools include chest radiograph (CXR), ABG analysis, D-dimer testing, and electrocardiogram (ECG) findings. The CXR cannot diagnose the presence of a PE, but it can exclude other reasons that may cause the same clinical manifestations. Patients with a PE may show PA distention, an elevation of the diaphragm, and small infiltrates or pleural effusions. ABG analysis can reveal respiratory alkalosis, low partial pressure of oxygen (PaO_2), and low partial pressure of CO_2 ($PaCO_2$). A D-dimer blood test detects clot fragments that have been produced from clot lysis. A negative D-dimer predicts a low likelihood of PE. Abnormal ECG findings usually involve transient, nonspecific ST-segment and T-wave changes.

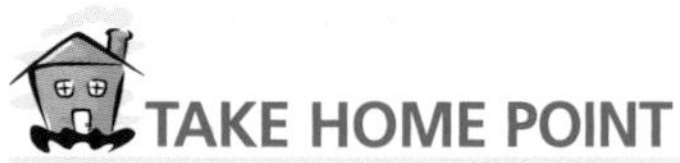

With a PICC constrast should only be given through a power PICC, not a regular PICC catheter.

Differential diagnostic studies include ventilation-perfusion (V/Q) scan, spiral computed tomographic (CT) scan, and pulmonary angiography. When compared with other diagnostic studies, V/Q scans can sometimes be inconclusive and other diagnostic studies need to be performed. Contrast-enhanced spiral CT scans are starting to replace V/Q scans as first line diagnostic studies to rule out PE, because they are quick and noninvasive. When intravenous contrast is given, vessels and thrombotic emboli can be visualized. Pulmonary angiography is the most definitive test for diagnosing a PE, but it is expensive, invasive, and not available in all settings.

What You DO

The best treatment for PE is prevention. When patients are at risk for developing PE, prophylactic measures should be instituted such as intravenous or subcutaneous heparin, low–molecular-weight heparin (Lovenox), and/or oral anticoagulants such as warfarin (Coumadin). The goal of therapy is to prevent thrombi formation, limit thrombi growth, and encourage breakdown of existing thrombi. Management of hypoxia may require supplemental oxygen, intubation, and mechanical ventilation.

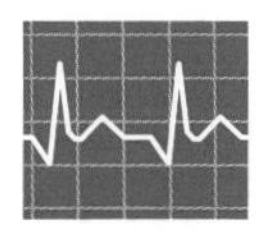

When injecting subcutaneous heparin or Lovenox, you do not wipe or rub the site post needle removal.

FIRST-LINE AND INITIAL TREATMENT FOR HYPOXIA

- Administer oxygen.
- Provide intubation.
- Provide mechanical ventilation.

Heparin therapy is started with a bolus (usually based on the patient's weight) and a continuous infusion adjusted every 4 to 6 hours, depending on institutional protocol. Activated partial thromboplastin time (aPTT) should be maintained at 1.5 to 2 times the normal value. Heparin therapy is generally continued for 7 to 14 days while the patient is on bedrest. If oral anticoagulant therapy such as Coumadin is used, it is generally started 2 to 3 days after heparin therapy has begun, once the aPTT levels have stabilized. A 5-day overlap of parenteral and oral anticoagulation is recommended. Oral anticoagulant doses are adjusted until the international normalized ratio (INR) is 2 to 3 times the normal value, then therapy is maintained for 3 to 6 months. Once discharged from the hospital, the INR should be checked frequently to maintain therapeutic anticoagulation.

The placement of an umbrella-type filter (i.e., Greenfield) is used for high-risk patients or whenever anticoagulant therapy is contraindicated. The filter is placed in the inferior vena cava to trap emboli before they can reach the lungs. Thrombolytic therapy may be used for patients who have had a major PE and those who are hemodynamically unstable. Drugs in this category include streptokinase, urokinase, and recombinant tissue plasminogen activator (rt-PA). Thrombolytic therapy is used to break down clots that have formed and are generally given within the first 24 to 48 hours of symptom onset. Heparin therapy should be started within 24 hours after the initial thrombolytic dose is given. Hemorrhage is a major concern with this type of therapy.

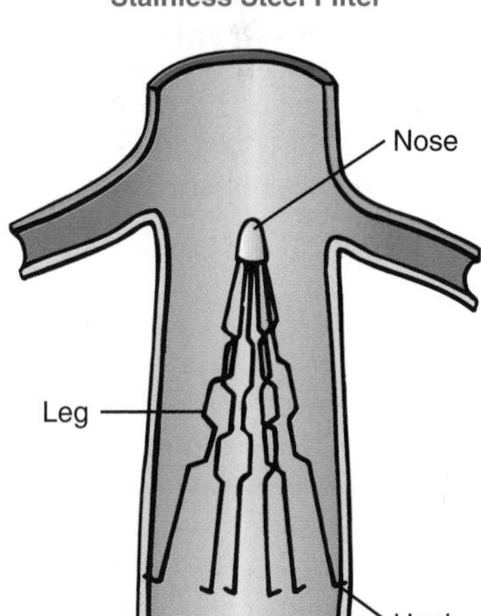

Placed in inferior vena cava of the heart. *(From Lewis SM, Heitkemper MM, Dirksen SR:* Medical-surgical nursing: assessment and management of clinical problems, *ed 5, St Louis, 2000, Mosby.)*

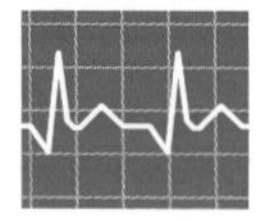

The therapeutic range for a patient taking heparin is based on the aPTT, which should be 1.5 to 2 times the normal value.

The reversal agent for unfractionated heparin is protamine sulfate; the reversal agent for warfarin (Coumadin) is vitamin K or fresh-frozen plasma (FFP).

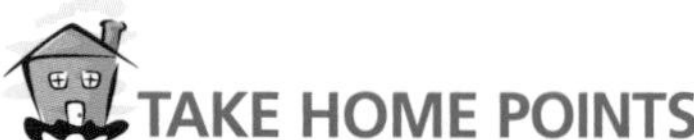

An inferior vena cava filter is not a treatment for PE; rather, it is a device to prevent a PE from occurring in patients with a known venous thrombus or at high risk for developing thrombi.

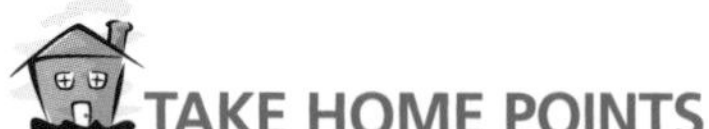

Administration of thrombolytics will break down the clots.

Hemorrhage is a major concern with the administration of thrombolytic therapy.

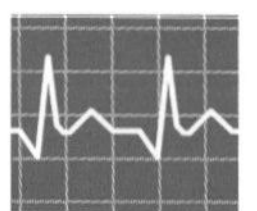

A large PE can result in increased PA pressures.

Surgical intervention is rarely used and is considered a last resort. Pulmonary embolectomy is the removal of a clot from a large vessel within the pulmonary vasculature. This surgery carries a high risk of death and is only used in patients who do not respond or have contraindications to other interventions.

Hemodynamic changes associated with PE stem from the development of pulmonary hypertension. Acute pulmonary hypertension causes increased PA pressures and a dilated RV. Interventions include the use of fluid to increase RV preload and improve contractility, and the use of inotropic agents to improve contractility and cardiac output. (For more information on heart failure, refer to the discussion in Chapter 4.)

Nursing Responsibilities

The main nursing goal is to prevent the development of DVT, which can lead to a thrombotic PE. Interventions to improve venous blood flow include early ambulation or use of intermittent pneumatic compression (IPC) devices in conjunction with elastic stockings and range-of-motion (ROM) exercises for those confined to bedrest. Monitor extremities for signs of DVT, such as pain, redness, warmth, or increased circumference. Although most DVTs originate in the calf, it is important to note that the upper arm is also a high-risk location.

Other nursing interventions include the following:

- Monitor extremities for signs and symptoms of DVT (calf pain or tenderness, redness, swelling, warmth, pain on dorsiflexion of foot [Homans' sign]).
- Maintain prescribed oxygen therapy and ask the patient to cough and deep breathe every 2 hours.
- Monitor for signs and symptoms of respiratory distress or worsening pulmonary status (heart failure, pulmonary edema), and notify the physician of any abnormal findings.
- Monitor ABGs and continuous pulse oximetry. Notify the physician of any changes in parameters ($SpO_2 < 90$, $PaO_2 < 80$, or $SaO_2 < 90$).
- Position patient for comfort and optimal oxygenation, and to promote secretion removal. If oxygenation is problematic, the patient should be turned to the unaffected side to improve ventilation and perfusion.
- Monitor for signs and symptoms of bleeding when anticoagulant or thrombolytic therapy is in progress (e.g.., blood in stool or urine,

pale mucous membranes, petecchiae, ecchymosis, complaints of back or flank pain, headache, or change in level of consciousness).

- Monitor anticoagulant laboratory values (complete blood count [CBC], aPTT, INR, fibrinogen) for abnormal or nontherapeutic range levels. Adjust anticoagulant dosing as prescribed to maintain therapeutic drug levels.
- Monitor for signs of cardiac arrhythmias such as atrial fibrillation and flutter; these may predispose the patient to thrombi formation.
- Administer medication to minimize anxiety and pain.
- Assess all skin puncture sites (e.g., venipuncture, lumbar puncture, bone marrow aspiration) for signs of bleeding, such as leakage, hemorrhage, and hematoma.

If Homans' sign is positive, then do NOT retest; doing so may dislodge the clot.

Patient Education

Topics to be covered in educating the patient and family include the following:

- Explain the cause, signs and symptoms, and interventions used to treat and prevent PE to the patient and family.
- If the patient is receiving anticoagulant or thrombolytic therapy, explain the signs and symptoms of bleeding to the patient and family.
- If the patient is receiving oral anticoagulant therapy when discharged, discuss medications, doses, side effects, food and drug interactions, importance of follow-up laboratory work, and physician visits.
- Instruct the patient on the application of elastic stockings, as well as the importance of avoiding crossing the legs, prolonged sitting (such as on airplanes or in the car), and wearing constrictive clothing.
- Discuss the importance of adequate hydration.

Do You UNDERSTAND?

DIRECTIONS: **Choose the correct answer to each of the following questions, and write the corresponding letter in the space provided.**

_____ 1. Which of the following is a risk factor for the development of a PE?

a. Anticoagulated blood
b. Early ambulation
c. Compression device
d. Injury to vessel wall

_____ 2. Which of the following is caused by decreased CO_2 related to ventilation-perfusion mismatch?
a. Bronchoconstriction
b. Decrease in pulmonary resistance
c. Increase in oxygenation
d. Shunting of blood to affected areas of lung

_____ 3. A clinical manifestation of PE includes which of the following?
a. Cardiac tamponade
b. Hypertension
c. Wheezing
d. Dyspnea

_____ 4. Heparin therapy is maintained at a therapeutic level that is _____________ times normal.
a. 1 to 1.5
b. 2 to 2.5
c. 1.5 to 2
d. 0.5 to 1.5

What IS Acute Respiratory Distress Syndrome?

Acute respiratory distress syndrome (ARDS), a severe form of acute lung injury (ALI), consists of a systemic inflammatory process that causes increased permeability of the alveolocapillary membrane and vasoconstriction of the pulmonary vasculature. This inflammation causes noncardiogenic pulmonary edema with severely impaired gas exchange. The mortality rate is greater than 40%, mostly from multisystem organ failure. Of those who survive, many have long-term impairment of lung function.

What You NEED TO KNOW

Causes

A multitude of possible causes for ARDS result from direct and indirect injury to the lungs. Some of the more common conditions that can

Answers: 1. d; 2. a; 3. d; 4. c.

precipitate ARDS are:

- Sepsis (18%-48%)
- Aspiration of gastric contents
- Pneumonia
- Near drowning
- Trauma or shock
- Pancreatitis
- Multiple blood transfusions
- DIC

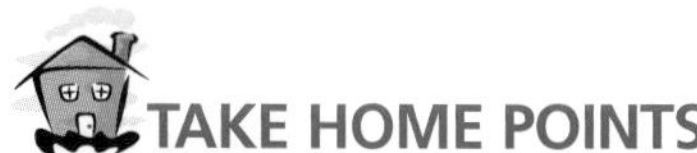

TAKE HOME POINTS

Increased risk of ARDS:

- >68 years old
- Female
- COPD
- Malignancy
- VRE infection
- Cigarette smoking
- ETOH abuse

Pathophysiologic Changes

When an injury occurs to the lungs, an inflammatory response is initiated by the immune system. This response stimulates the activation of neutrophils, macrophages, and endotoxins into the lungs and the release of protein mediators. Permeability of the alveolocapillary membrane is increased, allowing large molecules, such as protein-rich fluid, to enter into the lung tissue, which causes the alveoli to collapse and the lungs to become very stiff (decreased compliance). Severe hypoxia develops, leading to respiratory acidosis, narrowing of small airways, and pulmonary vasoconstriction. As hypoxia increases, the patient begins to hyperventilate, which creates fatigue and eventually respiratory failure. Pulmonary vasoconstriction can lead to pulmonary hypertension with RV dysfunction and decreased cardiac output.

Clinical Manifestations

A review of the patient's history and the potential risk factors related to ARDS is helpful for early assessment, diagnosis, and intervention. Most patients exhibit symptoms 24 to 48 hours after the initial insult to the lungs. Apprehension and restlessness, hyperventilation, hypertension, tachycardia, and SOB with the use of accessory muscle are some of the first signs leading to respiratory failure. Auscultation of lungs can reveal clear lung fields and crackles or rales. Other signs and symptoms of ARDS include intercostal retraction, cyanosis, and in some cases hyperthermia and cough.

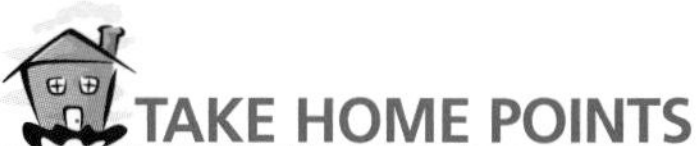

TAKE HOME POINTS

Patients with ARDS often exhibit symptoms within 24 to 48 hours after the initial insult to the lungs.

Diagnosis

ABG analysis reveals a low PaO_2, despite the increase in supplemental oxygen concentration. This is known as refractory hypoxemia; PaO_2/FiO_2 ratio less than 200 mm Hg is often used as a diagnostic criteria. $PaCO_2$ will decrease initially, related to hyperventilation, but as the patient becomes fatigued, the $PaCO_2$ will eventually increase, leading to respiratory acidosis. CXR findings can reveal bilateral infiltrates as

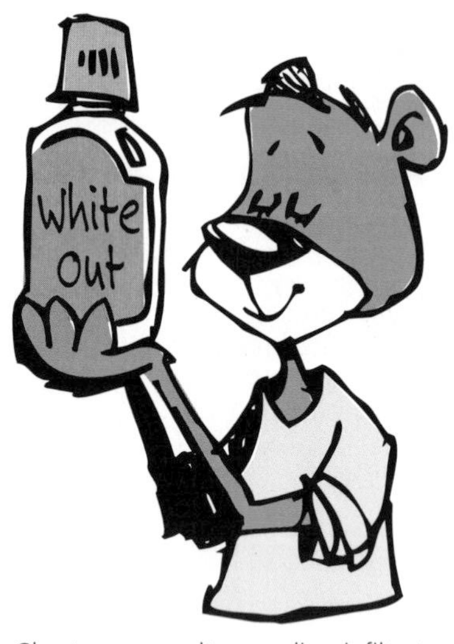

Chest x-ray results revealing infiltrates in the lungs is often called "white out" or "patchy" in appearance.

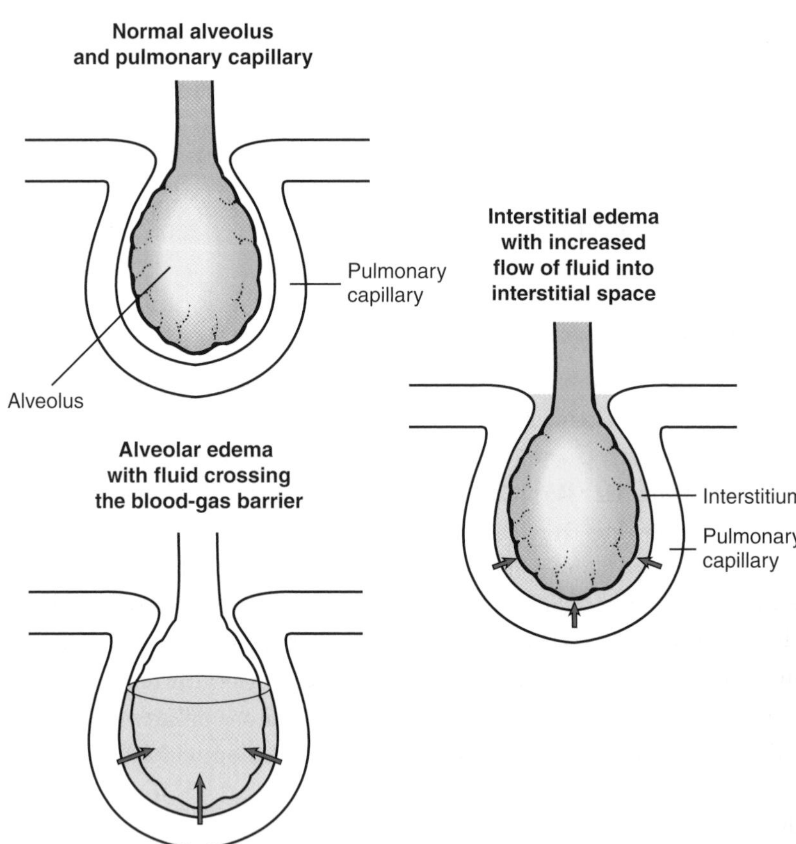

(*From Lewis SM, Heitkemper MM, Dirksen SR:* Medical-surgical nursing: assessment and management of clinical problems, *ed 5, St Louis, 2000, Mosby.)*

In patients with ARDS, PaO_2 is low, despite oxygen administration; $PaCO_2$ decreases initially as a result of hyperventilation.

a result of the increased alveoli permeability. Terms such as "patchy" infiltrates or "white out" may be associated with these CXR results. Hemodynamic monitoring with a PA catheter reveals a pulmonary artery occlusion pressure (PAOP) of less than 18 mm Hg.

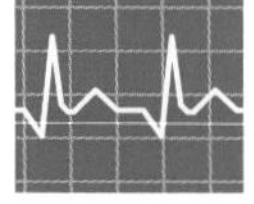

The PAOP reading from a PA catheter is normal (less than 18 mm Hg), which means that the pulmonary edema is not of cardiac origin.

What You DO

Treatment

The main goals in the treatment of ARDS include improving and maintaining oxygenation, maintaining fluid and electrolyte balances, providing adequate nutrition, and preventing respiratory and metabolic complications.

Supplemental oxygen is the first step in the treatment of patients with ARDS, who generally require intubation and mechanical ventilation to maintain adequate gas exchange. FiO_2 as high as 100% and intubation may be needed to help with tissue oxygenation. The main goal of oxygen therapy is maintaining a PaO_2 55 to 80 mm Hg or SpO_2 of 88 to 95 mm Hg using the lowest amount of FiO_2 possible. If FiO_2 greater than 60% is used for longer than 24 to 48 hours, oxygen toxicity may develop. Oxygen toxicity can increase damage to lung tissue by increasing membrane permeability and causing alveolar damage. It is important to establish specific treatment goals with medical and respiratory team members, because they may be individualized to the patient.

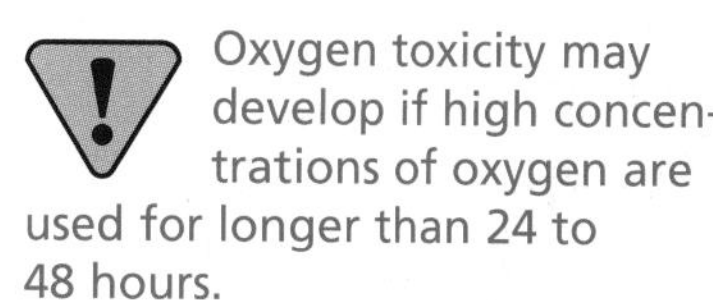

Oxygen toxicity may develop if high concentrations of oxygen are used for longer than 24 to 48 hours.

Mechanical ventilation is required following intubation in response to fatigue and respiratory failure, allowing for the underlying problem to be treated. The goal of mechanical ventilation is to improve ventilation function while decreasing the work of breathing and FiO_2. The use of PEEP between 5 and 24 cm H_2O generally leads to improved gas exchange (because it opens alveoli that have closed) and allows for lower concentrations of oxygen to be used. PEEP is typically increased when FiO_2 concentration is greater than 60% and is increased as necessary in an attempt to avoid using high levels of oxygen.

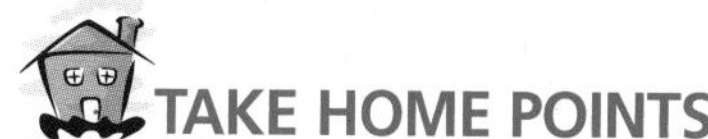

TAKE HOME POINTS

Ventilation with small tidal volumes (6.2 mL/kg) reduces ventilator-associated lung injuries.

Hypercapnia (elevated CO_2), may occur when alveoli are collapsed or full of fluid, decreasing their ability to participate in gas exchange, and can be exacerbated by ventilatory practice, such as low tidal volumes and IRV. Strategies such as increasing respiratory rates or using nonconventional methods of ventilation have been successful in lowering $PaCO_2$ levels. It is important to establish hypercapnia goals with the health care team because high levels of $PaCO_2$ can cause severe acidosis, which can lead to life-threatening hemodynamic complications.

Patients in respiratory failure from ARDS have a tendency to continue to hyperventilate and breathe against the ventilator. The use of sedation allows for the ventilator to take over the work of breathing; decreasing anxiety helps the patient rest. Neuromuscular-blocking agents may be used in conjunction with sedatives, allowing the relaxed respiratory muscles to achieve full lung expansion. Because neuromuscular-blocking agents and sedatives do not have analgesic effects, the nurse must continue to monitor the patient for signs of pain and provide analgesia as necessary.

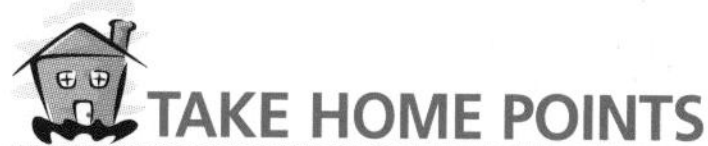

TAKE HOME POINTS

PEEP may need to be at high levels (greater than 7.5 cm H_2O); the astute nurse watches for possible complications such as a pneumothorax and decreased cardiac output.

Inverse-ratio ventilation (IRV) is a ventilatory strategy that has been used in ARDS to improve oxygenation. With normal, spontaneous breathing, the inspiratory-to-expiratory (I:E) ratio is 1:2. In IRV, the inspiratory time is lengthened and the expiratory time is shortened. It is recommended that inspiratory time remain less than or equal to expiratory time. Prolonged inspiratory time helps to reopen closed alveoli (alveolar recruitment) and lowers peak airway pressures. The increased inspiratory time also allows a longer period for gas exchange, thereby improving oxygenation. IRV has become less common in recent years as more advanced ventilatory strategies have become available. IRV is used in combination with a primary mode of ventilation, such as PRVC. This type of ventilation creates an abnormal breathing pattern, often necessitating the need for deeper levels of sedation or neuromuscular blockade to reduce anxiety and suppress spontaneous ventilation. One disadvantage of IRV is the potential for increased $PaCO_2$ levels caused by the shortened expiratory phase. Higher $PaCO_2$ levels (permissive hypercapnia) may be allowed, but in the event that hypercapnia causes severe acidosis, $PaCO_2$ may be decreased by increasing the respiratory rate.

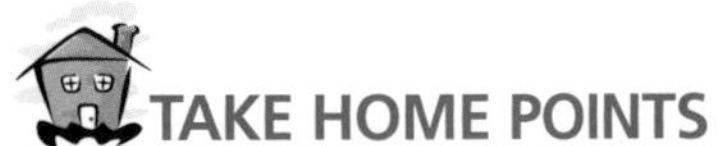

IRV ventilation improves oxygenation through increasing the inspiratory time.

The use of PPV can create complications such as increased airway pressures, increased inflammation, and alveolar hemorrhage by overdistending the lung tissue. These complications can increase lung injury and mortality rate. Ventilatory support with smaller tidal volumes (6 mL/kg) have been used to decrease airway resistance, decrease the stretch on lung tissue, and possibly reduce mortality. VILI can be limited by lowering tidal volumes and limiting airway plateau pressures to 30 cm H_2O or less.

When conventional modes of ventilation cause high peak airway pressures (greater than 30 cm H_2O) or the patient has refractory hypoxemia despite additional measures such as increased PEEP and IRV, nonconventional modes of ventilation may be used. Clinical research continues to be performed on these nonconventional modes to establish efficacy and long-term benefits. Nonconventional ventilatory modes include high-frequency ventilation, extracorporeal membrane oxygenation, and partial liquid ventilation. Nitric oxide, an additional method to improve oxygenation, can be used in combination with other ventilatory modes. Nonconventional modes often require greater levels of sedation and in some cases neuromuscular blocking agents.

High-frequency ventilation (HFV) describes modes of ventilation that deliver small tidal volumes at very high respiratory rates. Tidal volumes can range from 50 to 400 mL with respiratory rates from 60 to greater than 200 breaths/minute. Modes of HFV include jet ventilation and high-frequency oscillatory ventilation (HFOV). Smaller tidal volumes help minimize airway pressures, reducing the risk of VILI. HFV is generally used on patients who develop high peak airway pressures when conventional tidal volumes are used, although studies have shown inconclusive data to support this therapy.

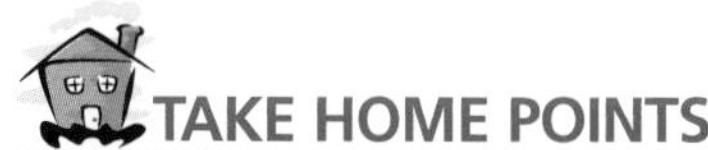

HFOV may not be the optimal rescue ventilation modality post inhalation (burn) injury (Cartotto et al., 2009).

HFOV has been used for severe respiratory failure when hypoxemia is refractory to conventional modes of ventilation. This mode and its terminology are very different from conventional ventilation because it does not provide breaths with measured tidal volumes. HFOV "shakes" the gas molecules, allowing for better transport of oxygen to the lungs and better transport of CO_2 from the lungs. HFOV helps prevent overdistention of alveoli and has more complete lung recruitment, facilitating better gas exchange than conventional ventilation modes.

Extracorporeal membrane oxygenation (ECMO) is another new treatment that is being investigated for use on patients with ARDS who experience refractory hypoxemia with conventional PPV. ECMO, like cardiopulmonary bypass, can be used for long-term support of a patient. It improves oxygenation and allows the lungs to rest and recover. The use of ECMO has not yet been shown to reduce mortality for patients with ARDS, and its use in research is limited to major institutions. A more recent method of ECMO, pumpless extracorporeal interventional lung assist (iLA), has demonstrated improved oxygenation and carbon dioxide removal.

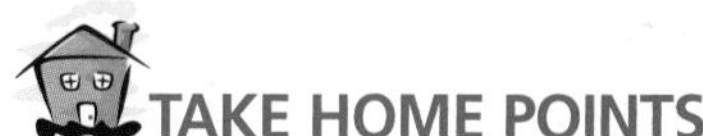

The words "Alveolar recruitment" refer to the opening of collapsed alveoli.

Liquid ventilation is a promising new treatment for patients with refractory hypoxemia. In partial liquid ventilation (PLV), liquid perfluorocarbons are instilled into the lungs through the endotracheal tube until the FRC is reached. A normal ventilator is then used to deliver oxygen and a tidal volume and to remove CO_2. Although there has been evidence of improved gas exchange, evidence to support this therapy for all patients remains inadequate. Liquid fluorocarbon has been shown to recruit closed alveoli, improve oxygen and carbon dioxide transport, and improve pulmonary blood flow.

Inhaled nitric oxide, a selective pulmonary vasodilating agent, has been shown to improve oxygenation but has had no effect on other outcomes, such as mortality. Nitric oxide can be delivered through the ventilatory system, along with either conventional or nonconventional ventilation. Patients must be monitored for formation of methemoglobin during treatment.

Hemodynamic Monitoring

The use of an arterial pressure line is commonly used to monitor blood pressure and sample ABGs. PA catheters may be used to measure cardiac output and monitor fluid management. The use of PEEP can cause a decrease in venous return (low central venous pressure [CVP]), cardiac output, and blood pressure. Pulmonary vasoconstriction that can occur with ARDS may lead to pulmonary hypertension and RV dysfunction. Although increased dysrhythmias have been reported with the use of PA catheters in ARDS, data suggest that this may be due to concurrent use of vasopressor agents. Recent guidelines discourage the routine use of PA catheters for ARDS management.

Mixed Venous Oxygen Saturation

Monitoring mixed venous oxygen saturation (SvO_2) indicates the amount of oxygen available after the tissues have been perfused. It provides valuable information about oxygen supply and demand. Specialized PA catheters can measure continuous SvO_2 or intermittent samples of mixed venous blood can be obtained from the PA lumen of all PA catheters. Four components are used to measure SvO_2: (1) SaO_2, (2) hemoglobin, (3) cardiac output, and (4) oxygen consumption (VO_2). Normal values of SvO_2 range between 60% to 80%. Values less than 50% indicate increased tissue oxygen demand. If a PA catheter is not available, a sample for central venous oxygen saturation ($ScvO_2$) can be obtained from the distal lumen of any central venous catheter (see Take Home Points).

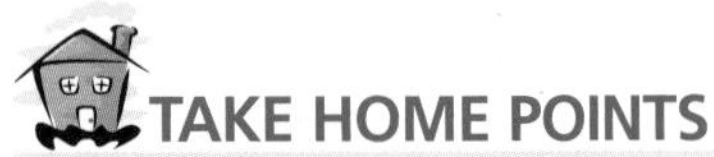

TAKE HOME POINTS

Distal lumen of CVC.

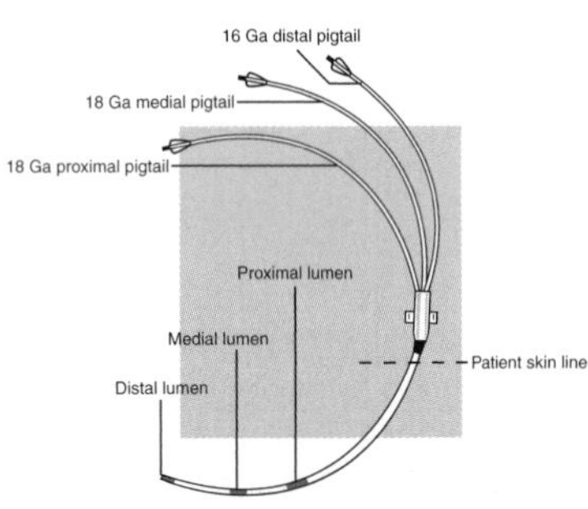

Fluid Management

The goal of fluid therapy is to maintain tissue perfusion. Conservative fluid management is recommended in the absence of shock to prevent further leakage of fluid into the alveoli. Mean arterial pressure (MAP) should be maintained above 65 mm Hg using a combination of fluids and vasopressors such as dopamine or norepinephrine, as appropriate. If hypotension is cardiac in origin, an inotropic agent such as dobutamine can be used.

TAKE HOME POINTS

Fluid restriction is necessary; however, tissue perfusion and cardiac output should not be compromised.

Positioning

Prone positioning has been shown to improve oxygenation when implemented early in ARDS. Conventional supine positioning delivers the majority of pulmonary blood flow to alveoli that are impaired by atelectasis or fluid, an effect of gravity. Although the mechanism behind improved oxygenation in prone positioning is not fully understood, it assists in alveolar recruitment. In a prone position, the healthier alveoli receive the best perfusion, improving intrapulmonary shunting. Prone positioning requires a team effort to safely reposition the patient; airway protection is of utmost concern. Hemodynamic instability and activity intolerance with increased oxygen consumption are contraindications to prone positioning. Patients remain at risk for pressure ulcers while prone and must be repositioned regularly.

Increased oxygen consumption and hemodynamic instability (unstable blood pressure) are contraindications for prone positioning.

Nutrition

Energy expenditure during respiratory failure is high, caused by the increased work of breathing. The goal of nutritional support is to provide the necessary nutrients to maintain the patient's current level of metabolism, energize the immune system, and maintain end organ function. Enteral feeding is the route of choice to provide the calories and nutrients needed and to assist in maintaining normal GI function. If the patient is unable to tolerate enteral feeding, total parenteral nutrition may be administered by the parenteral (intravenous) route until the patient can tolerate enteral feeding.

Corticosteroid Therapy

Corticosteroids may be prescribed as antiinflammatory agents to decrease the permeability of the alveolocapillary membrane and to prevent further leakage of fluid into the alveoli. Recent studies have shown that moderate-dose long-term glucocorticoids reduce inflammation and improve oxygenation. Although steroid therapy can increase the risk of infections related to immune suppression, the literature suggests that the risk can be reduced by maintaining tight glycemic control.

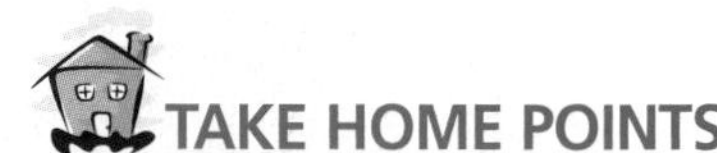

Enteral feeding is preferred over the parenteral route because it promotes the normal functioning of the GI tract.

Nursing Responsibilities

The main nursing goals are to optimize oxygenation, maintain tissue perfusion, provide adequate nutrition, and provide emotional support to the patient and family. Follow the expected practice for mechanical ventilation, including the following exceptions and additions:

- Assess respiratory status every 1 to 2 hours, documenting rate, rhythm, breathing pattern, and use of accessory muscles.
- Assess breath sounds at least every 4 hours for abnormal findings such as crackles or rales, or complications such as pneumothorax.
- Assess for restlessness, anxiety, change in level of consciousness, and tachypnea; any one of these symptoms can indicate a progression of respiratory distress.
- Reposition the patient for optimal gas exchange and comfort (prone position is recommended if not contraindicated).
- Monitor ABGs and notify the physician of any significant changes (goals of treatment should be individualized and clearly defined by the care team).
- Administer supplemental oxygen at the lowest percentage possible to provide adequate oxygen saturation.

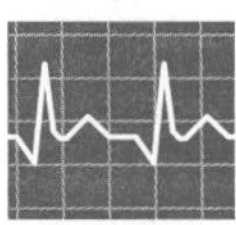
Patients taking steroids (i.e., glucocorticoids) have increased blood sugars and should have their blood sugars monitored.

- Provide adequate periods of rest, being mindful of activities such as routine nursing care that increase oxygen demands.
- Provide adequate nutrition. If enteral feeding is delivered through a tube with gastric (vs. small bowel) placement, measure the gastric residual volume (GRV) every 4 hours. Notify the physician if the GRV is greater than 100 mL or volume specified by institutional policy. Although high GRVs do not directly reflect gastric motility, the addition of a promotility agent such as metoclopramide (Reglan), or a temporary reduction in the formula rate may be required.

Patient and Family Education

Topics to be covered in educating the patient and family include the following:

- Provide an explanation of ARDS.
- Describe signs and symptoms of respiratory failure.
- Discuss typical interventions for ARDS with patient and family.
- Explain the rationale for frequent laboratory testing and ABG monitoring.
- Describe the role of sedation during ventilatory support.

Do You UNDERSTAND?

DIRECTIONS: **Choose the correct answer to each of the following questions, and write the corresponding letter in the space provided.**

_____ 1. The increased permeability that is seen in ARDS increases fluid accumulation in which of the following areas?
   a. RV
   b. Brain tissue
   c. Pericardial sac
   d. Alveoli

_____ 2. Symptoms of respiratory distress associated with ARDS begin within __________ hours of insult to lungs?
   a. 6 to 12
   b. 12 to 24
   c. 24 to 48
   d. 48 to 72

______ 3. High levels of PEEP can cause which of the following to occur?
   a. Increased venous return
   b. Decreased cardiac output
   c. Decreased oxygen saturation
   d. Increased work of breathing

______ 4. Which of the following medications can be used to maintain tissue perfusion during periods of hypotension that are not cardiac in origin?
   a. Dopamine
   b. Phenylephrine (Neo-Synephrine)
   c. Nitroglycerin
   d. Sodium nitroprusside (Nipride)

Answers: 1. d; 2. c; 3. b; 4. a.

References

Acute Respiratory Distress Syndrome Network: Ventilation with lower tidal volumes as compared with traditional tidal volumes for acute lung injury and the acute respiratory distress syndrome, *New England Journal of Medicine,* 342(18):1301-1308, 2000.

Adhikari N, Burns KEA, Meade MO: Pharmacologic therapies for adults with acute lung injury and acute respiratory distress syndrome, *Cochrane Database of Systematic Reviews,* (4):2007.

Alsaghir AH, Martin CM: Effect of prone positioning in patients with acute respiratory distress syndrome: a meta-analysis, *Critical Care Medicine,* 36(2):603-609, 2008.

American Association of Critical Care Nurses: AACN practice alert: ventilator-associated pneumonia, *AACN Clinical Issues: Advanced Practice in Acute & Critical Care,* 16(1):105-109, 2005.

American Association of Critical Care Nurses: Practice alert. Oral care in the critically ill, *AACN News,* 23(8):4-4, 2006.

American Association for Respiratory Care. AARC clinical practice guideline: capnography/capnometry during mechanical ventilation—2003 revision & update, *Respiratory Care,* 48(5):534-539, 2003.

Bein T, Weber F, Pilipp A, Prasser C, Pfeifer M, Schmid F, et al: A new pumpless extracorporeal interventional lung assist in critical hypoxemia/hypercapnia, *Critical Care Medicine,* 34(5):1372-1377, 2006.

Bourgault AM, Ipe L, Weaver J, Swartz S, O'Dea PJ: Development of evidence-based guidelines and critical care nurses' knowledge of enteral feeding, *Critical Care Nurse,* 27(4):17-29, 2007.

Brown JK, Haft JW, Bartlett RH, Hirschl RB: Acute lung injury and acute respiratory distress syndrome: extracorporeal life support and liquid ventilation for severe acute respiratory distress syndrome in adults, *Seminars in Respiratory & Critical Care Medicine,* 27(4):416-425, 2006.

Cartotto R, Walia G, Ellis S, Fowler R: Oscillation after inhalation: high frequency oscillatory ventilation in burn patients with the acute respiratory distress syndrome and co-existing smoke inhalation injury, *Journal of Burn Care & Research,* 30(1):119-127, 2009.

Chan EY, Ruest A, Meade MO, Cook DJ: Oral decontamination for prevention of pneumonia in mechanically ventilated adults: systematic review and meta-analysis, *BMJ: British Medical Journal,* 334(7599):889-893, 2007.

Dellinger RP, Levy MM, Carlet JM, Bion J, Parker MM, Jaeschke R, et al: Surviving Sepsis Campaign: international guidelines for management of severe sepsis and septic shock: 2008, *Critical Care Medicine,* 36(1):296-327, 2008.

Dong B, Jirong Y, Liu G, Wang Q, Wu T: Thrombolytic therapy for pulmonary embolism, *Cochrane Database of Systematic Reviews,* (2):CD004437, 2006.

Fessler HE, Derdak S, Ferguson ND, Hager DN, Kacmarek RM, Thompson BT, et al: A protocol for high-frequency oscillatory ventilation in adults: results from a roundtable discussion, *Critical Care Medicine,* 35(7):1649-1654, 2007.

Goldhill DR, Imhoff M, McLean B, Waldmann C: Rotational bed therapy to prevent and treat respiratory complications: a review and meta-analysis, *American Journal of Critical Care,* 16(1):50-62, 2007.

Granton JT, Slutsky AS: Ventilator-induced lung injury. In Hall JB, Schmidt GA, Wood LDH, eds: *Principles of critical care,* New York, McGraw-Hill, 2005.

Meduri GU, Golden E, Freire AX, Taylor E, Zaman M, Carson SJ, et al: Methylprednisolone infusion in early severe ARDS. Results of a randomized controlled trial, *Chest,* 131(4):954-963, 2007.

Oudega R, Hoes AW, Moons KG: The Wells rule does not adequately rule out deep venous thrombosis in primary care patients, *Annals of Internal Medicine,* 143(2):100-107, 2005.

Qaseem A, Snow V, Barry P, Hornbake ER, Rodnick JE, Tobolic T, et al: Current diagnosis of venous thromboembolism in primary care: a clinical practice guideline from the American Academy of Family Physicians and the American College of Physicians, *Annals of Family Medicine,* 5(1):57-62, 2007.

Schmidt GA, Hall JB: Management of the ventilated patient. In Hall JB, Schmidt GA, Wood LDH, eds: *Principles of critical care,* New York, McGraw-Hill, 2005.

Stapleton RD, Wang BM, Hudson LD, et al: Cause and timing of death in patients with ARDS, *Chest,* 128(2): 525-532, 2005.

Steinberg KP, Hudson LD, Goodman RB, Hough CL, Lanken PN, Hyzy R, et al: Efficacy and safety of corticosteroids for persistent acute respiratory distress syndrome, *New England Journal of Medicine,* 354(16):1671-1684, 2006.

Wratney AT, Cheifetz IM: AARC clinical practice guideline. Removal of the endotracheal tube—2007 revision & update, *Respiratory Care,* 52(1):81-93, 2007.

Wunsch H, Mapstone J, Takala J: High-frequency ventilation versus conventional ventilation for the treatment of acute lung injury and acute respiratory distress syndrome: a systematic review and Cochrane analysis, *Anesthesia & Analgesia,* 100(6):1765-1772, 2005.

NCLEX® Review

1. Which ventilation mode is the most appropriate for a patient who has decreased lung compliance?
   1 SIMV.
   2 PRVC.
   3 CPAP.
   4 ACV.
2. Recognizing that prolonged delivery of high oxygen concentrations can lead to oxygen toxicity, which strategy would be used first to increase oxygenation in an attempt to decrease FiO_2?
   1 Inverse ratio ventilation.
   2 Prone positioning.
   3 Increase PEEP.
   4 High-frequency ventilation.
3. Inadequate PEEP can increase the risk of:
   1 Barotrauma.
   2 Volutrauma.
   3 Atelectrauma.
   4 Pneumothorax.
4. Your patient has these ventilation settings: SIMV, FiO_2 0.50, TV 600, Rate 10, PEEP 5 cm H_2O, PSV 12 cm H_2O. The patient has taken four spontaneous breaths with an average tidal volume of 350 mL. Which statement best describes this situation?
   1 There is a possible equipment failure; prepare to manually ventilate.
   2 Spontaneous tidal volumes are often lower.
   3 Pressure support setting is too high.
   4 Monitor for low pressure alarms.
5. Which signs and symptoms in a patient with atrial fibrillation would indicate a pulmonary emboli?
   1 Palpitations, diaphoresis.
   2 Irregular heart beat, syncope.
   3 Hypertension, fever.
   4 Hypoxia, dyspnea.
6. Your patient receives a thrombolytic agent following diagnosis of a large pulmonary emboli. Which signs and symptoms might alert you to a major complication of this medication?
   1 Change in level of consciousness.
   2 Pink mucous membranes.
   3 Copious, dilute urine output.
   4 Increased cardiac output.
7. Your patient is being discharged on oral anticoagulation for pulmonary emboli. What is the best advice you can provide during discharge education?
   1 Regular aPTT monitoring is required.
   2 Regular dose adjustment is required.
   3 Regular INR monitoring is required.
   4 Continue heparin for 5 days.
8. A patient receiving continuous intravenous heparin for pulmonary embolus has an aPTT 1.2 times the normal value. What is the next nursing intervention?
   1 Begin oral anticoagulation.
   2 Increase heparin by protocol.
   3 Decrease heparin by protocol.
   4 Repeat aPTT in 4 hours.
9. A patient with ARDS has received a fluid bolus to increase mean arterial blood pressure (MAP) to 65 mm Hg. Following this, oxygen requirements increase to FiO_2 1.0 and blood pressure decreases to less than 65 mm Hg. What is the next anticipated intervention?
   1 Diuresis.
   2 Decrease FiO_2.
   3 Dopamine.
   4 Nitroprusside.
10. What is happening at the cellular level to cause hypoxia in ARDS?
    1 Respiratory acidosis.
    2 Pulmonary hypertension.
    3 Right ventricular failure.
    4 Leaking alveolocapillary membranes.

NCLEX® Review Answers

1.2 Pressure-regulated volume control (PRVC) is a pressure-cycled mode of ventilation that limits the airway pressures, reducing the risk of ventilator-associated lung injury, which can occur when plateau pressures are greater than 30 cm H_2O. SIMV and ACV are volume-cycled ventilation modes, which may allow airway pressures to exceed safe limits. CPAP is only for patients who are breathing spontaneously; it would not be appropriate to meet the ventilatory needs of a patient with decreased lung compliance.

2.3 Increasing PEEP to open alveoli is a first-line strategy to increase oxygenation if FiO_2 levels are becoming too high. Although inverse ratio ventilation, prone positioning, and high-frequency ventilation have all been shown to improve oxygenation, there are more risks associated with these interventions.

3.3 Inadequate levels of PEEP may cause the alveoli to collapse. Opening and closing of the alveoli can cause damage to the alveolar tissue, known as atelectrauma. Barotrauma occurs secondary to increased airway pressure. Volutrauma occurs secondary to increased volume, or overstretching of the alveoli. Pneumothorax is a complication of PPV that occurs when airway pressures become too high.

4.2 It is normal for spontaneous tidal volumes to be lower than tidal volumes preset in PPV modes. No intervention is necessary when this occurs. Once a patient is allowed to breathe spontaneously, adequate removal of CO_2 depends on the total minute volume (respiratory rate $\times$ tidal volume).

5.4 Patients with atrial fibrillation are at very high risk for thrombi formation and emboli. Signs and symptoms of hypoxia, including dyspnea, should alert the nurse to an acute change in respiratory status, requiring further investigation.

6.1 Thrombolytic agents are used to break up existing clots. Because of this "clot busting" action, bleeding is a major complication. A change in level of consciousness may indicate a cerebral hemorrhage, in which case a more thorough neurologic examination would be indicated. If bleeding is suspected, the thrombolytic agent should be stopped and the physician notified.

7.3 Coumadin is the drug of choice for oral anticoagulation for pulmonary emboli. Therapeutic anticoagulation levels for Coumadin are monitored by INR. It is necessary for patients to have regular blood work drawn to monitor INR. INR outside of the therapeutic range requires adjustments to Coumadin dosing. Frequency of blood work depends on changes to Coumadin dosing.

8.2 The therapeutic range for intravenous heparin therapy is an aPTT 1.5 to 2 times the normal range. If the aPTT is only 1.2 times normal, the nurse should increase the heparin rate (dose) per protocol and repeat the aPTT as indicated. Adjustment of heparin dosing followed by aPTT testing is necessary until the aPTT is within therapeutic range.

9.3 Fluids are administered cautiously in patients with ARDS due to the leaky alveolocapillary membranes. Goals of therapy should include maintaining MAP greater than 65 mm Hg with adequate tissue perfusion. If too much fluid is given, oxygen needs may increase. If BP and perfusion remain inadequate, a vasopressor such as dopamine or norepinephrine should be started.

10.4 One of the primary causes of hypoxia in ARDS is leaking alveolocapillary membranes secondary to a systemic inflammatory response. Respiratory acidosis and pulmonary hypertension may occur with ARDS, but they do not directly cause hypoxia.

Nervous System

What You WILL LEARN

After reading this chapter, you will know how to do the following:

- ✔ Recognize the signs and symptoms of a seizure.
- ✔ Differentiate between a seizure and status epilepticus.
- ✔ Describe the various types of seizures.
- ✔ Discuss the care of a patient who has a seizure.
- ✔ Explain the physiologic changes associated with meningitis.
- ✔ Discuss nursing interventions for the patient with meningitis.
- ✔ Describe the pathophysiology of spinal cord injury.
- ✔ Compare and contrast the signs and symptoms of the varying levels of spinal cord injury.
- ✔ Identify appropriate nursing interventions for caring for a patient with a spinal cord injury.
- ✔ Discuss relevant patient education topics.

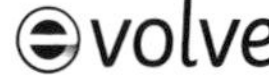

See http://evolve.elsevier.com/Schumacher/criticalcare for additional NCLEX® review questions.

What IS a Seizure?

A seizure is a sudden, abnormal, excessive discharge of electrical activity within the brain that disrupts the brain's usual system for nerve conduction. A seizure is a nonchronic disorder. Epilepsy is a chronic disorder, characterized by recurrent seizure activity.

TAKE HOME POINTS

- A seizure is an outward sign of the disruption of the brain's electrical activity.
- A seizure is a symptom, not a disease.
- A seizure will frequently result in changes in behavior, movements, sensation, perception, or consciousness.

A patient may experience an aura before seizing.

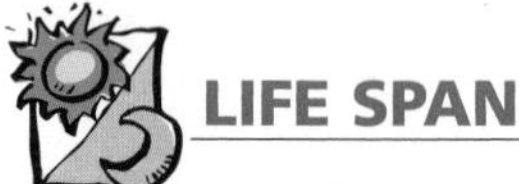

- Absence, or petit-mal, seizures are most common in children.
- Head trauma and injury is a common cause of seizures in young adults.

TAKE HOME POINTS

- Unclassified seizures are idiopathic; they occur for an unknown reason and do not fit into the partial or generalized classifications.
- Seventy-five percent of seizures are idiopathic.
- A seizure can occur in isolation or with an acute problem within the central nervous system (CNS) (e.g., low blood sugar, drug or alcohol withdrawal, head injury, hypoxia).
- Brain tumors are the most common cause of seizures. Seizures are often the first manifestation of an intracranial mass.

What You NEED TO KNOW

Three phases of seizure activity exist. The first phase is the *prodromal phase.* It consists of mood or behavior changes that can precede the seizure by hours or days. An aura occurs in some individuals before the seizure. It is a sensory warning such as an unusual taste or smell, metallic taste, or flash of lights. The second phase is the *ictal phase,* which is the seizure activity itself. The third phase is the *postictal phase,* which follows the seizure. Behavior changes, lethargy, or confusion can also occur.

Classification of Seizures

The International Classification of Epileptic Seizures recognizes three broad categories of seizure disorders. Seizures are classified as (1) *partial (focal) seizures,* (2) *generalized seizures,* or (3) *unclassified seizures.* Simple partial seizures occur in about 15% of patients with seizures. Symptoms may be motor, cognitive, sensory, autonomic, or affective, depending on the area of cerebral cortex involved. Consciousness is not impaired with this type of seizure. Complex partial seizures occur in approximately 35% of patients with seizures. Consciousness is partially or completely impaired, but no initial generalized tonic-clonic activity occurs.

Clinical presentation does vary, but patients usually experience an aura, automatism, postictal confusion, or tiredness. They will have no memory of the events during the seizure.

Generalized seizures occur in 40% of patients with epilepsy. The manifestations of generalized seizures indicate involvement of both hemispheres, most commonly impairment of consciousness with bilateral motor involvement. Patients usually have amnesia of the event.

Types of Generalized Seizures and Signs and Symptoms

Type of Seizure	Signs and Symptoms
Absence (petit-mal)	Occurs in 5% of patients with seizures Occurs primarily in children Vacant, blinking stare Some body movements may occur No convulsions or postictal signs or symptoms
Atonic (drop attacks)	Sudden loss of postural muscle tone
Myoclonic	Brief symmetric jerking of the extremities that usually involve the upper extremities
Clonic	Repetitive, rapid motor activity
Tonic	Rigidity

Types of Generalized Seizures and Signs and Symptoms—cont'd

Type of Seizure	Signs and Symptoms
Tonic-clonic (grand-mal)	Occurs in 25% of patients with seizures Most common type of generalized seizures in adults
	Tonic stiffening (extension) followed by jerking movements (clonic phase)
	May produce cyanosis, labored respirations, bowel or bladder incontinence (or both), involuntary tongue biting, and postictal fatigue, confusion, or stupor

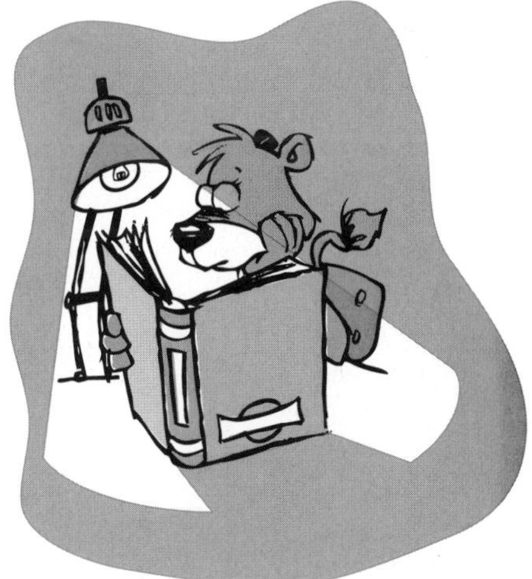

Myth: Persons with epilepsy are stupid.

Cause of Seizures

Seizures can be triggered by toxic states, electrolyte imbalances, anoxia, cerebral tumors, inflammation of the CNS tissue, cerebrovascular disease, hyperpyrexia, increased intracranial pressure (ICP), trauma, hypoxia, Huntington's disease, multiple sclerosis, Alzheimer's disease, or idiopathic causes.

Myths and Stigmas Associated with Seizures

Many myths and stigmas are associated with seizures, all of them untrue:

- Epilepsy is synonymous with stupid.
- Epilepsy is contagious.
- Seizures are an act of the supernatural.
- Epileptics have psychiatric problems.
- Epileptics cannot participate in sports or other normal activities of daily living.
- Epileptic employees have a higher rate of on-the-job injuries and absenteeism.

Diagnostic Tests

Blood tests should include a sodium, potassium, calcium, phosphorus, magnesium, blood urea nitrogen (BUN), glucose level, and a toxicology screen. Other laboratory tests that can be used to look for abnormalities that can result in seizures include oxygen tension in the arterial blood (PaO_2) (hypoxemia), low anticonvulsant medication therapeutic levels, and associated blood identifying disorders (lead poisoning, leukemia, sickle cell anemia). An EEG is the definitive test to diagnose seizure activity. An EEG can determine the presence of a seizure focus; it measures electrical activity of the brain through electrodes placed on the

TAKE HOME POINTS

For a routine electroencephalogram (EEG) test, the patient should not receive any medicines for 24 to 48 hours before the test, except medicines prescribed by the physician. Tranquilizers, stimulants (including tea, coffee, colas, and cigarettes), and alcohol all cause changes in brain patterns. The patient should have normal meals because hypoglycemia can cause changes in brain patterns. The patient's hair should be shampooed the day before the EEG, and no oils, lotions, or sprays should be applied to the hair.

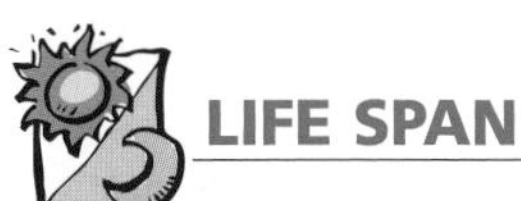

LIFE SPAN

- Adults are usually instructed to stay up late the night before the EEG and to awaken early.
- For a sleep-deprived EEG, children and infants should not be allowed to nap before the scheduled test.

scalp. The standard 21-lead, 30-minute EEG can be falsely negative; it has a sensitivity of only 50% to 60%. A 24-hour EEG may be necessary to establish a definitive diagnosis.

Sleep-deprived EEG can be prescribed because sleep deprivation can evoke abnormal brain patterns. Most EEGs require the patient to sleep during the last part of the EEG test.

A computed tomography (CT) scan of the head with contrast is particularly useful in the setting of a focal seizure, neurologic deficit, absence of a history of alcohol abuse, or possible trauma. Magnetic resonance imaging (MRI) of the head is indicated after a tonic-clonic seizure. MRI shows an abnormality in 10% to 20% of patients with a generalized tonic-clonic seizure and a normal CT scan. Single photon emission computed tomography (SPECT) scans also help diagnose seizure disorders. This scan uses several of the common commercially prepared radionuclides. A SPECT scan is the scan of choice for a diagnostic evaluation of certain types of CNS disorders; it provides information about the metabolism of and the blood flow through the brain tissue. A cerebral arteriogram may be prescribed to visualize vascular abnormalities not seen on the CT scan. Skull radiographs may be done if head trauma is involved. Finally, a lumbar puncture (LP) is indicated if infection or hemorrhage is suspected as the cause of the seizure activity, and a bone marrow aspiration is conducted if leukemia is suspected.

The only specific nursing care required after an EEG is to shampoo the patient's hair to remove the electrode gel from the hair.

Treatment

Medication therapy is the hallmark of seizure management. However, less than 75% of seizures are fully controlled by anticonvulsant drug therapy. Seizure type and the patient's tolerance for side effects determine drug choice. Combination therapy results in total control of seizures in 10% of patients whose condition is not controlled with monotherapy, and an additional 40% have a reduction in seizure frequency. The doses of the anticonvulsant medication are determined by clinical response, not serum drug level. If the patient is seizure-free, increasing the dose does not reduce the risk of future seizures but does increase toxicity, even if the drug level is subtherapeutic. Finally, the normally effective plasma concentration may be exceeded to achieve seizure control if the patient is not having significant drug toxic effects.

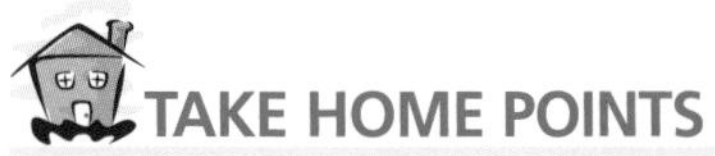

A brain SPECT scan costs about as much as a CT brain scan.

Antiepileptic Drugs

Drug	Therapeutic Serum Drug Level (micrograms/mL)	Indication for Use	Common Side Effects
Acetazolamide (Diamox)	Not established	Second choice for myoclonic seizures	Lethargy, paresthesias, appetite suppression, renal calculi, metabolic acidosis
Carbamazepine (Tegretol)	6-12 Toxic is >14	First choice for partial simple and complex and tonic-clonic	Dizziness, diplopia, leukopenia
Clonazepam (Klonopin)	0.02-0.08	Second choice for myoclonic seizures	Sedation, confusion, ataxia, depression
Ethosuximide (Zarontin)	40-100	First choice for typical absence seizures Second choice for atypical absence seizures	Gastrointestinal side effects: nausea/vomiting; lethargy, anorexia, skin rash
Gabapentin (Neurontin)	Not established	Second choice for partial simple and complex seizures	Somnolence, ataxia, dizziness, fatigue, weight gain, nausea
Lamotrigine (Lamictal)	Not established	Second choice for partial simple and complex seizures, typical and atypical absence seizures, and tonic-clonic seizures	Weight gain, somnolence, rash, ataxia, dizziness, diplopia, headache, nausea/vomiting, rhinitis
Levetiracetam (Keppra)	Not established	Second choice for partial complex seizures	Psychiatric symptoms, somnolence, asthenia, sedation, incoordination
Oxcarbazepine (Trileptal)	Not established	First choice for partial complex and tonic-clonic seizures	Diplopia, ataxia, dizziness, somnolence, tremors
Phenobarbital	10-40 Toxic level >60	Second choice for tonic-clonic seizures	Dizziness, ataxia, rash, sedation, cognitive impairment, drowsiness
Phenytoin sodium (Dilantin)	10-20 Toxic level >40	First choice for partial simple and complex seizures and tonic-clonic seizures	Gingival hyperplasia, gastric distress, rash, ataxia, nystagmus, osteomalacia, lymphadenopathy, macrocytosis, hypertrichosis
Primidone (Mysoline)	5-12	Second choice for tonic-clonic seizures	Nystagmus, ataxia, nausea, dizziness, sedation, vertigo
Topiramate (Topamax)	Not established	Second choice for tonic-clonic seizures	Weight loss, nervousness, somnolence, ataxia, confusion, dizziness
Valproic acid (Depakene)	50-100 Toxic level >150	First choice for partial simple and complex seizures and for typical and atypical absence seizures and tonic-clonic and myoclonic seizures	Somnolence, nausea/vomiting, anorexia, hair loss, increased liver enzymes, bruising
Zonisamide (Zonegran)	Not established	Second choice for partial complex and myoclonic seizures	Headache, dizziness, ataxia, somnolence, renal calculi

Surgical management is another consideration for some patients experiencing seizures. Resective procedures to remove the brain tissue that is the focus of the seizure activity is one type of surgical treatment. The goal is to remove the maximal amount of seizure-producing tissue without causing any neurologic deficit. Another surgical treatment is a palliative corpus callosotomy. The corpus callosum is a fibrous network of nerves

TAKE HOME POINTS

- Monotherapy (or the use of one anticonvulsant) is preferred; in some cases, however, combination therapy is needed.
- Clinical response to medication, not serum drug levels, is key for dosing and managing the seizure patient.
- Most seizures decrease in frequency but are not totally eliminated when a corpus callosotomy is done.

that join the brain hemispheres; this procedure stops the spread of seizures and thus prevents loss of consciousness.

The use of vagal nerve stimulation (VNS) is achieving more attention in the treatment of seizures. The VNS is a pacemaker-like device connected to a programmable generator. It stimulates the left vagus nerve (the nerve that affects parts of the brain that propagate seizures) in the neck and can modestly reduce seizure frequency. The patient can also trigger it with a hand-held device (magnet) if he or she experiences an aura, and often the seizure is prevented or the severity of the seizure is lessened.

What You DO

Seizure Precautions

Seizure precautions vary from institution to institution and are performed to prevent injury to the patient if a seizure does occur. In most institutions, it is recommended that oxygen (O_2) and suction equipment with an airway be readily available in the patient's room. It is also appropriate to have intravenous (IV) access at all times for a patient with a history of seizures, which allows IV medication to be given if needed. The usefulness of padded side rails is debatable because side rails are rarely a source of significant injury for the patient with seizures. Because of the social stigma that is attached to seizures, the padded side rails can be a source of embarrassment for the patient and the family. However, side rails should always be left up to prevent a fall from the bed. The bed must be in the lowest position at all times in case the patient falls out of bed.

FIRST-LINE AND INITIAL TREATMENTS FOR SEIZURES

- Have O_2, suction equipment, and an airway ready for use if a patient is placed on seizure precautions.

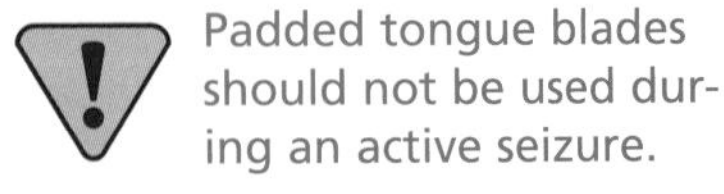

Padded tongue blades should not be used during an active seizure.

Padded tongue blades are rarely kept at the bedside, and they should not be inserted into the patient's mouth after the seizure begins. Because the jaw can clench down after the onset of a seizure, forcing a tongue blade or airway into the mouth is more likely to chip the teeth and cause aspiration of tooth fragments than it is to prevent the patient from biting the tongue. In addition, improper placement of a padded tongue blade can obstruct the airway.

In determining the best plan of care, nurses must note the type of seizure activity, whether the patient experienced an aura, and the events that surrounded the seizure. Current research shows health-related quality of life improves after epilepsy surgery, including seizure free and aura free time (Spencer et al., 2007). The following nursing interventions should be completed when a patient has a seizure:

- The patient should be protected from injury, and his or her movements should be guided if necessary.
- Objects that are in the patient's way should be removed to prevent injury.
- The patient should never be restrained.
- Any restrictive clothing worn by the patient should be loosened.
- A tongue blade or airway should not be forced into the patient's mouth.
- The patient should be turned onto his or her right side.
- The patient should be suctioned as needed to maintain the airway.

At the end of the seizure, the medical team should:

- Assess the patient's vital signs.
- Perform neurologic checks.
- Keep the patient on his or her right side.
- Allow the patient to rest.
- Document the seizure.

When documenting a seizure, the nurse should include the following;

- Onset: Was it sudden or preceded by an aura? (If an aura was present, describe it.)
- Duration: What time did the seizure start and end?
- Frequency and number: Did the patient have one or several seizures?
- State of consciousness: Was the patient unconscious? If so, for how long? Could he or she be aroused? (Any changes in consciousness should be noted.)
- Eyes and tongue: Did the pupils change in shape, size, equality, or in their reaction to light? Did they deviate to one side?
- Teeth: Were they opened or clenched?
- Motor activity: Where did the motor activity begin? What parts of the body were involved? Was there a pattern of progression of the activity? Describe the patient's movements.
- Body activities: Did the patient become incontinent of urine or stool? Did he or she have any oral bleeding, or vomit, or salivate?
- Respirations: What was the respiratory rate and quality? Was there any cyanosis?

- Drug response: If any drugs were given during the seizure, how did the patient respond? Did the seizures stop or worsen?
- Seizure awareness: Is the patient aware of what happened? Did he or she immediately go into a deep sleep after the seizure? Did he or she seem upset or ashamed? How long did it take for the patient to return to preseizure status?

The nursing interventions outlined in the section that follows should be performed if the patient develops status epilepticus.

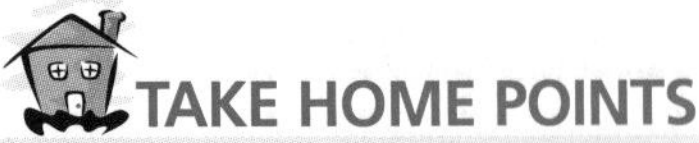

TAKE HOME POINTS

An airway is inserted into the patient's mouth wrong side up and then turned onto the correct side once it is in the middle of the mouth. This prevents the tongue from being pushed back and occluding the airway.

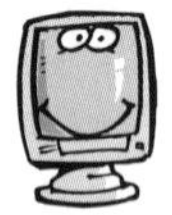

www.epilepsy.com
www.neurologychannel.com/seizures/index.shtml
www.epilepsyfoundation.org

What IS Status Epilepticus?

Status epilepticus is defined as (1) two or more consecutive seizures without the patient regaining consciousness between them or (2) continuous seizure activity that lasts 5 minutes or more. It is a potential complication of all seizure types. Principal concerns with convulsive status epilepticus are anoxia, arrhythmias, and acidosis. The usual causes of status epilepticus are as follows:

- Withdrawal from anticonvulsant medication
- Acute alcohol withdrawal
- CNS infections
- Metabolic disturbances
- Head injuries
- Brain tumors
- Cerebral edema
- Cerebrovascular disease

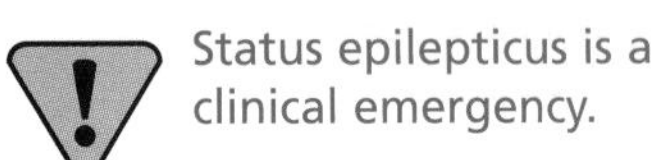

Status epilepticus is a clinical emergency.

What You DO

If status epilepticus occurs, the nurse must notify the physician immediately and support the airway, breathing, and circulation of the patient. Immediate interventions include providing O_2 via nasal cannula or facemask, preparing for intubation, protecting the patient from injury, establishing IV access, and begin infusing an IV of normal saline (NS). In addition, inserting a nasogastric (NG) tube and connecting it to gastric suction helps prevent the patient from vomiting and avoids possible aspiration. Cardiac rate and rhythm, along with continuous blood pressure (BP), should also be monitored.

FIRST-LINE AND INITIAL TREATMENTS FOR STATUS EPILEPTICUS

- Monitor ABCs (airway, breathing, circulation).
- Notify the physician.
- Establish IV access.
- Prevent injury.
- Monitor heart rate, ECG rhythm, and BP.
- Prepare to administer medications.

Medications should be administered as prescribed. Lorazepam (Ativan) may be prescribed at 4 mg IV over 2 to 5 minutes every 10 to 15 minutes if seizures persist. Onset of action of Lorazepam is approximately 15 minutes. Because this medication induces respiratory depression, the patient's vital signs must be monitored closely. Flumazenil (Romazicon) can be administered if the patient's respiratory status becomes compromised. Flumazenil is a benzodiazepine receptor antagonist that helps decrease the respiratory depression of the patient. It is administered IV to adults in doses as follows: 0.2 mg given over 30 seconds; wait 30 seconds, and then give 0.3 mg over 30 seconds; further doses of 0.5 mg can be given over 30 seconds at intervals of 1 minute up to a cumulative dose of 3 mg. Phenytoin (Dilantin) may also be prescribed, total dose of 15 to 18 mg/kg slow IV push (no more than 50 mg/min). The onset of action is 10 to 20 minutes; the duration of action is 24 hours.

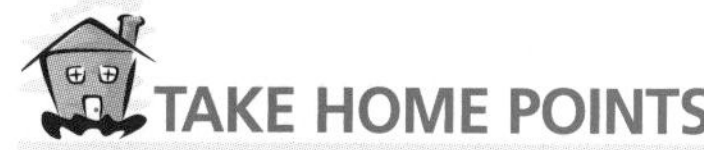

TAKE HOME POINTS

Phenytoin should be administered via a central venous line.

Phenytoin can infiltrate easily and is caustic to tissues. Current treatment of infiltrated tissue with phenytoin includes to elevate the extremity and apply dry heat then cool compresses. The use of topical nitroglycerine is also suggested to increase intravascular absorption and relieve vasospasms. Because of the possible infiltration and hemodynamic side effects (hypotension, bradycardia) of phenytoin, sometimes fosphenytoin is administered. Action of fosphenytoin is like that of phenytoin without the potentially detrimental side effects. Fosphenytoin is administered IV at 15 to 20 mg/kg or up to 150 mg/min. Phenobarbital (Luminal) can also be given IV at a dose of 5 to 8 mg/kg at 60 mg/min. The onset of action is 5 to 20 minutes; the duration of action is about 24 hours.

If seizure activity is not stopped with the previously mentioned medications, high-dose pentobarbital therapy can be used. Loading dose is 5 to 10 mg/kg over 1 hour and then 5 mg/kg per hour three times. Maintenance dose is 1 to 3 mg/kg per hour. Continuous EEG monitoring is required, along with monitoring serum levels (therapeutic level is 25 to 40 mg/dl).

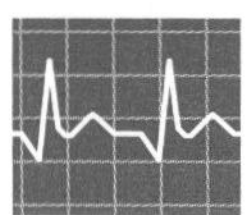

When administering phenytoin, one must assess for hypotension, bradycardia, or development of heart blocks.

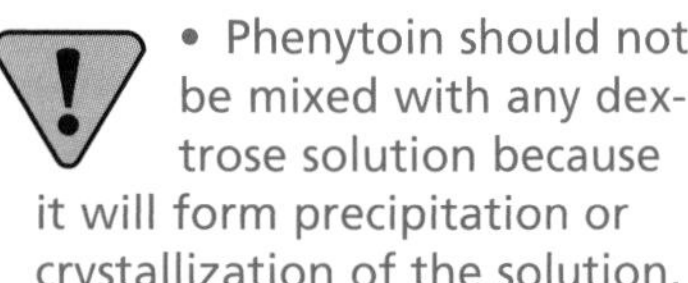

- Phenytoin should not be mixed with any dextrose solution because it will form precipitation or crystallization of the solution.
- Because of the adverse side effects of phenytoin, fosphenytoin is an alternative medication.

Respiratory depression, hypotension, and depression of consciousness may occur with phenobarbital; therefore, one must also monitor vital signs and neurologic status.

For status epilepticus, the nurse or other members of the medical team should do the following:

- Maintain the patient's airway. A nasal airway lubricated with water-soluble lubricant can be inserted while someone else is notifying the physician.
- Administer O_2 via nasal cannula or facemask; prepare for intubation.
- Turn the patient on his or her right side to allow for secretions to drain from the oral cavity.
- Suction the airway as needed.
- Start an IV of NS solution to keep the vein open. The IV insertion site should not be in the wrist or antecubital area, because the catheter could become dislodged.
- Remove any objects that can harm the patient.
- Connect the patient to a cardiac monitor, BP monitor, and O_2 saturation via telemetry pulse oximetry (SpO_2) monitor and automatic BP device.
- Administer medications as prescribed.
- Insert an NG tube and connect to suction.
- Plan for transfer to the intensive care unit (ICU), if not already there.
- Remember that patient education is vital for any patient diagnosed with a seizure disorder.

The Patient Should be Educated to do the Following:

DOs	DON'Ts
• Stay well hydrated. • Follow proper nutrition, and eat a balanced diet. • Learn to identify an aura and assume a safe position. • Tell the important people in his or her life, so they may react calmly and safely when a seizure occurs. • Take anticonvulsant medications as prescribed and on time; never miss a dose. • Wear a medical alert necklace or bracelet. • Contact the Epilepsy Foundation of America (www.epilepsyfoundation.org) or other organized epilepsy groups. • Join a seizure support group. • Investigate local and state laws covering driving as an epileptic.	• Ingest too much caffeine. • Use illegal drugs or alcohol. • Get excessively fatigued. • Tackle too many stressful activities at once. • Take any medications that the physician is unaware of, including over-the-counter and herbal medications.

Do You UNDERSTAND?

DIRECTIONS: **Choose the best answer for the question or statement.**

1. Mr. Dill has suffered a closed head injury secondary to a motor vehicle accident. He has begun to experience tonic-clonic (grand-mal) seizures. Which nursing action is **MOST** appropriate for Mr. Dill?
   1. Pad the bedside rails.
   2. Be sure someone is with Mr. Dill at all times.
   3. Place a padded tongue blade at Mr. Dill's bedside.
   4. Place oxygen and suction equipment in Mr. Dill's room.
2. You are at Mr. Dill's bedside when he has another grand-mal seizure. To avoid aspiration, you should immediately:
   1. Summon the physician.
   2. Turn him on his right side.
   3. Force a padded tongue blade between his teeth.
   4. Restrain him.
3. Following Mr. Dill's seizure, nursing interventions should include:
   1. Keeping him awake for several hours.
   2. Giving him phenytoin immediately.
   3. Offering him comfort and reassurance.
   4. Doing neurology checks every 5 minutes for 6 hours.
4. Tom is a young man who is being placed on long-term seizure treatment with phenytoin (Dilantin). The importance of regular medical follow-up is emphasized. Which instruction is critical to include in the teaching for this client?
   1. The drug should always be taken on an empty stomach.
   2. Constipation is a common side effect, so he should increase his intake of fiber and fluids.
   3. Good oral hygiene and gum massage should be incorporated into his daily routine.
   4. Hyperactivity and insomnia are common early effects, but these should gradually decrease with time.
5. Mrs. Smith is admitted with a diagnosis of partial occlusion of the left common carotid artery. She is an epileptic and has been taking

phenytoin for 10 years. In planning her care, it is most important that the nurse:
1. Place an airway, suction, and restraints at her bedside.
2. Ask her to remove her dental bridge and eyeglasses.
3. Observe her for evidence of increased restlessness and agitation.
4. Obtain a history of seizure incidence.

TAKE HOME POINTS

- Meningitis is an inflammation of the brain's membranes and involves the subarachnoid space and CSF.
- Meningococcal meningitis is the only type of bacterial meningitis that occurs in outbreaks.

What IS Meningitis?

Meningitis is an inflammation of the membranes covering the brain and spinal cord (arachnoid and pia mater). Viruses, bacteria, fungi, chemicals, trauma, or tumors are causes. The infective agent can be introduced by way of the sinuses or ear canal. Other possible causes of infection include a basilar skull fracture resulting in dural tears with cerebrospinal fluid (CSF) leak; otitis media or sinusitis; disruption at the blood-brain barrier through a penetrating head wound, gunshot wound, depressed skull fracture; ICP monitoring device; dental abscess or recent dental therapy; septicemia or septic emboli; ruptured cerebral abscess; or surgical procedure. The organism can then migrate throughout the CNS via the subarachnoid space, producing an inflammatory response in the arachnoid, pia mater, CSF, and ventricles. The exudates, which are formed during the inflammatory response, may spread to both the cranial and spinal nerves, thus causing further neurologic deterioration.

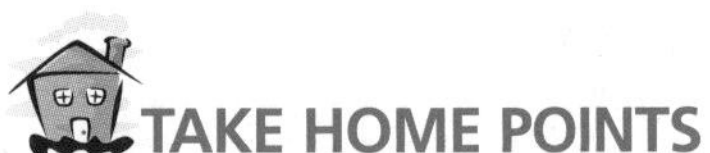

TAKE HOME POINTS

A vaccine is available to prevent some bacterial meningitis and is highly recommended for teenagers.

What You NEED TO KNOW

Bacterial Meningitis

In 80% to 90% of cases, bacterial meningitis is caused by streptococcal pneumonia, *Haemophilus influenzae,* or *Neisseria meningitidis.* Bacterial meningitis is seen most frequently in the fall and winter, when upper respiratory tract infections are more common.

Bacterial meningitis largely occurs in areas of high population density, such as refugee groups, college dormitories, military barracks, prisons,

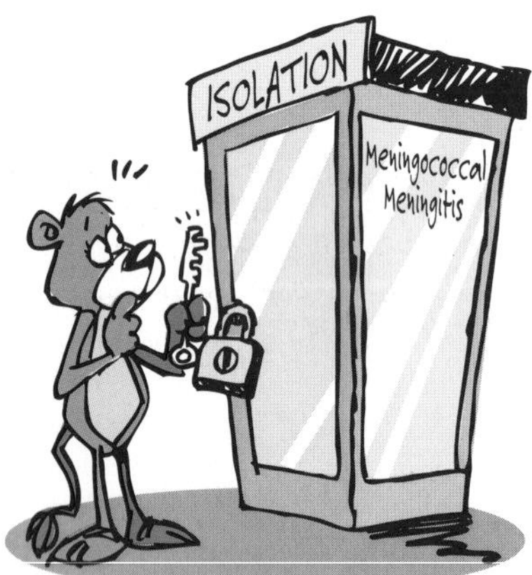

Treatment of meningococcal meningitis includes isolation.

Answers: 1. 4; 2. 2; 3. 3; 4. 3; 5. 4

and crowded living areas. Transmission occurs through direct contact with infectious respiratory secretions. More often the patient who develops bacterial meningitis has a predisposing condition, such as otitis media, pneumonia, acute sinusitis, or sickle cell anemia. A fractured skull or spinal or brain surgery may also contribute to the development of meningitis. Treatment is focused on antimicrobial therapy. Patients with meningococcal meningitis must be kept in isolation to prevent the spread of the disease. Ten percent to 15% of patients with meningococcal meningitis will die; of those who recover, as many as 10% will have long-term effects such as arthritis, myocarditis, and hearing loss.

Vulnerable populations include patients with infections elsewhere in the body, those who are immunosuppressed or have immunocompromised disorders, and older adults, especially those with chronic debilitating diseases.

Viral or Aseptic Meningitis

Viral or aseptic meningitis often occurs as a sequela to a variety of viral illnesses. For example, respiratory or gastrointestinal (GI) illnesses that are common with enteroviruses can cause viral meningitis. Enteroviruses, which include echoviruses and coxsackieviruses, account for most cases of viral meningitis in the United States. Other viral causes include measles, mumps, herpes simplex, and herpes zoster. Transmission of viral meningitis most often occurs through contact with respiratory secretions, but mode of transmission, communicability, and incubation times vary with the infecting virus.

Symptoms of viral meningitis are usually milder than those of bacterial meningitis, including headache, muscle aches and pains, and abdominal and chest pain, but most patients recover without permanent neurologic deficits.

TAKE HOME POINTS

- The causative virus is unidentified in approximately 50% of cases.
- Prevention of some types of viral meningitis is accomplished by vaccines for polio, varicella, and measles-mumps-rubella.

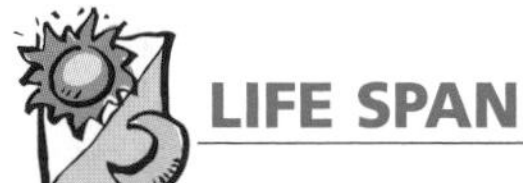

LIFE SPAN

The majority of patients with viral meningitis (70%) are younger than 5 years old.

Fungal Meningitis

Cryptococcus neoformans is the most common cause of fungal meningitis in patients with immune deficiency disorders (e.g., acquired immunodeficiency syndrome [AIDS]), reticuloendothelial system disorders (e.g., sarcoidosis), and those who are on corticosteroid therapy. Fulminant invasive fungal sinusitis is also a cause of fungal meningitis. Clinical manifestations vary among patients because of their compromised immune systems, which affects the inflammatory response. Some patients have a fever while others do not. Almost all patients have nausea, vomiting, headache, and a decline in mental status. Transmission is suspected to occur by inhalation. The fungus can be isolated from the bark and foliage of some eucalyptus trees, pigeon nests, and soil. The patients can have symptoms of kidney, lung, prostate, and bone infections. Untreated patients die within weeks to months.

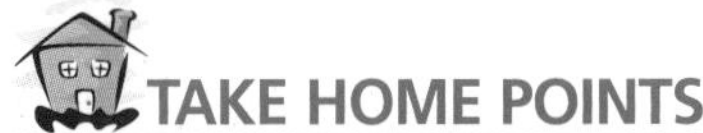

TAKE HOME POINTS

Fungal meningitis is not transmitted between people and can best be prevented by removal of accumulations of pigeon droppings from populated areas.

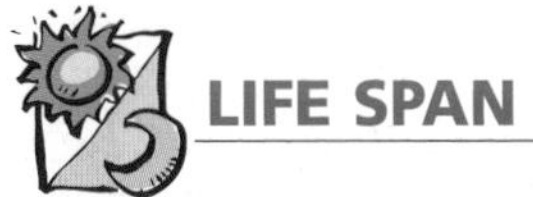

LIFE SPAN

Typically, *Haemophilus* meningitis is seen in patients 1 month old to 6 years of age.

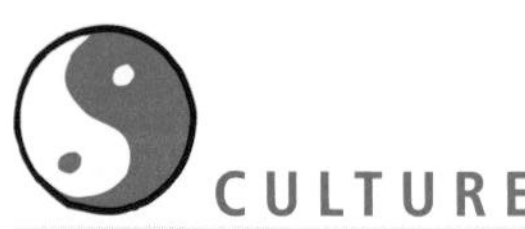

The incidence rate of *Haemophilus* meningitis is three times higher in Native Americans and Eskimos than in the general population.

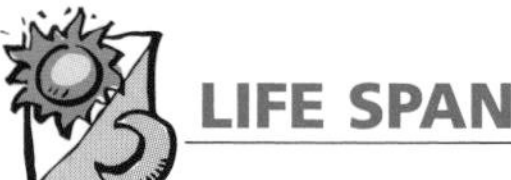

Pneumococcal meningitis is the most common meningitis in adults.

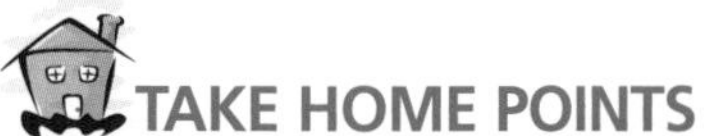

Pneumococcal meningitis is not transmitted from person to person.

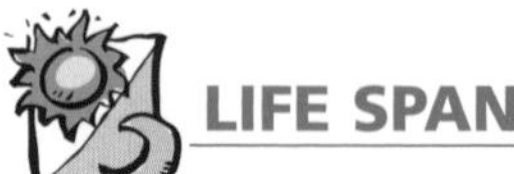

Neonatal meningitis is an infection that develops at 2 weeks to 2 months of life and could be related to birth or a nosocomial infection.

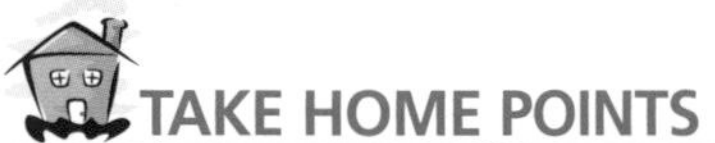

Syphilitic meningitis cannot be transmitted from person to person.

Haemophilus Meningitis

Haemophilus meningitis is caused by *Haemophilus influenzae.* Transmission occurs through droplets and contact with nasal and throat secretions during the communicable period of the disease (until the patient has 24 to 48 hours of effective antibiotic therapy). Infection can follow otitis media or an upper respiratory tract infection. Treatment is centered on antimicrobial therapy, but the use of corticosteroids can reduce the risk of hearing loss. The disease has a 5% mortality rate, even for those patients who are treated. Fifty percent of patients have neurologic defects, including learning disorders and abnormal speech and language development.

Pneumococcal Meningitis

Pneumococcal meningitis is caused by *Streptococcus pneumoniae.* Transmission and incubation are linked to the underlying disease or condition, which typically is otitis media, bacteremia, mastoiditis, pneumonia, infective endocarditis, or basilar skull fracture. The mortality rate for this type of meningitis is approximately 25%.

Neonatal Meningitis

Neonatal meningitis is often caused by group B streptococcus, as well as monocytogenes and *Escherichia coli.* Infants are thought to become infected when passing through the birth canal or nosocomially. Infections within the first week of life are usually due to transmission via the birth canal. Incubation of disease acquired nosocomially usually takes 2 weeks to 2 months. Neonatal meningitis is not usually transmitted through normal social contact between people. The mortality rate for this type of meningitis is high—50%.

Syphilitic Meningitis

Treponema pallidum causes syphilitic meningitis; the risk factor for developing this disease is having a previous infection with syphilis. It is a potential consequence of untreated secondary or early latent syphilis. Clinical manifestations include psychologic changes, altered vision or sensation, cerebrovascular accident, tremors, ataxia, or seizures.

Tuberculous Meningitis

Tuberculous meningitis is caused by *Mycobacterium tuberculosis;* the risk factor for developing this disease is a history of tuberculosis. Clinical manifestations include a loss of appetite and weight loss.

Regardless of the cause of meningitis, the signs and symptoms are usually similar. For adults, they are severe headache, fever, nausea, vomiting, nuchal rigidity, positive Kernig's sign (see p. 200), positive Brudzinski's sign (see p. 200), photophobia, seizures, mental status changes, skin rash, and petechiae or purpura. Neurologic abnormalities will reflect which cranial nerve (CN) is involved. Potential complications of meningitis include Waterhouse-Friderichsen syndrome (adrenal hemorrhage) with resulting hemorrhage and shock, encephalitis, hydrocephalus, cerebral edema, hearing or vision loss, brain damage, muscle paralysis, and disseminated intravascular coagulation (DIC).

TAKE HOME POINTS

Tuberculous meningitis results from the spread of tuberculosis infection from another site of the patient's body; it cannot be transmitted from person to person.

Diagnostic Tests

LP for a specimen of CSF is used to diagnose most cases of meningitis. The result will depend on the type of organism causing the meningitis. An LP is not usually done if increased ICP is suspected.

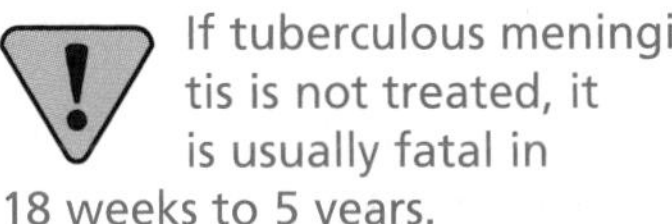

If tuberculous meningitis is not treated, it is usually fatal in 18 weeks to 5 years.

Cerebrospinal Fluid (CSF) Findings in Meningitis

CSF Finding	WBCs (cells/mm³)	Protein (mg/dl)	Glucose (mg/dl)	Differential Cell Count	Gram Stain	Culture
Viral meningitis	Increased (6-1000)	Elevated (40-150)	Normal (50-75)	Mostly lymphocytes	Negative	Viruses may be isolated
Meningococcal meningitis	Increased (>100)	Elevated	<40% of simultaneous blood glucose level	Mostly polymorphonuclear cells	Gram-negative diplococci	*Neisseria meningitidis*
Haemophilus meningitis	Increased (>100)	Elevated (50-1000)	<40% of simultaneous blood glucose level	Mostly polymorphonuclear cells	Gram-negative bacilli	*Haemophilus influenzae*
Pneumococcal meningitis	Increased (>100)	Elevated (50-1000)	<40% of simultaneous blood glucose level	Mostly polymorphonuclear cells	Gram-positive cocci	*Streptococcus pneumoniae*
Neonatal meningitis	Increased or decreased	Elevated (50-1000)	<40% of simultaneous blood glucose level	Mostly polymorphonuclear cells	Gram-negative bacilli	Usually group B streptococci, may be *Listeria monocytogenes* or *Escherichia coli*
Cryptococcal meningitis	Increased (10-500)	Elevated (50-1000)	<40% of simultaneous blood glucose level	Mostly lymphocytes	May resemble leukocytes	Negative
Tuberculosis meningitis	Increased (25-500)	Elevated (50-1000)	Normal (50-75)	Mostly lymphocytes	Negative	*Mycobacterium tuberculosis*

CSF, Cerebrospinal fluid.

Blood tests also help diagnose meningitis. A complete blood count (CBC) that reveals a white blood cell (WBC) count being elevated well above normal can indicate meningitis. Serum electrolytes may also be obtained with the focus on the sodium level.

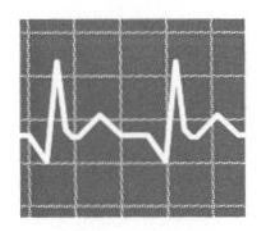

Petechiae or purpura is most common in meningococcal meningitis.

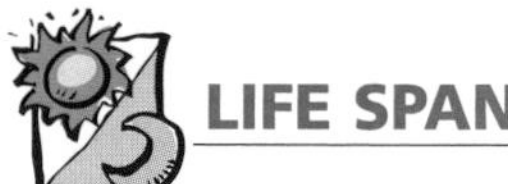

LIFE SPAN

Signs and symptoms of young children with meningitis include fever, behavioral changes, lethargy, refusal of feeding, vomiting, arching of the back or neck retraction, blank-stare facial expression, bulging fontanels, seizures, and pale or blotchy skin.

- Performing an LP on a patient with increased ICP could be detrimental and cause herniation of the brainstem as a result of the sudden release of ICP.
- Dilutional hyponatremia may be present due to syndrome of inappropriate antidiuretic hormone (SIADH), which is a common complication of bacterial meningitis.

CT scan may be normal in acute uncomplicated meningitis, but it may show hydrocephalus and diffuse enhancement in severe cases. Radiographic films of the air sinuses, mastoids, and chest determine the presence of infection or a basilar skull fracture. MRI may be prescribed to identify the presence of a brain abscess or increased ICP. An EEG may show generalized slow wave activity.

Medical Management

The physician prescribes antibiotics specific to the bacterial or fungal causative agent. Rifampin (Rifadin) is the medication of choice for household contacts; nursery, preschool, and school contacts; and health care providers who have been exposed to bacterial meningitis.

Empiric Therapy for Meningitis

Organism	Antibiotic/Agent
Virus	Acyclovir (Zovirax)
Neisseria meningititis	Penicillin Cephalosporins
Haemophilus influenzae	Ceftriaxone (Rocephin) Cefotaxime (Claforan)
Streptococcus pneumoniae	Penicillin Cefotaxime (Claforan) Ceftriaxone (Rocephin) Rifampin (Rifadin) Vancomycin (Vancocin)
Treponema pallidum (causing syphilitic meningitis)	Penicillin G Procaine penicillin plus probenecid
Fungus *(Cryptococcus neoformans)*	Amphotericin B with 5-fluorocytosine Fluconazole (Diflucan)
Mycobacterium tuberculosis	Four-drug therapy with isoniazid (INH), rifampin (Rifadin), ethambutol (Myambutol), and pyrazinamide (Tebrazid)
Staphylococcus	Vancomycin Ceftazidime (Fortaz)

FIRST-LINE AND INITIAL TREATMENTS FOR BACTERIAL MENINGITIS

- Rifampin (Rifadin) is prescribed for individuals exposed to someone with bacterial meningitis.

Treatment of viral or aseptic meningitis is mainly supportive, although acyclovir can be used to treat herpes virus and varicella-zoster virus, along with IV hydration.

FIRST-LINE AND INITIAL TREATMENTS FOR HAEMOPHILUS MENINGITIS

- Rifampin is prescribed for individuals exposed to someone with *Haemophilus* meningitis.

Treatment for pneumococcal meningitis is based on antimicrobial therapy, and prevention of this type of meningitis is achieved through vaccination with the pneumococcal vaccine to prevent pneumonia. Treatment for neonatal meningitis is also based on antimicrobial therapy, and prevention is aimed at screening pregnant women for group B streptococcus and then initiating group B streptococcus prophylaxis by administering antibiotics before delivery of the infant. If indicated, the mother should also be prepared for cesarean section.

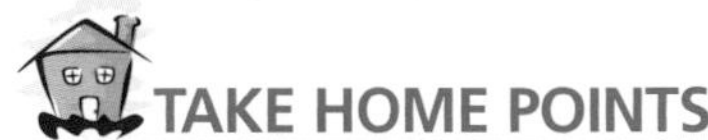

The incidence of pneumonia is not reduced by pneumococcal conjugate vaccine.

How to Prevent Meningitis

Vaccines are available against pneumonia, *Haemophilus influenzae* type b (Hib), pneumococcal meningitis, and other bacteria that can lead to meningococcal meningitis. The Centers for Disease Control and Prevention recommends that adolescents between 11 to 18 years of age receive the MCV4 vaccine against meningococcal meningitis. The MCV4 vaccine is also recommended for military recruits, first-year college students, anyone with a damaged spleen (or postsplenectomy), persons exposed to a meningitis outbreak, and anyone traveling to a country where meningitis is endemic (sub-Saharan and African countries from December to June). Meningococcal vaccines protect against most types of meningococcal disease, although they do not prevent all cases. There are two vaccines against *Neisseria meningitidis* available in the United States: meningococcal polysaccharide vaccine (MPSV4 or Menomune) and meningococcal conjugate vaccine (MCV4 or Menactra).

What You DO

To help decrease morbidity and mortality, it is vital that an accurate and immediate assessment be made of a patient with suspected meningitis. This can be accomplished by gathering a good nursing history. Subjective and objective findings may include the following:

- Headache that has grown progressively worse
- Nausea and vomiting

- Photophobia
- Neck or back pain upon flexion
- Seizures
- Irritability, confusion
- Medications, such as immunosuppressant drugs
- Presence of causative or precipitating factors: a highly suspect injury, procedure, or pathologic condition
- Social history, such as IV drug abuse

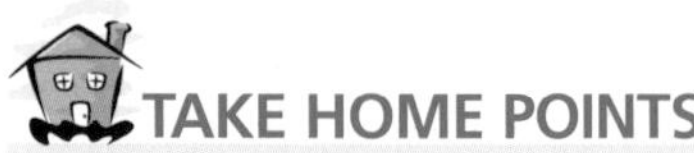

Kernig's reflex = flex patient's hip 90°, then extend the patient's knee. If this causes pain, it is a positive sign.
Brudzinski's reflex = flex patient's neck. If this causes flexion of the patient's hips and knees, it is a positive sign.

The nurse must then examine the patient for the following:

- Signs of infection: Chills, fever, tachycardia, skin rash, petechiae or purpura (most common in meningococcal meningitis)
- Meningeal irritation: Headache, nuchal rigidity, Brudzinski's reflex, Kernig's sign
- Neurologic abnormalities: Decreased level of consciousness (LOC), seizures, focal neurologic signs (hemiplegia, hemiparesis)

CN involvement:

- Optic (CN II): Papilledema may be present; blindness can occur
- Oculomotor, trochlear, abducens (CN III, CN IV, CN VI): Impairment of ocular movement, ptosis and unequal pupils, and diplopia commonly found
- Trigeminal (CN V): Photophobia
- Facial (CN VII): Facial paresis
- Acoustic (CN VIII): Tinnitus, vertigo, deafness
- Complications: Waterhouse-Friderichsen syndrome (adrenal hemorrhage) with resulting hemorrhage and shock (sometimes seen in fulminating meningococcal meningitis), DIC, hydrocephalus, cerebral edema, brain abscess, subdural effusions, encephalitis

The nurse must then examine the laboratory and radiologic findings of the patient:

- CSF: Results depend on type of organism
- Protein levels: Higher level in bacterial than in viral meningitis
- Glucose levels: Low glucose levels in most cases of bacterial meningitis; may be normal in viral meningitis
- Purulent and turbid in most cases of meningitis; may be clear with some viruses
- Cells: Mostly lymphocytes in viral form and polymorphonuclear leukocytes in bacterial form
- Cultures: Specimens from CSF, blood, drainage from sinuses or wounds to help identify the organism; nurse should make sure that

specimens are transported to laboratory expeditiously (prompt culturing necessary for certain organisms)

- EEG: May show generalized slow wave activity
- Electrolytes: Hyponatremia may be present
- Nasopharyngeal smear: Causative bacteria may be present
- Radiologic findings: CT scan may be normal in acute uncomplicated meningitis but show diffuse enhancement in some types or reveal hydrocephalus; skull radiographs may reveal infected sinuses or basilar skull fracture

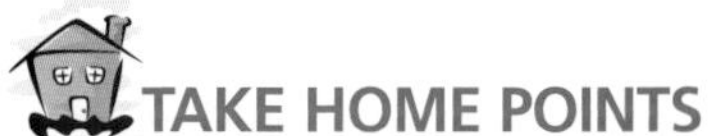

TAKE HOME POINTS

Collect naspharyngeal swab by using a Dacron swab (not cotton). Pass swab through nare until resistance is met. Remove after a few seconds as the patient usually coughs.

Nursing interventions are focused on the accurate monitoring and recording of the patient's neurologic status, vital signs, and vascular assessment. The nurse should do the following:

- Assess vital signs and perform gross neurologic examinations every 2 to 4 hours, or as prescribed.
- Assess cranial nerves with particular attention to CN II, III, IV, V, VI, VII, VIII.
- Provide interventions to treat or prevent increased ICP (see Increased Intracranial Pressure).
- Protect the patient from injury from potential seizures (see previous section on seizures).

Manage pain through nursing interventions, such as:

- Assess symptoms of pain and administer pain medications as prescribed.
- Monitor and record side effects and effectiveness of pain medications.
- Perform comfort measures to promote restfulness.
- Plan activities that provide distraction, such as allowing for radio, television, visitors, or reading as appropriate.
- Manipulate the environment to promote periods of uninterrupted rest, such as turning down lights (this would assist in decreasing irritability [photophobia]) and placing the patient in a comfortable position.

Manage hyperthermia by the following actions:

- Administer antibiotic therapy as prescribed and at the first suspicion of infection, even before CSF results are obtained from the cultures.
- Monitor temperature every 2 to 4 hours, or as prescribed.
- Administer antipyretic medications, such as acetaminophen (Tylenol).
- Use cooling measures as indicated (e.g., remove blankets; use a hypothermia blanket; use tepid water, alcohol sponges, ice bags under armpits, or a fan for ambient cooling).

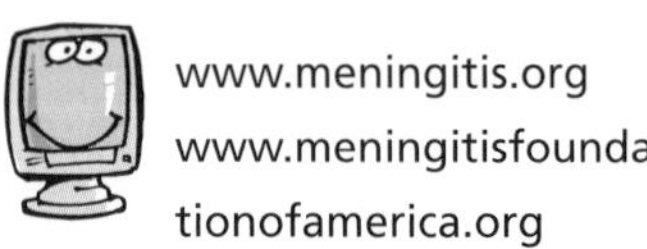

www.meningitis.org
www.meningitisfoundationofamerica.org
www.nmaus.org
www.ninds.nih.gov

- Monitor systemic response to infection or fever such as vital signs, respiratory rate, LOC.
- Perform vascular assessment and monitor for vascular changes that may be caused by septic emboli. The patient's temperature, color, pulses, and capillary refill of all extremities should be assessed.
- Maintain isolation precautions in accordance with the health care institution's policy.
- Make sure that those individuals exposed to the patient with bacterial meningitis are treated prophylactically with rifampin.

Do You UNDERSTAND?

DIRECTIONS: **Unscramble the letters in italics to form types of meningitis or meningitis management, treatment, or terminology.**

1. ______________________________
   (niifrmpa)
2. ______________________________
   (zbdiinkur'ss xfeelr)
3. ______________________________
   (bphhooopiat)
4. ______________________________
   (hnclau iiiygtdr)
5. ______________________________
   (vylccroia)

What IS Spinal Cord Injury?

Spinal cord injury occurs when a force is exerted on the vertebral column, resulting in damage to the spinal cord.

Injuries to the spinal cord are classified by the area and mechanism of injury. The area of injury refers to the level of the spine where the injury occurred (cervical, thoracic, lumbar, or sacral). The higher the spinal level, the greater the degree of injury. The mechanism of injury includes hyperflexion, hyperextension, axial loading and vertical compression,

Answers: 1. rifampin; 2. Brudzinski's reflex; 3. photophobia; 4. nuchal rigidity; 5. acyclovir or penetrating injury. The spinal cord may remain intact or undergo a destructive process.

Spinal Segments and Nerve Supply

Spinal Segments/Roots	Nerve Supply
Cervical	C4—diaphragm C5—deltoid and biceps C6—wrist extensors C7—triceps C8—hand
Thoracic	T2-T7—chest muscles T9-T12—abdominal muscles
Lumbar	L1-L5—leg muscles
Sacral	S2-S5—bladder, bowel, and sexual functioning

Mechanisms of Injury

Hyperflexion/Flexion Injury

Cervical flexion injury: Head is suddenly and forcefully accelerated forward

Lower thoracic/lumbar: Flexion injury when trunk is suddenly flexed on itself, as with a fall on the buttocks

- Posterior ligaments are stretched or torn
- Vertebrae may fracture or dislocate
- Causes hemorrhage, edema, necrosis

Hyperextension Injury

- Occurs most often with auto accidents (hit from behind) or falls where chin is struck
- Head is suddenly accelerated and then decelerated
- Anterior longitudinal ligaments are stretched or torn
- Vertebrae may fracture or subluxate
- Intervertebral disks may possibly rupture

Axial Loading/Vertical Compression Injury

- Most often caused by diving or fall from a ladder
- Vertebrae shatter with the blow
- Pieces of bone enter spinal canal and damage the spinal cord

Penetrating Injury

- Low velocity (knife): Causes damage directly at the site; localized damage to cord or spinal nerves
- High velocity (gunshot wound): Causes direct and indirect damage; spinal cord edema develops; necrosis of cord from compromised capillary circulation and venous return

The *anatomic level of injury* refers to damage of the upper and lower motor neurons. The upper motor neurons descend from the brain to the spinal cord and begin and end with the CNS. The lower motor neurons originate in the anterior horns of the spinal cord and end in the muscles and tissues. If damage to an upper motor neuron occurs above the level of decussation (crossing) at the medulla,

Spinal Cord Injury Functional Activity Chart

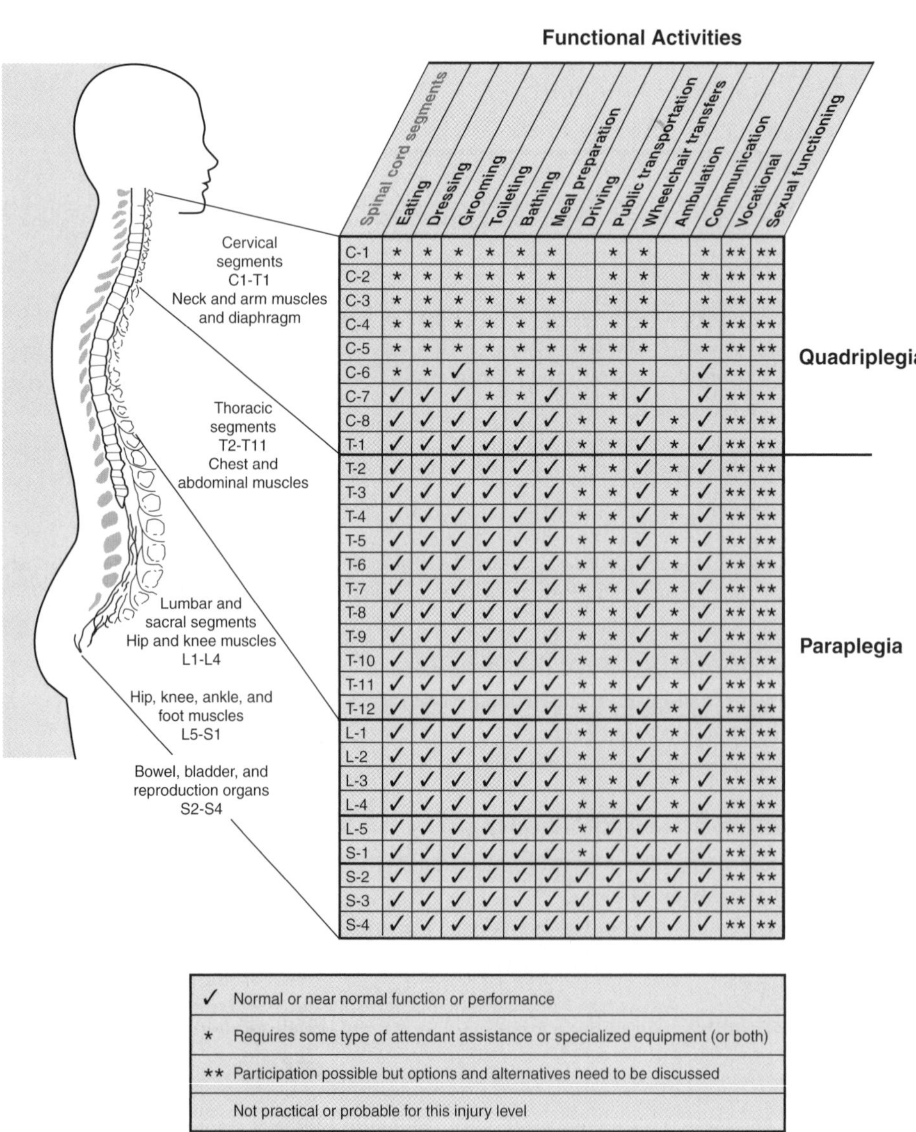

Spinal cord segments	Eating	Dressing	Grooming	Toileting	Bathing	Meal preparation	Driving	Public transportation	Wheelchair transfers	Ambulation	Communication	Vocational	Sexual functioning
C-1	*	*	*	*	*	*		*	*		*	**	**
C-2	*	*	*	*	*	*		*	*		*	**	**
C-3	*	*	*	*	*	*		*	*		*	**	**
C-4	*	*	*	*	*	*		*	*		*	**	**
C-5	*	*	*	*	*	*	*	*	*		*	**	**
C-6	*	*	✓	*	*	*	*	*	*		✓	**	**
C-7	✓	✓	✓	*	*	✓	*	*	✓		✓	**	**
C-8	✓	✓	✓	✓	✓	✓	*	*	✓	*	✓	**	**
T-1	✓	✓	✓	✓	✓	✓	*	*	✓	*	✓	**	**
T-2	✓	✓	✓	✓	✓	✓	*	*	✓	*	✓	**	**
T-3	✓	✓	✓	✓	✓	✓	*	*	✓	*	✓	**	**
T-4	✓	✓	✓	✓	✓	✓	*	*	✓	*	✓	**	**
T-5	✓	✓	✓	✓	✓	✓	*	*	✓	*	✓	**	**
T-6	✓	✓	✓	✓	✓	✓	*	*	✓	*	✓	**	**
T-7	✓	✓	✓	✓	✓	✓	*	*	✓	*	✓	**	**
T-8	✓	✓	✓	✓	✓	✓	*	*	✓	*	✓	**	**
T-9	✓	✓	✓	✓	✓	✓	*	*	✓	*	✓	**	**
T-10	✓	✓	✓	✓	✓	✓	*	*	✓	*	✓	**	**
T-11	✓	✓	✓	✓	✓	✓	*	*	✓	*	✓	**	**
T-12	✓	✓	✓	✓	✓	✓	*	*	✓	*	✓	**	**
L-1	✓	✓	✓	✓	✓	✓	*	*	✓	*	✓	**	**
L-2	✓	✓	✓	✓	✓	✓	*	*	✓	*	✓	**	**
L-3	✓	✓	✓	✓	✓	✓	*	*	✓	*	✓	**	**
L-4	✓	✓	✓	✓	✓	✓	*	*	✓	*	✓	**	**
L-5	✓	✓	✓	✓	✓	✓	*	✓	✓	*	✓	**	**
S-1	✓	✓	✓	✓	✓	✓	*	✓	✓	✓	✓	**	**
S-2	✓	✓	✓	✓	✓	✓	✓	✓	✓	✓	✓	**	**
S-3	✓	✓	✓	✓	✓	✓	✓	✓	✓	✓	✓	**	**
S-4	✓	✓	✓	✓	✓	✓	✓	✓	✓	✓	✓	**	**

Symbol	Meaning
✓	Normal or near normal function or performance
*	Requires some type of attendant assistance or specialized equipment (or both)
**	Participation possible but options and alternatives need to be discussed
	Not practical or probable for this injury level

(*From Phipps WJ, et al:* Medical-surgical nursing: health and illness perspectives, *ed 7, St Louis, 2003, Mosby.*)

ipsilateral (same side) dysfunction is seen; if damage occurs below the level of decussation for upper or lower motor neurons, contralateral (opposite side) dysfunction occurs.

The functional level of injury refers to the extent of disruption of normal spinal cord function; they are classified as *complete* or *incomplete* injuries. Complete injuries, where the cord is completely transected, occur infrequently. They usually result in total loss of motor, sensory, and reflex activity below the level of injury. Complete injuries can result in spinal or neurogenic shock, which lasts between 1 and 6 weeks, at which point 50% of patients regain some degree of spinal cord function. In incomplete lesions, a mixed pattern of motor, sensory, and reflex function is preserved. Five syndromes exist that are secondary to incomplete spinal cord lesions.

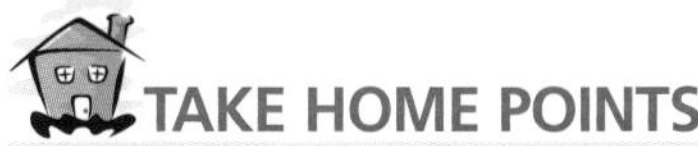

- The *anatomic area* refers to the level of the spine where the injury occurred.
- Same side dysfunction is called *ipsilateral.*
- Opposite side dysfunction is called *contralateral.*

Syndromes Secondary to Incomplete Spinal Cord Injuries

Incomplete Lesion	Associated with	Loss of Function	Intact Function
Anterior cord syndrome	Flexion and dislocation injuries of the cervical cord	Pain and temperature sensations and motor function Babinski reflex pathologically positive and spastic paralysis seen	Touch, proprioception, pressure, and vibration senses
Posterior cord syndrome	Hyperextension of the cervical spine	Proprioception and sensation of light touch	Pain and temperature sensations and motor function
Central cord syndrome	Hyperextension of the cervical spine and in older patients in whom degenerative changes of the vertebrae and disks allow central cord compression to occur	Upper extremity motor function with an accompanying but less significant loss of lower extremity motor function	Some patients do not experience loss of lower extremity motor function Sensory function, varying degrees remain intact
Brown-Séquard syndrome	Penetrating wounds, such as knife or bullet wounds, that cause hemisection of the cord; also seen in surfers who suffer traumatic injury caused by the surfboard hitting them in the neck	Ipsilateral (same side of the lesion) motor, proprioception, vibration, and deep touch Contralateral (opposite side of the lesion) pain, temperature, and light touch	Contralateral motor, proprioception, vibration, and deep touch Ipsilateral pain, temperature, and light touch
Cauda equina or conus medullaris	Damage to spinal nerve roots in the sacral area from trauma-induced fracture dislocation	Variable pattern of motor or sensory loss results in neurogenic bowel and bladder	Neurologic deficits specific to the nerve roots involved

TAKE HOME POINTS

- Total loss of all reflex activity occurs below the level of injury in complete spinal cord injuries.
- A mixed loss of reflex activity or a preservation of some reflexes is found with incomplete injury.

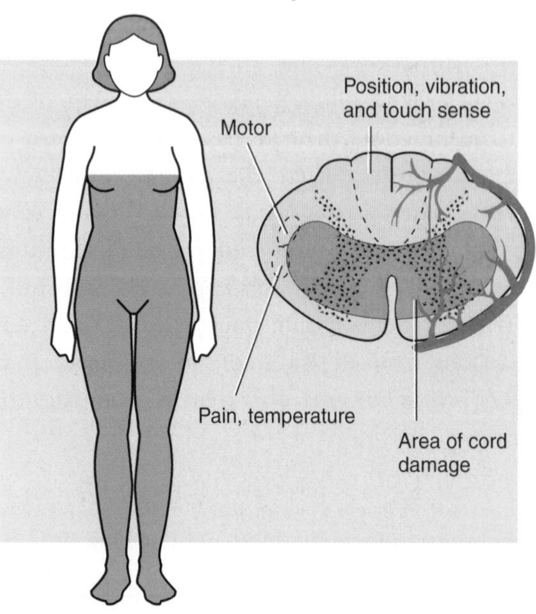

(From Ignatavicus DD, Workman ML: Medical-surgical nursing: critical thinking for collaborative care, *ed 4, Philadelphia, 2002, WB Saunders.)*

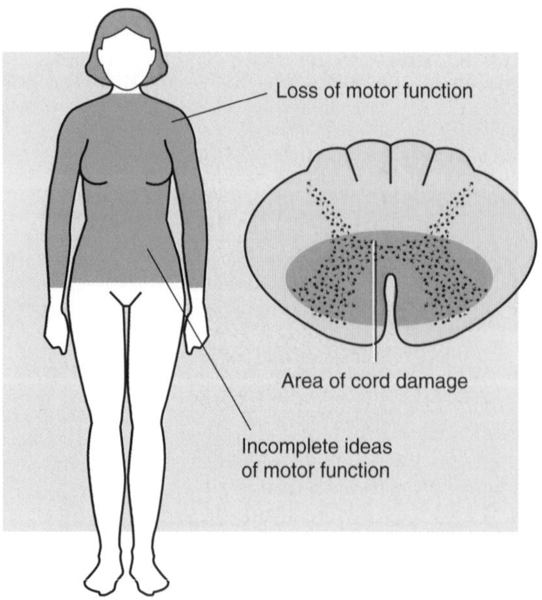

(From Ignatavicus DD, Workman ML: Medical-surgical nursing: critical thinking for collaborative care, *ed 4, Philadelphia, 2002, WB Saunders.)*

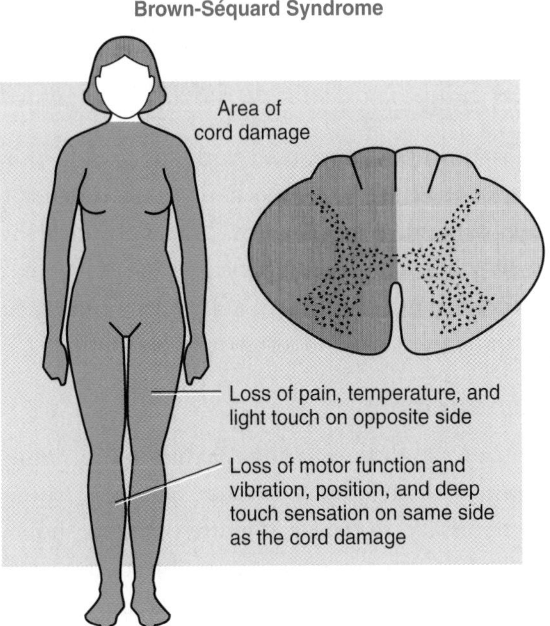

Brown-Séquard Syndrome

Area of
cord damage
Loss of pain, temperature, and
light touch on opposite side
Loss of motor function and
vibration, position, and deep
touch sensation on same side
as the cord damage

(From Ignatavicus DD, Workman ML: Medical-surgical nursing: critical thinking for collaborative care, *ed 4, Philadelphia, 2002, WB Saunders.)*

Conus Medullaris and Cauda Equina Syndromes

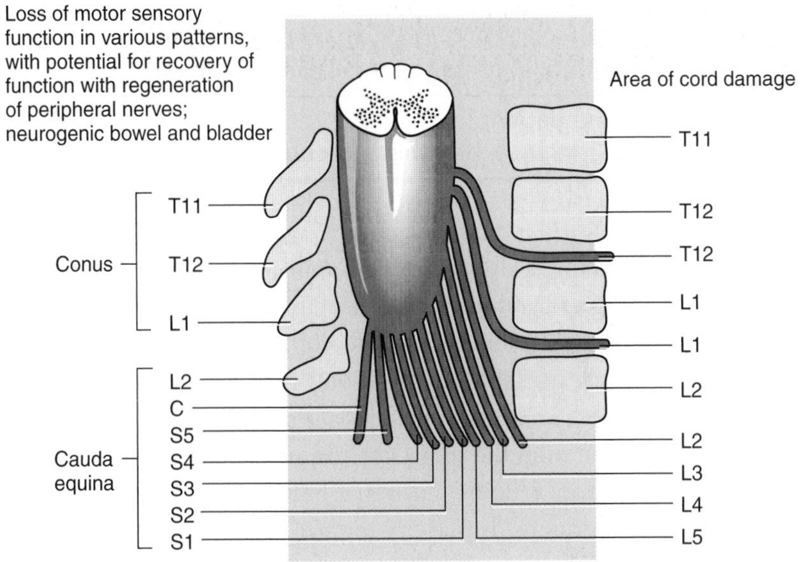

Loss of motor sensory
function in various patterns,
with potential for recovery of
function with regeneration
of peripheral nerves;
neurogenic bowel and bladder
Area of cord damage
T11
T12
T12
L1
L1
L2
L2
L3
L4
L5
Conus
T11
T12
L1
Cauda
equina
L2
C
S5
S4
S3
S2
S1

(From Ignatavicus DD, Workman ML: Medical-surgical nursing: critical thinking for collaborative care, *ed 4, Philadelphia, 2002, WB Saunders.)*

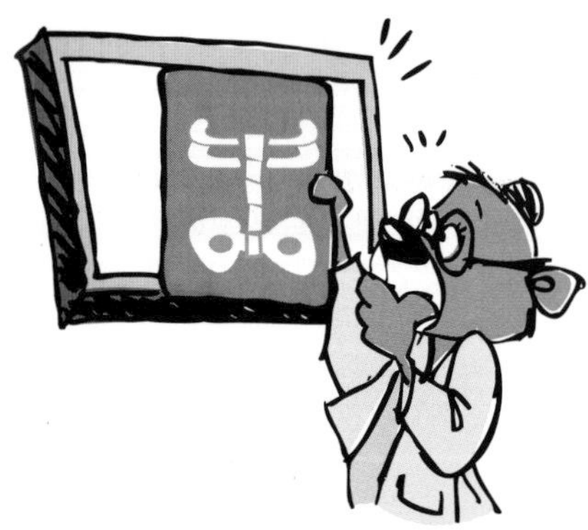
Spinal x-ray is one diagnostic test performed in patients with spinal cord injuries.

What You NEED TO KNOW

Diagnostic Tests

A variety of diagnostic tests are used with spinal cord injuries. Spinal radiographs assess for fractures, dislocations, and degenerative changes of the vertebral column. A CT scan may demonstrate bony pathology, myelography may show cord compression, and MRI may show soft tissue injury. In addition, in patients with gunshot or stab wounds, an angiography can be prescribed to assess vascular injuries.

Medical Management

Immobilization or stabilization of the spinal injury is the priority of initial care along with treatment of acute symptoms. Emergency surgery may be necessary to repair fractures, remove bone fragments, evacuate hematomas, remove penetrating objects (bullet), or decrease pressure on the spinal cord. For cervical spine injuries, Gardner-Wells tongs or a halo fixation device with jacket can be applied to the patient's head to help immobilize the cervical-spinal column. Spinal fusion with bone plugs or wires and rods may be required to stabilize spinal injuries.

FIRST-LINE AND INITIAL TREATMENTS FOR SPINAL CORD INJURY

- Immobilize the patient.
- Monitor ABCs (airway, breathing, circulation).

Medication therapy is also used after a spinal cord injury. Atropine is used to treat bradycardia; dopamine (Intropin) is used to treat hypotension; and methylprednisolone (Solu-Medrol), a steroid, is given as a bolus dose of 30 mg per kg over 15 minutes followed by 5.4 mg per kg per hour for the next 23 hours if diagnosis is made in less than 3 hours; if the period of time from the spinal cord injury to treatment is between 3 hours and less than 8 hours, an initial bolus of methylprednisolone is given and a continuous drip at 5.4 mg per kg per hour is given over 48 hours (2 days). This is used to decrease cord swelling, inflammation, glutamate release, and free-radical accumulation, thereby limiting spinal cord injury.

FIRST-LINE AND INITIAL TREATMENTS FOR SPINAL CORD INJURY

- Methylprednisolone may be started within hours after the injury in an attempt to decrease the edema associated with the destructive process that occurs in a spinal cord injury.

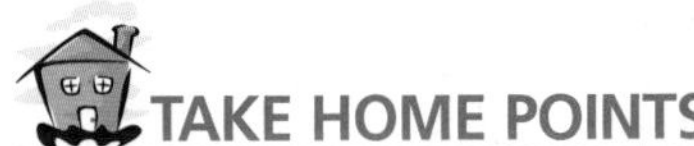

Stabilization of the spinal cord is important to preserve any possible function.

Crystalloid and colloid fluid replacement is used to maintain normal BP, along with vasopressors. Plasma expanders such as dextran increase capillary blood flow within the spinal cord.

Hyperbaric oxygenation is used in some facilities after 12 to 24 hours of injury. It supplies 100% O_2 in a pressurized chamber, which allows the blood to carry more O_2 and is thought to improve O_2 perfusion to the spinal cord, thus decreasing ischemic injury.

Autonomic Dysreflexia

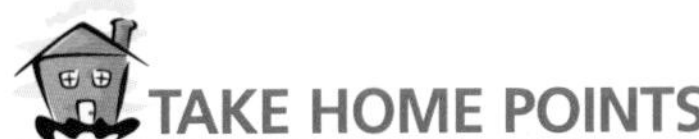

Autonomic dysreflexia is a clinical emergency that can happen at any time after injury.

Damage to the spinal cord at T6 or above can lead to autonomic dysreflexia, an emergency clinical condition that can occur after the period of spinal shock is completed. It results in uninhibited sympathetic discharge to a noxious stimulus below the level of the spinal cord injury. The spinal cord injury prevents the message from reaching the brain, so the response of the sympathetic nervous system (SNS) is unopposed, resulting in life-threatening hypertension. Symptoms of this sympathetic discharge include diaphoresis and flushing above the level of injury, with chills and severe vasoconstriction below the level of injury. The dramatic increase in BP produces a pounding headache. Other signs and symptoms include nasal congestion, nausea, bradycardia, and unusually frequent spasms of the lower extremities or abdomen.

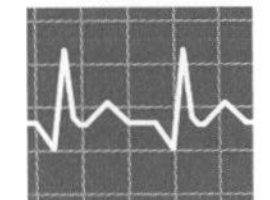

Patients with autonomic dysreflexia have severe, life-threatening hypertension.

The noxious stimulus that most frequently triggers this response is a distended bladder or bowel. Other triggers are a hot or cold stimulus (sitting in a drafty hall), skin pressure (e.g., tight clothing or staying in one position too long), pressure ulcers, ingrown toenail, or bowel and bladder stimulation during bowel and bladder training regimens. Autonomic dysreflexia usually occurs suddenly.

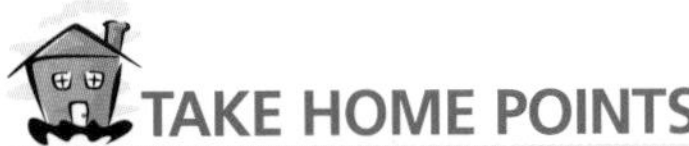

A noxious stimulus is the triggering event for autonomic dysreflexia.

Physicians treat autonomic dysreflexia by removing the noxious stimulus and administering antihypertensive medications to avoid a stroke from the hypertension. If the noxious stimulus is relieved immediately, the dysreflexia may resolve on its own. If the physician is unable

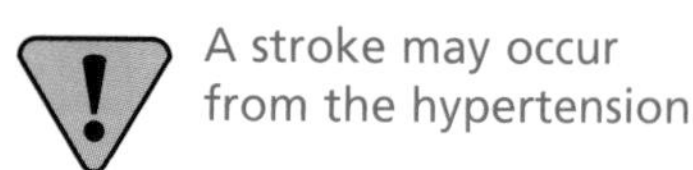

A stroke may occur from the hypertension.

to relieve the noxious stimulus, he or she may order topical 2% nitroglycerine ointment. Caution should be taken if the patient has taken sildenafil citrate (Viagra) or similar medications in the past 24 hours; combining these drugs with a nitrate could cause dangerous hypotension. Additionally, oral immediate-release nifedipine or IV hydralazine hydrochloride is given to reduce the BP.

FIRST-LINE AND INITIAL TREATMENTS FOR AUTONOMIC DYSREFLEXIA

- Remove the noxious stimulus (e.g., urinary catheterization, manual rectal decompaction).
- Administer antihypertensive medications.

What You DO

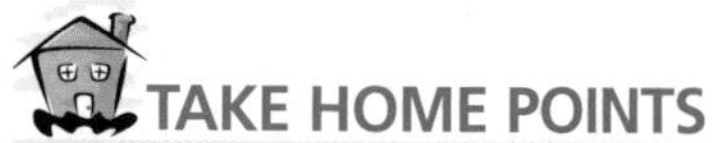

TAKE HOME POINTS

Pin infections may be decreased with the use of chlorhexidine gluconate-impregnated polyurethane dressings (Wu et al., 2008).

If the patient's spinal cord has been immobilized by Gardner-Wells tongs (see the figure on the next page), which consist of two tongs inserted in the outer aspect of the skull with traction added, nursing care is focused on the traction of this device and on infection control. To accomplish this, the nurse should do the following:

- Ensure that the prescribed weights are on the device and are hanging freely at all times.
- Make sure the patient is in proper alignment and that the ropes remain in the pulley device.
- Assess neurologic signs at least every 4 hours or more frequently as prescribed.
- Inspect pins for signs and symptoms of infection, and administer pin care with ½ hydrogen peroxide and ½ NS solution every shift (or as the hospital policy and procedure manual dictates).

If the patient is in a halo fixation device with jacket, four pins are inserted into the skull with the fixation device and then the jacket is applied, which stabilizes the halo from the chest. To maintain cervical stability and patient safety, the nurse must do the following:

- Assess the skin and jacket to make sure no pressure areas are present. One should be able to insert one finger easily under the jacket.

- Assess pins for a secure tight fit, administer pin care, assess for signs and symptoms of pin infection, and perform neurologic assessment as previously discussed.
- Ensure that a "key" or Allen wrench is taped to the outer chest of the jacket for easy removal in the event of a cardiac arrest.

The nurse should remember that immobilization places the patient at increased risk for hypoventilation, pneumonia, and pulmonary embolism. To avoid these complications the nurse should:

- Perform respiratory assessment and breath sounds assessment every 2 hours or as prescribed.
- Suction as necessary to keep airway clear using aseptic technique.
- Provide chest physical therapy per unit protocol.
- Monitor sputum cultures, PT, PTT, INR.
- Ensure adequate hydration to help liquefy secretions.
- Apply antiembolic stockings, sequential/pneumatic compression devices, or both.
- Get the patient out of bed three to four times a day when the spinal cord is stabilized.
- Encourage deep breathing and use of incentive spirometry every hour while the patient is awake (coughing may increase spinal cord pressure).
- Measure vital capacity and tidal volumes, and monitor pulse oximetry and arterial blood gases.

If the patient had a surgical intervention to immobilize a portion of the spinal cord with bone plugs or wires and rods, the nurse should initiate the following postoperative measures:

- Empty Jackson Pratt (JP) drains and record drainage at least every shift.
- Assess neurologic signs (motor and sensory) based on the level of the spinal cord injury to detect changes from baseline values.
- Change spinal cord dressing as prescribed, usually after a few days it is left open to air.
- Prevent further damage by immobilizing the area, using special beds and equipment.
- Logroll the patient from side to side, and use additional help as needed.
- Assess for hypotension, bradycardia, and vasovagal reflex, which may result in cardiac arrest; be prepared to institute advanced cardiovascular life support (ACLS).

Gardner-Wells tongs

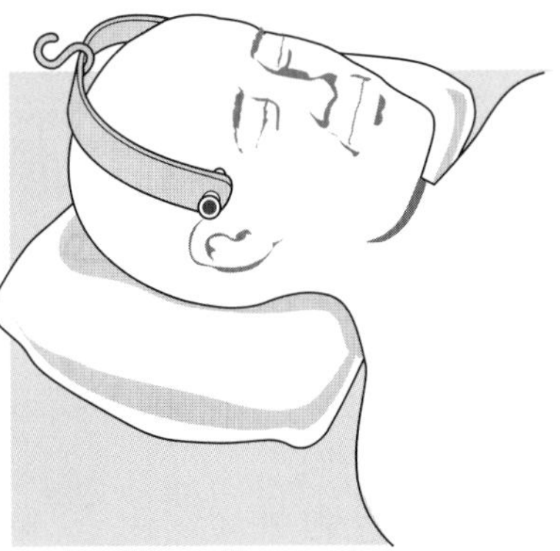

Halo Fixation Device with Jacket

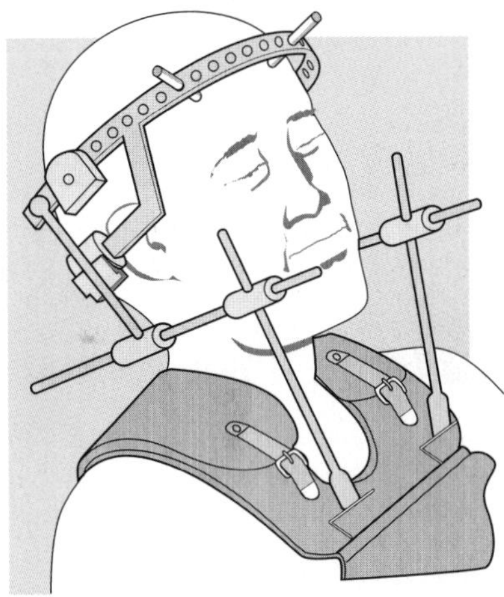

- Hyperoxygenate before and after suctioning to prevent hypoxia and vasovagal reactions.
- Avoid placing peripheral IV lines in paralytic limbs.
- Prevent deep vein thrombosis (DVT) and skin breakdown with proper positioning, frequent turning, therapeutic range-of-motion exercises, antiembolism stockings, and prophylactic anticoagulant therapy as prescribed.
- Apply splints or high-top tennis shoes to feet on a 2-hours-on and 2-hours-off schedule to maintain normal alignment and prevent foot drop.

Fluid volume deficit may result from hemorrhage, gastric dilation (vomiting), or gastric ulceration. Urine retention may occur due to anatomic bladder or areflexia and can result in urinary tract infections (UTIs), stone formation, or renal deterioration. The nurse needs to consider the following interventions when addressing these issues:

- Administer histamine-2 antagonists, antacids, gastric lavage, and fluids as prescribed.
- Inspect the abdomen for distention.
- Place indwelling urinary catheters during hemodynamic instability.
- Monitor urine cultures as necessary.
- Initiate intermittent catheterization or self-catheterization programs when the patient's condition stabilizes.
- Begin patient teaching regarding self-catheterization as soon as feasible.
- Provide supportive care and treatment of complications resulting from the injury, such as arrhythmias, especially tachycardia and bradycardia, which are common in patients with spinal cord injuries. Respiratory disturbances are also common and associated with the level of injury. High cervical neck injuries result in respiratory nerve paralysis; therefore, the patient is ventilator dependent.

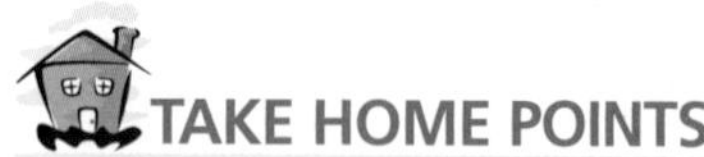

Women who experience a spinal cord injury should be taught that they can conceive and deliver, and that they should consider a method of birth control that does not increase the risk of clot formation, such as a diaphragm, foam, or condom.

For patients with T6 or above lesions who are susceptible to autonomic dysreflexia, one must be aware of the algorithm (www.pva.org) to follow:

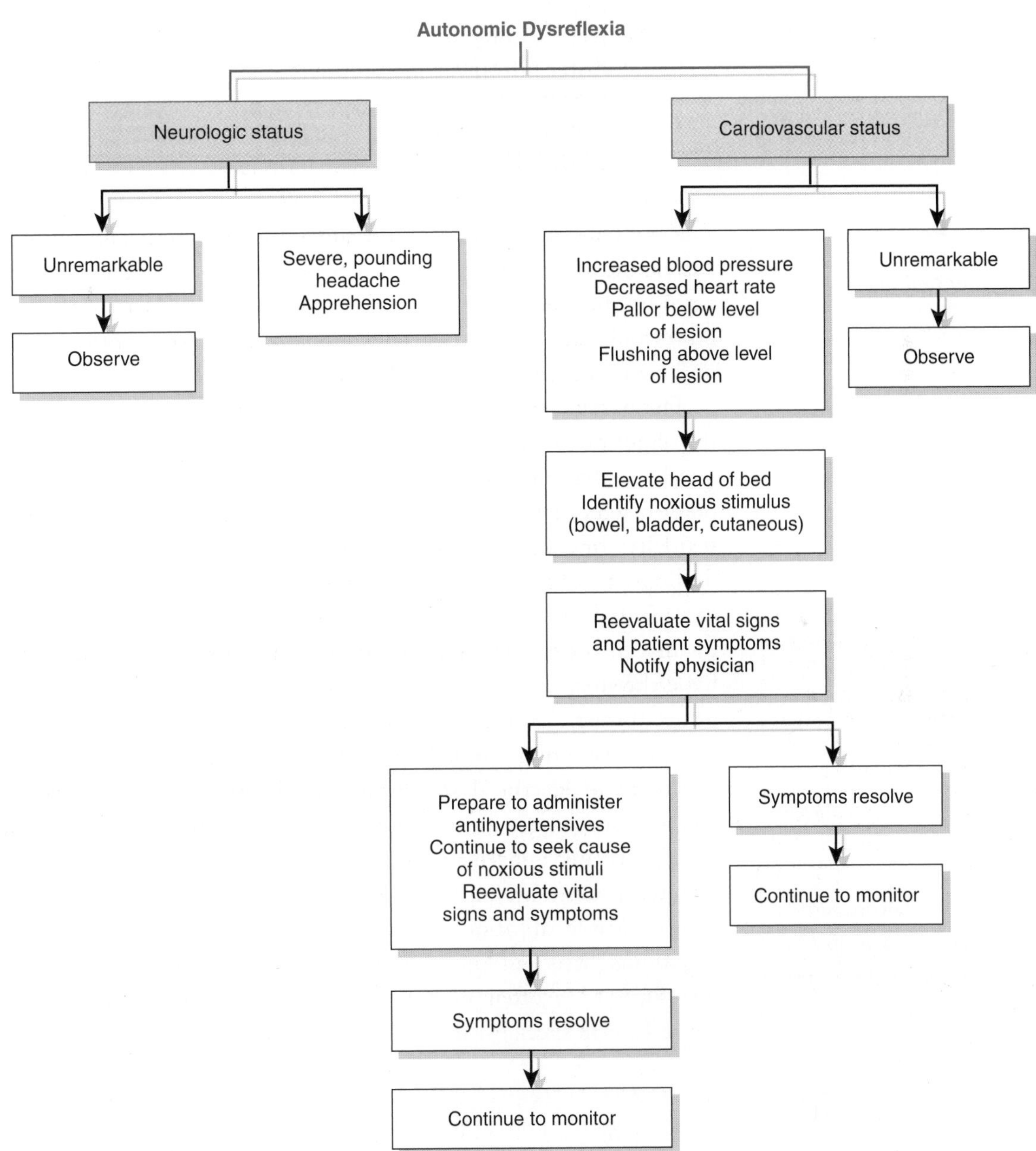

FIRST-LINE AND INITIAL TREATMENTS FOR AUTONOMIC DYSREFLEXIA

- Identify and remove noxious stimulus.
- Elevate HOB.
- Administer antihypertensives.
- Administer nitroglycerine ointment.
- Administer nifedipine.
- Administer hydralazine IV.

Intrauterine devices (IUDs) are not recommended because of decreased sensation in the pelvis of spinal cord–injured women.

Patient and family education regarding how to prevent an episode of autonomic dysreflexia is essential. The patient and family should be educated on the elimination of drafts, good skin and nail care, and regular bowel and bladder regimens. They should also be given written material on how to identify and remove noxious stimuli.

The patient and family members will need assistance coping with the emotional repercussions of these devastating injuries. Patient issues involve impaired adjustment related to depression, change in body image, or role performance. Disrupted self-concept, related to sexuality issues and feeling of powerlessness, are also common patient findings. Fertility is an especially important component of postinjury care. In men, erectile and ejaculatory dysfunction is present. Semen quality and motility is reduced secondary to recurrent UTIs, scrotal hyperthermia, drugs, prostatic fluid stasis, spermatozoan contact with urine through retrograde ejaculation, testicular denervation, and changes in seminal fluid. It should be explained to the patient that treatment of erectile dysfunction includes mechanical interventions and pharmacologic interventions, and that ejaculatory dysfunction can be treated pharmacologically. Assisted reproductive methods include intrauterine insemination, intracytoplasmic sperm injection, and in-vitro fertilization. Family coping may be ineffective, given the situational crisis and long-term burden of care. Professional consultative support is often needed from a psychologist, psychiatrist, or clinical nurse specialist in psychiatric mental health.

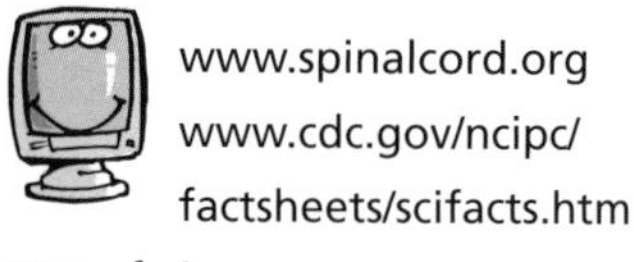
www.spinalcord.org
www.cdc.gov/ncipc/factsheets/scifacts.htm
www.fscip.org

Do You UNDERSTAND?

DIRECTIONS: Select the BEST answer to the question or complete the statement.

1. Jack, a 20-year-old college student, suffered a complete C3 transverse cord injury following an automobile accident involving a drunk driver. Which nursing diagnosis is the highest priority for Jack?
   1. Potential for impaired skin integrity due to paralysis
   2. Alteration in urinary elimination due to paralysis and immobility
   3. Impaired physical mobility due to paralysis
   4. Ineffective airway clearance due to high cervical spinal cord injury
2. Jack experiences autonomic dysreflexia 1 week after his injury. All of the following nursing interventions are appropriate **EXCEPT**:
   1. Checking for the source of irritation.
   2. Relieving his urinary obstruction.
   3. Placing him in a supine position.
   4. Monitoring his blood pressure.
3. Mr. Smith has fallen from a ladder and experienced an axial loading injury to L4-5. After surgery to remove the fragments of bone, which of the following assessments is vital to include in his nursing care?
   1. Assess cranial nerves II, III, IV, and VI, and assess dressing.
   2. Assess arm strength and arm sensation; assess dressing.
   3. Assess pupils and check for bladder distention; assess dressing.
   4. Assess leg strength, motion, position sense and sensation, and dressing.
4. Sam Jones is admitted to the hospital after falling off his motorcycle. A fracture in the cervical area of the spine is suspected. What is the first priority of nursing care?
   1. Immobilize his cervical spine.
   2. Perform neurologic examinations every 10 minutes.
   3. Restrict movement of his extremities.
   4. Keep him on a nothing-by-mouth regimen.
5. Your patient has had a C4 spinal cord injury and is suffering from autonomic dysreflexia. Which of the following would not be a symptom of dysreflexia?
   1. Severe headache
   2. Tachycardia
   3. Profuse sweating
   4. Rapidly increasing blood pressure

Answers: 1. 4; 2. 3; 3. 4; 4. 1; 5. 2

References

Alspach JG, ed: *Core curriculum for critical care nursing,* ed 6, St Louis, 2006, Elsevier.

Abrahm JL, Banffy MB, Harris MB: Spinal cord compression in patients with advanced metastatic cancer, *The Journal of the American Medical Association,* 299(8):937-946, 2008.

Burnet S, Huntley A, Kemp KM: Meningitis the inflamed brain, *Nursing2007 Critical Care,* 2(4):28-36, 2007.

Carlson KK, ed: *AACN advanced critical care nursing,* St Louis, 2009, Elsevier.

Centers for Disease Control and Prevention. *Vaccines and preventable diseases: meningococcal vaccination.* Retrieved May 22, 2008, from www.cdc.gov/vaccines/vpd-vac/mening/default.htm#vacc.

Fagley MU: Taking charge of seizure activity, *Nursing* 2007*,* 37(9):42-47, 2007.

Hickey JV: *The clinical practice of neurological and neurosurgical nursing,* ed 5, Philadelphia, 2003, Lippincott Williams & Wilkins.

Kaplow R, Hardin SR: *Critical care nursing: synergy for optimal outcomes,* Sudbury, MA, 2007, Jones and Bartlett Publishers.

Lowey SE: Spinal cord compression: an oncologic emergency associated with metastatic cancer: evaluation and management for the home health clinician, *Home Healthcare Nurse,* 24(7):439-446, 2006.

Marini JJ, Wheeler AP: *Critical care medicine: the essentials,* ed 3, Philadelphia, 2006, Lippincott Williams & Wilkins.

Marino PL: *The ICU book,* ed 3, Philadelphia, 2007, Lippincott Williams & Wilkins.

Matthews C, Miller L, Mott M: Getting ahead of acute meningitis & encephalitis, *Nursing 2007,* 37(11):36-41, 2007.

Newberry L: *Sheehy's emergency nursing: principles and practice,* ed 5, St Louis, 2003, Mosby.

Spencer SS, Berg AT, Vickrey BG, Sperling MR, Bazil CW, Haut S et al.: Health-related quality of life over time since resective epilepsy surgery, *Annals of Neurology,* 62(4):327-334, 2007.

Urden LD, Stacy KM, Lough ME: *Thelan's critical care nursing: diagnosis and management,* ed 5, St Louis, 2006, Elsevier.

Vacca VM: Action stat: acute paraplegia, *Nursing,* 2007, 37(6):64, 2007.

Vacca VM: Action stat: autonomic dysreflexia, *Nursing2007,* 37(9):72, 2007.

Vacca VM: Action stat: status epilepticus, *Nursing,* 2007 37(4):80, 2007.

Wiegand DJL, Carlson KK, eds: *AACN procedure manual for critical care,* ed 5, St Louis, 2005, Elsevier.

Wu SC, Crews RT, Zelen C, Wrobel JS, Armstrong DG: Use of chlorhexidine-impregnated patch at pin site to reduce local morbidity: the ChIPPS Pilot Trial, *International Wound Journal,* 5(4):416-422, 2008.

NCLEX® Review

1. A 49-year-old man is brought to the unit with a diagnosis of status epilepticus. He is having generalized tonic-clonic seizures every 5 minutes. Each seizure lasts 30 to 90 seconds. He is receiving a total of 50 mg diazepam before arriving at the ICU. In accordance with accepted safety precautions, which medication should you ensure is available at the patient's bedside?
   1 Flumazenil (Mazicon).
   2 Phenobarbital.
   3 Naloxone (Narcan).
   4 Phenytoin (Dilantin).
2. Ms. Coletta has suffered a closed head injury secondary to a motor vehicle accident. She has begun to experience tonic-clonic (grand-mal) seizures. Which nursing action is *most* appropriate?
   1 Pad the bedside rails.
   2 Ensure that someone is with the patient at all times.
   3 Place a padded tongue blade at the patient's bedside.
   4 Place oxygen and suction equipment in the patient's room.
3. If you come upon a patient having a seizure, you should:
   1 Protect his or her head from injury and turn him or her to the right side if possible.
   2 Place an object between the teeth, and move the patient to an upright position.
   3 Restrain the patient to prevent injury.
   4 Move the patient to the floor and hold the patient down.
4. Which intervention would be most effective in minimizing the risk of seizure activity in a patient with tonic-clonic seizures?
   1 Maintain the patient on bedrest.
   2 Close the door to the room to minimize stimulation.
   3 Administer sedatives as prescribed.
   4 Administer anticonvulsant medications on schedule.
5. Which assessment finding would the nurse expect in the patient after a tonic-clonic (grand-mal) seizure?
   1 Drowsiness.
   2 Inability to move.
   3 Hypotensive.
   4 Memory recall.
6. Tom is a young man who is being placed on long-term seizure treatment with phenytoin (Dilantin). The importance of regular medical follow-up is emphasized. Which instruction is critical to include in the teaching for this patient?
   1 The drug should always be taken on an empty stomach.
   2 Diarrhea is a common side effect, so he should increase his intake of fiber and fluids.
   3 Good oral hygiene and gum massage should be incorporated into his daily routine.
   4 Hyperactivity and insomnia are common early effects, but these should gradually decrease with time.
7. A high temperature often accompanies meningitis. A nursing intervention most helpful in relieving febrile delirium is to:
   1 Apply a warm water bottle to the posterior neck.
   2 Restrain the patient to prevent self-injury.
   3 Apply cool compresses or an ice bag to the forehead.
   4 Increase fluid intake to prevent dehydration.

8. With a diagnosis of acute bacterial meningitis, it is likely that the laboratory data of the CSF will reveal:
   1 Glucose 70 mg/dL.
   2 Protein 450 mg/dL.
   3 White blood cells (WBCs) 4 cells/mm.^{3}
   4 Specific gravity 1.007.

9. When caring for a person with meningitis, the critical care nurse should be alert for the development of which complication?
   1 Cerebral dehydration.
   2 Deafness.
   3 Hypothermia.
   4 Hypervigilance.

10. A physician performs a lumbar puncture on a 4-year-old with suspected meningitis. The CSF is then sent to the laboratory for testing. The nurse should then:
    1 Assess the child for discomfort at the insertion site and administer narcotics as ordered.
    2 Make sure the child lies flat for at least 8 hours.
    3 Encourage the parents to hold the child.
    4 Place a sandbag over the puncture site for 3 hours.

NCLEX® Review Answers

1.1 Flumazenil is a benzodiazepine antagonist that reverses the effects of diazepam. It should be administered if respiratory distress is noted, secondary to an overdose of diazepam (Valium). Although phenobarbital can effectively control seizure activity, the nurse must be aware of the amount of medication that has already been given because this medication may further suppress respiration. Naloxone is used to reverse the effects of opioids. Phenytoin does not reverse the effects of benzodiazepines.

2.4 Airway, breathing, and then circulation are the priorities in patient care. Padding the bed's siderails is a controversial nursing intervention because of the social stigma associated with seizures. Ensuring that the patient is never alone is not necessary. Although a padded tongue blade is used before a seizure starts, it is not a priority for patient care.

3.1 Protecting the head from trauma and decreasing the risk of aspiration are the priorities for patient safety. Forcing something into his or her mouth after the seizure has begun is also likely to cause injury; a piece of tooth may break off and be aspirated. Restraints and holding the patient down can cause any injury that may occur to become more serious.

4.4 Anticonvulsant medications administered as scheduled help prevent further seizures. Bedrest and closing the door are not interventions that help minimize the risk of seizures. Sedation is also not an intervention that helps minimize the risk of seizures.

5.1 A patient is often drowsy after a seizure. Despite this drowsiness, the patient is usually able to move and speak. Hypotension is not a frequent problem after a seizure. The patient may not remember what, if anything, triggered the seizure.

6.3 A common side effect of long-term phenytoin (Dilantin) therapy is an overgrowth of gingival tissues; problems may be minimized with good oral hygiene. Dilantin should always be taken with meals to decrease gastrointestinal upset; however, diarrhea is not a frequent side effect. Hyperactivity is not a common early side effect; rather, drowsiness may occur but may decrease with time.

7.3 Cool compresses or ice bags to the forehead help relieve febrile delirium. Warmth may increase the fever, and restraints often cause injury to the patient. Fluid intake does not relieve the fever, although it may help prevent dehydration.

8.2 In acute bacterial meningitis, the CSF analysis reveals increased protein (100 to 500 mg/dL); normally, CSF protein is between 15 and 45 mg/dl. Glucose is usually decreased (40 mg/dL); normally, CSF contains glucose levels between 60 and 80 mg/dL. The CSF will reveal an increase in WBCs (1000 to 2000 mm^3 or more); normally, CSF WBCs is between 0 and 5 mm^3. The CSF is also cloudy; normally, specific gravity of CSF is 1.007.

9.2 Persistent neurologic deficits may occur with meningitis. If the cranial nerve VIII is involved, deafness may result. Cerebral edema occurs rather than dehydration. Hyperthermia, not hypothermia, may result. Hypervigilance is a sign found in selected psychiatric disorders.

10.3 The child needs to be comforted after an invasive procedure by individuals he or she trusts. Little discomfort is experienced at the insertion site after a lumbar puncture. Narcotics are not the drugs of choice because they hinder the assessment of neurologic status. A young child does not need to lie flat for any length of time after a lumbar puncture; it is difficult to persuade a 4-year-old to lie flat for any period. Applying a small bandage after applying pressure for a short time is usually sufficient to stop any leaking and to prevent infection of the site.

Chapter 7

Gastrointestinal System

What You WILL LEARN

After reading this chapter, you will know how to do the following:

- ✔ Differentiate between gastrointestinal bleeding, pancreatitis, and liver failure.
- ✔ Describe the pathophysiologic process associated with gastrointestinal bleeding, pancreatitis, and liver failure.
- ✔ Discuss complications associated with gastrointestinal alterations in a critically ill patient.
- ✔ Identify appropriate nursing interventions for caring for a patient with gastrointestinal alterations.
- ✔ Describe prevention approaches that can be instituted in the critical care environment when caring for a patient with gastrointestinal alterations.
- ✔ Describe relevant patient education topics.

evolve

See http://evolve.elsevier.com/Schumacher/criticalcare for additional NCLEX® review questions.

What IS Gastrointestinal Bleeding?

Gastrointestinal (GI) bleeding is a symptom of an underlying disease. Bleeding can result from a variety of diseases that occur in the esophagus, stomach, small intestine, large intestine, or rectum, such as peptic ulcer disease, Mallory-Weiss syndrome, esophageal or rectal varices, neoplasms, esophagitis, stress ulcers, or inflammatory bowel disease. GI bleeding can also result from underlying clotting disorders, such as those with liver disease.

Bleeding can be chronic or acute. Symptoms of GI bleeding can occur without warning and be sudden and severe or have a slow onset. Acute GI bleeding can be a life-threatening condition if the cause of bleeding cannot be treated or controlled. Assessment of the patient for the underlying cause of the bleeding and his or her hemodynamic stability are key factors in the initial care of the patient.

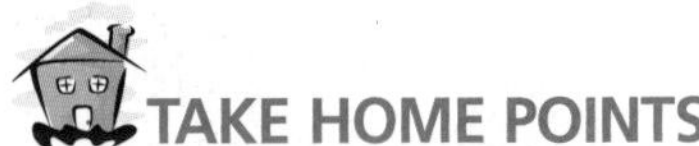

Bleeding from the GI tract is a symptom, not a disease.

Uncontrolled or unmanaged GI bleeding can cause death.

What You NEED TO KNOW

Clinical Manifestations

Clinical manifestations such as anorexia, nausea, vomiting, constipation, diarrhea, weakness, fatigue, weight loss, abdominal pain, and discomfort may precede GI bleeding and indicate the underlying disease.

The feces and vomitus often are the first clues that reveal evidence of GI bleeding. The presence of blood in the stomach is an irritant and a stimulus for vomiting. Hematemesis is bright-red, bloody vomitus or vomitus with a coffee ground appearance. Bright-red vomitus is associated with fresh bleeding. Coffee ground vomitus is blood that has been exposed to the acid and pepsin action of the stomach for a period of time.

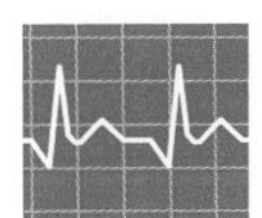

Bright red blood indicates fresh bleeding; secretions appearing like coffee grounds indicate old bleeding.

Examination of the stool in a patient with GI bleeding can reveal hematochezia, a bright, red or maroon blood passed via the rectum. Black, tarry stool is called *melena*. The black appearance of melena is caused by the breakdown of blood by intestinal bacteria and digestive enzymes. Occult blood is another clinical manifestation of GI bleeding. It cannot be identified on visual examination and is detected by guaiac testing.

Hematemesis and melena are associated with upper GI diseases that cause bleeding. Hematochezia is generally associated with diseases of the lower GI tract. If hematochezia is caused by an upper GI bleed, the loss of blood is usually significant. The amount of blood found in the vomitus or stool depends on the volume and rate of blood loss, the cardiovascular status of the patient, and the underlying disease state causing the bleeding.

TAKE HOME POINTS

- The appearance of melena in the stool means that the blood has gone through the digestive tract.
- Signs of shock include hypotension; tachycardia; decreased capillary refill; cool, clammy skin; shortness of breath; changes in level of consciousness; anxiety; and decreased urine output.
- Clinical manifestations of chronic blood loss include weakness, fatigue, shortness of breath, lethargy, and faintness.
- Povidone-iodine (i.e., Betadine) causes a false positive guaiac (i.e., hemoccult) test.

Causes

Peptic ulcer disease is caused by an imbalance of defensive and aggressive factors found in the stomach. The mucosal lining of the stomach forms a protective barrier against the acid-pepsin action of the stomach contents.

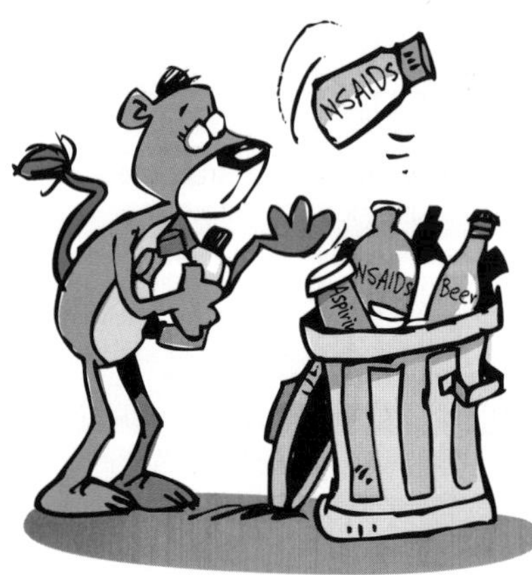

Causes of peptic ulcer disease

This lining has the ability to renew and regenerate. Adequate blood flow is necessary for the mucosal layer to regenerate. Any alteration in mucosal blood flow can cause decreased cellular renewal and weaken the defensive barrier. Chronic ingestion of aspirin, alcohol, and nonsteroidal anti-inflammatory drugs (NSAIDs) weakens the gastric mucosal barrier against the acid and pepsin action of the stomach. Aspirin and NSAIDs cause gastric mucosal irritation and inhibit prostaglandin synthesis, which increases gastric secretion. Other defensive factors include the secretion of bicarbonate and the production of prostaglandins. Bicarbonate balances the acid secretion of the stomach. Prostaglandins protect the stomach by suppressing gastric acid secretion, promoting the secretion of bicarbonate and mucus, and maintaining submucosal blood flow.

Aggressive factors include the presence of *Helicobacter pylori. H. pylori* are bacteria found in the majority of patients with gastric and duodenal ulcerations. The bacteria thrive in an acidic environment and can cause injury to the mucosal barrier of the stomach. This disruption makes the underlying layers of the stomach more susceptible to the acid and pepsin action of the stomach. Acid, pepsin, stress, and smoking are also thought to be aggressive factors that can lead to peptic ulcer disease. The three stimuli that promote the secretion of gastric acid by the parietal cells of the stomach are (1) acetylcholine, (2) histamine, and (3) gastrin. Vagal stimulation causes the release of acetylcholine for which a parietal cell muscarinic receptor exists that promotes hydrochloric acid release. Mast cells release histamine. Histamine 2 (H_2) receptors are found on the parietal cell and respond with the release of hydrochloric acid. G cells release gastrin, which is received by parietal cell G-cell receptors and results in hydrochloric acid release. The enzyme pepsin is responsible for the breakdown of proteins. Chief cells in the stomach release pepsinogen and, in the presence of the acidic stomach environment, form pepsin. Without an adequate mucosal protective barrier, pepsin will break down proteins found in the underlying layers of the stomach wall.

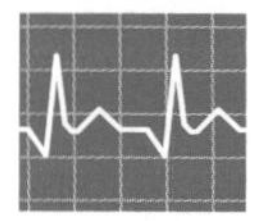
Patients who have acute blood loss will exhibit progressive signs of hemorrhagic shock.

An imbalance in the defensive or aggressive factors in the stomach can create conditions that promote cellular damage and cause erosion and ulceration. Progressive erosion into the underlying vascular layers of the stomach can result in GI bleeding. The treatment of peptic ulcer disease consists of pharmacologic and nonpharmacologic management. If this treatment is not effective and GI bleeding results, surgical intervention may be needed. Surgical intervention for peptic ulcer disease can include procedures such as total or partial gastrectomy, Billroth I or Billroth II procedures, antrectomy, vagotomy, or pyloroplasty.

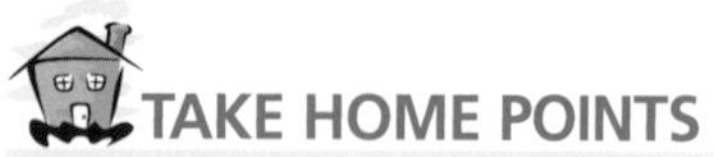

Anything that destroys or weakens the mucosal stomach lining can contribute to GI bleeding.

Mallory-Weiss syndrome is characterized by a linear tear of the gastric mucosa found at the stomach and esophageal junction, which is caused by retching during vomiting. Mild-to-massive GI bleeding is a result. Associated findings that can contribute to the development of Mallory-Weiss syndrome include aspirin or NSAID use, alcohol abuse, bulimia, hiatal hernia, gastritis, or esophagitis. Surgical intervention is used to repair the tear. Angiography may be useful in identifying the site of bleeding and in control of hemorrhage through the infusion of pharmacologic vasoconstrictors.

A superficial erosion of the gastric mucosa usually characterizes stress ulcers, which are often seen in the critically ill population. Patients who are diagnosed with immunosuppression, acute respiratory distress syndrome, sepsis, shock, burns, trauma, acute head injury, or multisystem organ failure are at risk for the development of stress ulcerations. Stress ulceration is caused by mucosal ischemia, which results in the loss of the defensive, mucosal barrier. As the mucosal barrier erodes, stomach lining becomes susceptible to the acid and pepsin action of the stomach contents. The treatment of stress ulceration focuses on the underlying cause of the mucosal ischemia.

Both benign and malignant neoplasms of the esophagus, stomach, and small and large intestine can lead to GI bleeding. Tumors that are not caught in their early stages can spread and erode into the vascular layers of the GI tract, resulting in GI bleeding. Treatment of GI neoplasms includes surgical removal, chemotherapy, and/or radiation. The type of treatment depends on the location, type, and progression of the cancer.

Gastritis, a diffuse inflammation of the gastric mucosa, can be acute or chronic. Factors that can cause acute gastritis include the ingestion of alcohol, aspirin, and bacterial endotoxins. Chronic gastritis is thought to be caused by inflammation associated with *Helicobacter pylori.* Acute or chronic gastritis can result in GI bleeding. Treatment of gastritis consists of removal of the irritant causing the inflammatory process such as cessation of alcohol consumption and treatment of positive *H. pylori* with appropriate antibiotics.

Esophageal Varices

Varices are engorged, distended veins that are susceptible to hemorrhage. They result from portal hypertension, an increase in pressure within the liver's portal circulation, usually related to chronic alcoholism. These distended esophageal veins result in esophageal varices. Rupture of the

Persons who are immunosuppressed have an increased risk of developing ulcers, and treatment requires proactive treatment.

TAKE HOME POINTS

- Smoking is thought to promote a decrease in mucosal blood flow and slow the mucosal renewal process.
- Peptic ulcer disease must be managed in an attempt to prevent GI bleeding.

A Mallory-Weiss tear is an arterial bleed.

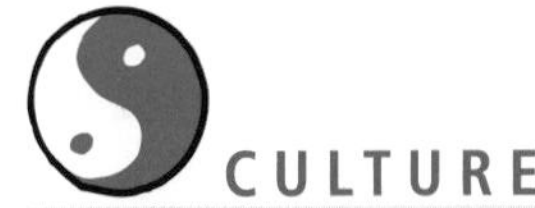

Mallory-Weiss syndrome is most commonly seen in men.

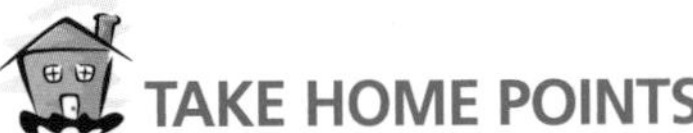

- Bleeding from a Mallory-Weiss tear is treated through surgery.
- Because of the stress of illness and hospitalization, stress ulcers can readily form in the critically ill patient.

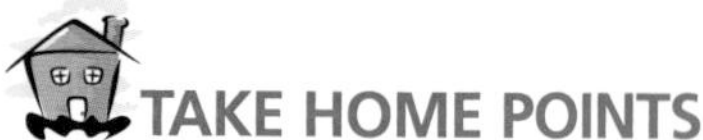

Esophageal varices are a symptom of cirrhosis and portal hypertension. Mortality is between 40%-70% on the first bleed event.

friable veins can cause life-threatening GI bleeding. Treatment of varices focuses on the reduction of portal pressures through the use of pharmacologic therapy and changes in behavior such as no ingestion of alcohol. Pharmacologic agents such as vasopressin (Pitressin), octreotide acetate (Sandostatin), beta-blockers, and nitrates are used to reduce portal pressures. Endoscopy is used as a diagnostic tool (i.e., to identify the site of bleeding) and as a form of treatment (e.g., endoscopic sclerosis or ligation (banding) of the fragile, distended veins to treat varices). Endoscopic ligation (banding) involves the suctioning of the vein into a chamber in the endoscope. The vein is ligated with a small band. A loss of blood flow occurs through the banded vein and, over time, thrombosis and fibrosis occur and the banded vein sloughs off. Sclerosis involves the injection of an agent that causes initial thrombosis and hemostasis. Repeated injections of a sclerosing agent results in mucosal fibrosis and less venous bleeding.

FIRST-LINE AND INITIAL TREATMENTS FOR ESOPHAGEAL VARICES

- Administer vasopressin (Pitressin), octreotide acetate (Sandostatin), beta-blockers, and nitrates.
- Treat with endoscopy, sclerosis, ligation (banding), and balloon tamponade.
- Use Sengstaken-Blakemore, Minnesota, or Linton-Nachias tubes.

Another esophageal varices treatment involves the use of balloon tamponade. Several types of tubes are used for the procedure: Sengstaken-Blakemore, Minnesota, and Linton-Nachias. In general, the tubes have three ports: (1) a gastric balloon port, (2) gastric aspiration port, and (3) an esophageal balloon port. The tube is anchored in the stomach via a gastric balloon. The stomach balloon exerts pressure on the fundus of the stomach and causes compression of esophageal blood flow. The esophageal balloon is then inflated, placing direct pressure on the varices. The balloon pressures are monitored and maximum inflation time is identified. Once placed, it is essential to prevent upward tube migration. The migration could lead to airway occlusion. Oropharyngeal and gastric secretions must also be managed.

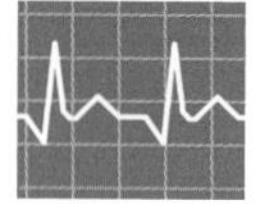

Because of the pressures exerted from the tubes for balloon tamponade, it is crucial that airway patency be continually assessed.

If these treatment modalities do not effectively manage esophageal varices, radiographic or surgical intervention is considered. The radiographic

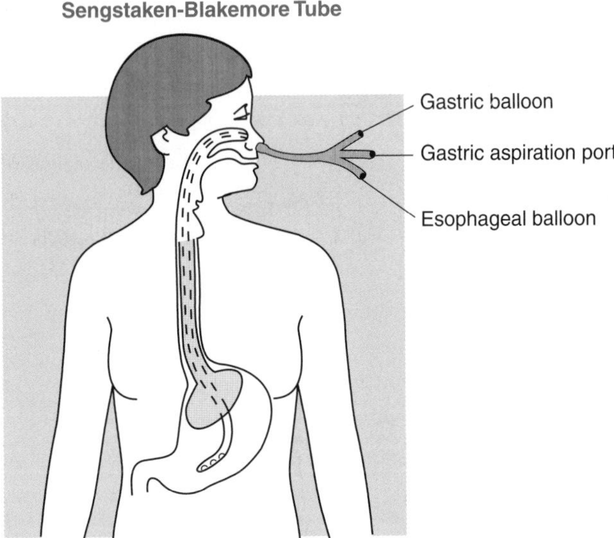

Sengstaken-Blakemore Tube

Gastric balloon
Gastric aspiration port
Esophageal balloon

(From Urden L, Stacy K, Lough M: Thelan's critical care nursing: diagnosis and management, *ed 4, St Louis, 2002, Mosby.)*

Minnesota Tube

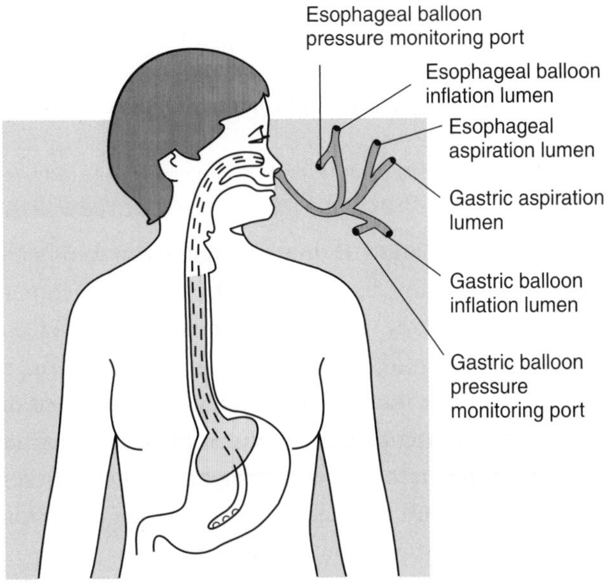

Esophageal balloon pressure monitoring port
Esophageal balloon inflation lumen
Esophageal aspiration lumen
Gastric aspiration lumen
Gastric balloon inflation lumen
Gastric balloon pressure monitoring port

(From Urden L, Stacy K, Lough M: Thelan's critical care nursing: diagnosis and management, *ed 4, St Louis, 2002, Mosby.)*

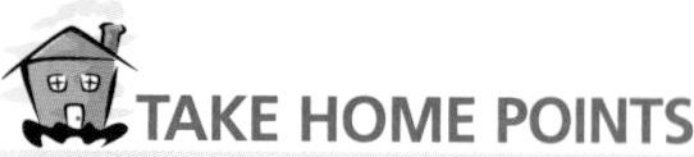

TAKE HOME POINTS

All treatment modalities for varices can have side effects and complications such as variceal hemorrhage, hypovolemic shock, rebleeding after treatment, and airway occlusion from migration of a balloon tamponade tube.

Linton-Nachias Tube

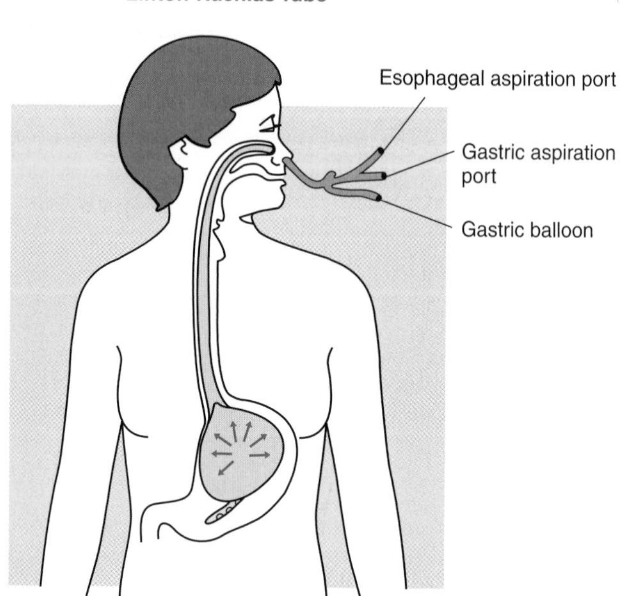

procedure involves the placement of a stent that creates a portosystemic shunt and reduces portal pressures. Surgical techniques to reduce portal hypertension include the placement of portacaval, mesocaval, or splenorenal shunts. The surgical shunts divert blood flow and result in a reduction of portal pressures.

Inflammatory Conditions of the Gastrointestinal Tract

Esophagitis is an inflammation of the esophagus often seen in association with gastroesophageal reflux disease (GERD). The acidic contents of the stomach flow back into the esophagus through the lower esophageal sphincter. Severe forms of GERD can result in esophageal tissue erosion and ulceration, which can lead to GI bleeding. The treatment of esophagitis focuses on suppressing gastric acidity, improving gastric emptying, and decreasing pressure on the lower esophageal sphincter. In some cases, surgical intervention to strengthen the lower esophageal sphincter may be needed.

Ulcerative colitis and Crohn's disease are two types of inflammatory bowel disease that can result in GI hemorrhage. Ulcerative colitis is commonly found in the colon and rectum and is characterized by abdominal pain, diarrhea, and rectal bleeding. Crohn's disease is an inflammatory process that affects the proximal colon and the terminal ileum. Ulcers form that extend into all the layers of the GI wall. Clinical manifestations of Crohn's disease include abdominal pain, diarrhea, and GI bleeding. Treatment of both inflammatory bowel processes focuses on reduction of the inflammatory process by pharmacologic intervention, diet, and in some cases surgical intervention. In patients with GI bleeding from inflammatory bowel disease, the diseased portion of the colon or small intestine is removed.

Diagnostics

Endoscopy is a diagnostic tool that provides direct visualization of the GI tract and the bleeding site. Esophagogastroduodenoscopy (EGD) is visualization of the esophagus, stomach, and duodenum. Colonoscopy provides for visualization of the colon, and sigmoidoscopy allows for rectal visualization. Enteroscopy is used for visualization of the small bowel. Endoscopy can also be used to treat and control bleeding by obtaining biopsies and for electrocoagulation, ligation, sclerosis, or laser therapy.

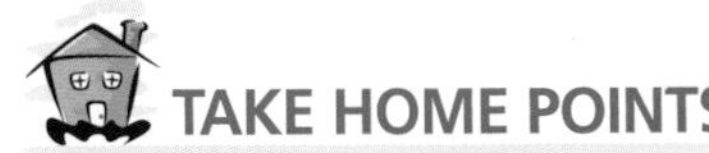

Endoscopy is considered the "gold standard" for diagnosis of GI bleeding.

Radiographic procedures, such as an upper GI series and barium enema, can be used to diagnose GI bleeding. An upper GI series can be used to detect varices, ulcers, neoplasms, and inflammation of the upper GI tract. A barium enema can help identify underlying disease processes such as neoplasms and inflammatory bowel disease, all of which can be a bleeding source.

Dye can be injected via angiography to identify the site of a bleeding vessel when the source of bleeding is not accessible to an endoscope. Medications, such as vasoconstrictors, can also be administered directly via angiographic means to assist in controlling hemorrhage.

Radionuclide scanning is a noninvasive diagnostic tool. A small amount of a radioactive substance is injected into the patient. Scans are then completed that locate the site of bleeding.

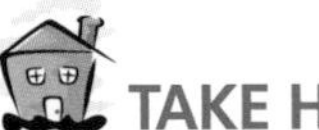

TAKE HOME POINTS

- The elevation of BUN is the result of the breakdown of blood proteins in the GI tract by bacteria and digestive enzymes.
- The elevation in WBCs and platelets reflects the body's attempt to achieve homeostasis after blood loss.
- Guaiac is a chemical reagent test that turns blue in the presence of blood. Note: Betadine (povidone-iodine) causes a false-positive result.

Complete blood counts (CBC), basic and complete metabolic profiles, coagulation profiles, liver function tests, arterial blood gases (ABGs), and gastric or stool aspirate for guaiac are diagnostic tests used for patients with GI bleeding. Hemoglobin and hematocrit laboratory values may not be helpful when obtained immediately after blood loss. An elevation in blood urea nitrogen (BUN) may be seen up to 24 hours after a GI bleed that results in hematemesis or melena. Coagulation studies should be assessed for any abnormalities. Platelets and WBCs can initially be elevated after a GI bleed, as can blood glucose levels. The glucose elevation is seen because of the stress response. Because the liver plays a role in the metabolism of clotting factors, liver function tests should be obtained to rule out any underlying liver abnormality that could be contributing to the GI bleeding. If the patient is vomiting, hypokalemia and a metabolic alkalosis may result from the loss of hydrogen ions with vomiting. Patients who are suspected of having chronic GI bleeding should have guaiac testing for occult blood in the feces and vomitus.

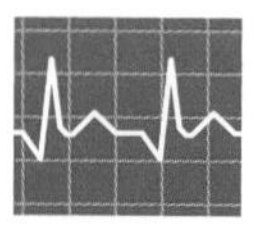

The patient's creatinine should be monitored for any signs of inadequate renal perfusion associated with hypovolemia and hemorrhagic shock—a complication associated with massive GI bleeding. An elevated creatinine indicates a slowing of the glomerular filtration rate (GFR) and a decrease in the functioning of the renal nephrons.

Patients with peptic ulcer disease and chronic gastritis should be tested for the presence of the *H. pylori* bacteria. Invasive and noninvasive tests are available for determining the presence of the bacteria. Blood and breath tests are available as noninvasive means, and tissue samples can be taken via endoscopy as an invasive means.

Complications

To care for the patient with GI bleeding, it is important to understand the potential complications including hemorrhagic shock, perforation, and obstruction.

For patients with massive hemorrhage, the lactic acid will elevate, indicating the body's conversion from aerobic to anaerobic metabolism and inability to meet cellular needs.

If GI bleeding is massive, hemorrhagic shock can occur. Hemorrhagic shock is characterized by a decrease in preload (venous return) to the heart, caused by the loss of blood volume. Losses of at least 15% of blood volume occur before the clinical manifestations of hemorrhagic shock are apparent.

Peptic ulcer disease, neoplasms, varices, and inflammatory bowel disease can cause perforation. Perforation occurs when an erosion of all the layers of the GI wall occurs and the contents of the GI tract spill into the peritoneum, resulting in peritonitis. Clinical manifestations of perforation include sudden onset of severe abdominal pain, tenderness, and distention. The abdomen often becomes rigid and boardlike. Other results include nausea, vomiting, fever, tachycardia, hypotension, paralytic ileus, and fluid and electrolyte imbalances. If perforation occurs, the area is surgically closed or patched; otherwise, the peritonitis can progress to sepsis, septic shock, and death. GI obstruction can also be an associated complication of GI bleeding.

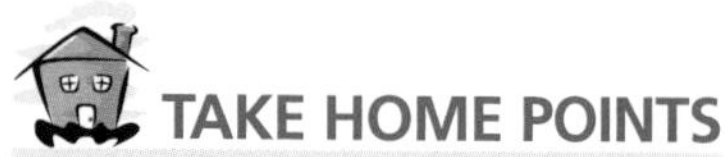

TAKE HOME POINTS

Perforation of the GI wall results in peritonitis.

What You DO

In addition to the traditional patient history, particular questions should be directed to the patient with GI bleeding. Questions should include:

- *Are you taking any medications that could be compounding the bleeding problem?* The patient should be assessed for use of anticoagulants

(Warfarin), NSAIDs, antiplatelets (aspirin), or recent use of thrombolytic medications.

- *Do you have any previous history of GI disease or surgery?* Bleeding from an operative site can be a postoperative complication.
- *Do you have any known liver disease?* One of the functions of the liver is to metabolize clotting factors. In the presence of liver disease, these factors are not metabolized and can result in coagulopathies.
- *Do you have any known bleeding or coagulation problems?* Other associated diseases such as thrombocytopenia, leukemias, multiple myeloma, and lymphomas can result in bleeding and coagulation defects. An assessment for the presence of these disorders helps rule each out as a possible underlying cause of the bleed.
- *What types of medications (prescribed, over the counter, and herbal) are you currently taking?* Of particular interest would be the use of NSAIDs. The nurse should remember to ask about herbal supplements when taking a medication history. Garlic, feverfew, Chinese fungus, Ganoderma lucidum, and *Ginkgo biloba* can suppress platelet aggregation and increase the risk of bleeding when taken in association with anticoagulant or antiplatelet drugs.
- *Do you drink alcohol and if so, how often?* Alcohol is a known irritant to the defensive mucosal barrier and an associated cause for bleeding.

The nurse should also perform a physical examination in addition to the history. A complete abdominal assessment should be performed, including inspection, percussion, auscultation, and palpation. Clues may be found on the physical examination that may identify the underlying cause of GI bleeding. For example, the presence of spider nevi, petechiae, and bruising in the presence of a palpable nodular liver may indicate liver cirrhosis. A rigid, boardlike, tender abdomen can indicate perforation. The presence of blood in the gut often stimulates peristalsis; on auscultation, hyperactive bowel sounds can be heard.

The goals for the care of a patient with GI bleeding include control of the hemorrhage, achievement and maintenance of hemodynamic stability, control of gastric acid secretion, observation for complications, preparation for surgical interventions if necessary, and patient and family education about the treatment and control of GI bleeding.

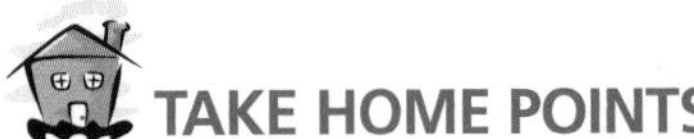

- It is important to take a focused patient history concerning factors pertaining to GI bleeding.
- Physical assessment findings can indicate certain underlying conditions that are the cause of the GI bleed.

FIRST-LINE AND INITIAL TREATMENTS FOR DECREASING GI BLEED

- Provide oxygen (O_2).
- Ensure IV access.
- Monitor vital signs and hemodynamic readings.
- Administer fluids (crystalloids, colloids) and blood.
- Insert nasogastric (NG) tube.
- Consider possible gastric lavage.
- Prepare for endoscopy.

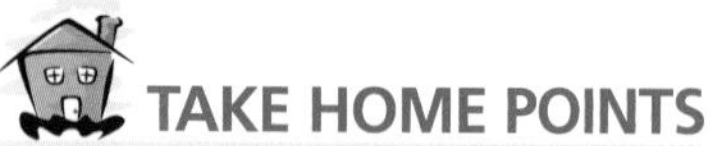

The treatment for hemorrhagic shock is volume replacement.

To achieve hemodynamic stability, venous and arterial lines are inserted to allow access for volume infusion and continuous monitoring of hemodynamic parameters such as pulse, blood pressure (BP), mean arterial pressure (MAP), and central venous pressures (CVPs). A pulmonary artery catheter may be inserted to monitor pulmonary capillary wedge pressure (PCWP) and cardiac output (CO).

Volume should be administered to the patient in the form of crystalloids, colloids, and blood (the best form of volume replacement), as well as packed red blood cells (RBCs) and coagulation factors. RBCs promote O_2-carrying capacity, whereas coagulation factors promote hemostasis. O_2 therapy should be initiated to compensate for the decrease in O_2-carrying capacity of the blood associated with the loss of RBCs and hemoglobin; O_2 saturation should be assessed via pulse oximetry. A nasogastric (NG) tube should be inserted to remove blood from the upper GI tract and to allow for an assessment of the amount of blood lost. Gastric lavage may be used to cleanse the stomach in preparation for endoscopy. A Foley catheter should be inserted to evaluate renal perfusion and urine output. The electrocardiogram (ECG) tracing should be assessed for any signs of myocardial ischemia that could be associated with decreased coronary perfusion, often associated with hemorrhagic shock.

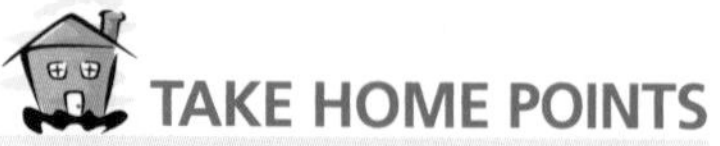

If massive volume replacement is required, the replacement products should be warmed to prevent hypothermia.

Once hemodynamic stability is achieved in patients with peptic ulcer disease, gastritis, stress ulcerations, and esophagitis, control of gastric acid secretion and pepsin action is accomplished through pharmacologic agents to promote healing. H_2-receptor antagonists, proton pump inhibitors, antacids, and mucosal protective agents are examples of the medications commonly used.

H_2-receptor antagonists act on the H_2-receptors found on the gastric parietal cells and decrease acid production. Examples of H_2-receptor antagonists include cimetidine (Tagamet), ranitidine (Zantac), famotidine (Pepcid), and nizatidine (Axid).

Proton pump inhibitors suppress gastric acid secretion by inhibition of the H^+K^+–ATPase enzyme. This category of drugs is thought to be the most effective in the suppression of gastric acid secretion. The H^+K^+–ATPase enzyme is responsible for the production of gastric acid in the parietal cell. Examples of proton pump inhibitors include omeprazole (Prilosec), lansoprazole (Prevacid), pantoprazole (Protonix), and rabeprazole (AcipHex).

Mucosal protective agents promote healing by creating a protective barrier around a known ulcer against the acid and pepsin action of the stomach. Mucosal protective agents are activated in the presence of the acidic environment of the stomach. If used in combination with antacids, the mucosal protective agents should be administered 30 to 60 minutes before antacids. An example of the mucosal protectant is sucralfate (Carafate).

Antacids are used to neutralize stomach acid, inactivate the effects of pepsin by raising the pH of stomach contents, and stimulate the production of prostaglandins that can enhance the mucosal barrier. Antacids come in four forms: (1) magnesium hydroxide (milk of magnesia), (2) aluminum hydroxide (Amphojel), (3) calcium carbonate (Caltrate, Tums), and (4) sodium bicarbonate. Magnesium and aluminum hydroxide preparations are most commonly used. Antacids should be taken on a regular schedule after meals and at bedtime.

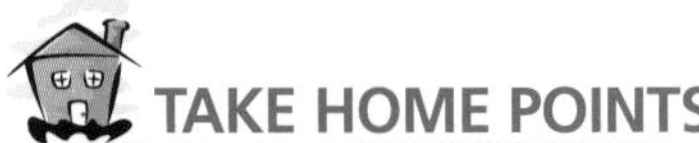

- Abuse of antacids can cause metabolic alkalosis.
- Misoprostol is an agent used in the prevention of ulcers specifically caused by the use of NSAIDs.

Patients with documented *Helicobacter pylori* infection are treated with combination antibiotics. Clarithromycin (Biaxin), tetracycline, amoxicillin (Amoxil), and metronidazole (Flagyl) are the most common.

The patient should be assessed for complications associated with GI bleeding with specific emphasis on hemodynamic status. If surgical intervention is required, the patient should be monitored for postoperative complications such as infection, peritonitis, fluid and electrolyte disturbances, and hemodynamic complications.

The nurse should also assess patency of the NG tube to ensure decompression of the upper GI tract and prevent vomiting. Patients who are experiencing GI bleeding should receive nothing by mouth, and gastric or enteral feeding should be discontinued until the source of bleeding is identified. When recovering from a bleeding episode, the patient's diet is increased and prescribed as tolerated. The nurse should ensure patient comfort throughout the course of treatment. Comfort measures include both pharmacologic and nonpharmacologic measures.

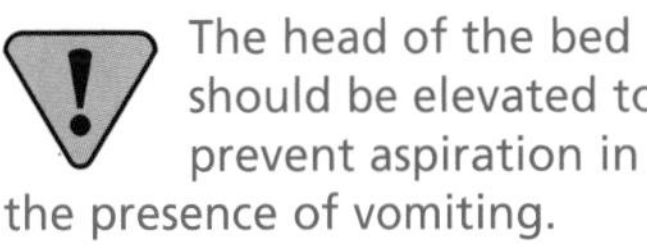
The head of the bed should be elevated to prevent aspiration in the presence of vomiting.

When medical management cannot stop GI bleeding, surgical intervention is indicated. Such situations would include hemorrhagic shock unresponsive to medical treatment, the need to transfuse a patient with more than eight units of blood in a 24-hour period, and the presence of GI perforation.

The patient and family must receive education throughout the course of an episode of GI bleeding. Patients who require transfer to an intensive care unit (ICU) need an explanation of why the transfer is occurring. Once in the ICU, the patient and family should be oriented to the environment, including being given an explanation of equipment and procedures. Once a source of bleeding is identified, the treatment plan should be reviewed with the patient and family and they should be given an opportunity to ask questions and voice concerns. As the patient is recovering, the nurse should review and reinforce the treatment plan for the underlying cause of the bleeding.

TAKE HOME POINTS

No specific diet prescriptions are available for a patient who is recovering from GI bleeding. The diet should be geared to the treatment of the disease that is the underlying cause of the bleeding.

TAKE HOME POINTS

The purpose of surgical intervention in a GI bleed is to prevent the patient from exsanguination.

Do You UNDERSTAND?

DIRECTIONS: **Select the best answer, and place the appropriate letter in the space provided.**

1. The nurse is reviewing the ABG results for a patient admitted for GI bleeding who is in hypovolemic shock. The patient's ABG results are pH, 7.27; pCO_2, 38; pO_2, 78; HCO_3, 14; and O_2 saturation, 94%. The nurse understands that the **MOST** probable cause of the ABG result is the following:
   1. Tachypnea associated with compensatory mechanisms in response to shock.
   2. The conversion from aerobic to anaerobic metabolism caused by cellular injury and damage.
   3. The increased production of bicarbonate by the kidney as a compensatory mechanism by the body in response to the shock state.
   4. Cellular destruction releasing an excessive amount of potassium into the vascular space.

Answer: 1. 3.

DIRECTIONS: Match the treatment in Column A with the appropriate disease process in Column B.

Column A	Column B
_____1. Balloon tamponade tube such as a Sengstaken-Blakemore is used to place direct pressure on the site of bleeding.	a. Gastroesophageal reflux
_____2. Surgical intervention is used to repair this arterial tear.	b. Mallory-Weiss tear
_____3. Antibiotic combinations are used to treat the inflammation caused by *Helicobacter pylori.*	c. Esophageal varices
_____4. Pharmacologic agents such as vasopressin and octreotide acetate are used to decrease portal pressures.	d. Peptic ulcer disease
_____5. That patient is instructed not to eat immediately before bedtime to prevent pressure on the lower esophageal sphincter.	

What IS Pancreatitis?

Pancreatitis is a serious illness caused by the inflammation of the pancreas. An episode of pancreatitis can be identified as either an acute or chronic condition. Acute pancreatitis can be severe, causing life-threatening conditions. The sudden onset of symptoms resulting in an acute situation can last for a short time; if the symptoms are promptly treated, the patient will have a full recovery. The severity is usually unpredictable and unrelated to the patient's age group. The most common causes of acute pancreatitis include alcoholism, drug toxicity, abdominal trauma, and biliary duct obstruction. Viral infections can also contribute to inflammation of the pancreas.

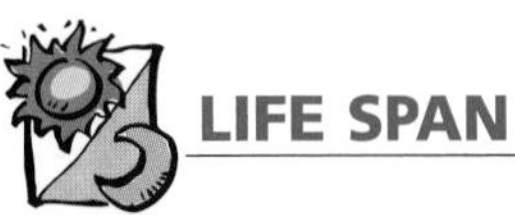

LIFE SPAN

Alcohol-related pancreatitis can develop in patients in their 30s after 4 to 7 years of drinking, whereas biliary pancreatitis usually occurs in an older adult population.

Answer: 1. c; 2. b; 3. d; 4. c; 5. a.

What You NEED TO KNOW

TAKE HOME POINTS

Chronic pancreatitis progresses slowly and does not resolve itself. Chronic pancreatitis severely impairs the function of the pancreas and causes permanent damage to the gland.

The pancreas is a large gland located behind the stomach close to the duodenum (the first part of the small intestine). The pancreas' tadpole shape is divided into three parts: (1) head, (2) body, and (3) tail. The head of the pancreas is located right of the midline of the abdominal cavity with the body and tail pointing upward, so the tail is found lying close to the edge of the left side of the ribs.

The head of the pancreas is attached to the duodenum and shares this space with the liver. The bile duct from the liver drains bile into the bowel at the same place that pancreatic fluids enter the bowel from the head of the pancreas via the pancreatic duct. Because of the many blood vessels behind the pancreas and the general positioning of the pancreas in the body, any surgical procedure involving the pancreas is difficult and challenging for the surgeon.

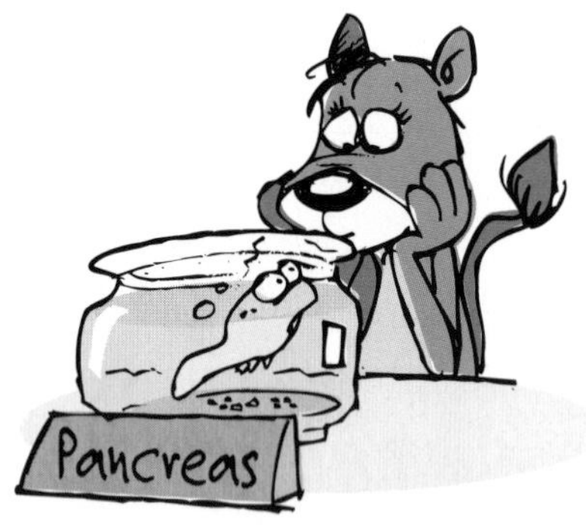

Pancreas is a tadpole-shaped gland.

The pancreas is considered a gland because of its unusual combination of endocrine and exocrine functions. Endocrine cells, found in the islets of Langerhans, produce several hormones that pass directly into the bloodstream. These hormones include insulin, glucagon, and vasoactive intestinal polypeptide (VIP). The pancreas also produces a variety of chemical digestive enzymes that pass into the duodenum, thus the label *exocrine.* Exocrine secretions are produced by the acini cells. The most commonly known digestive enzymes produced by the pancreas include trypsin, chymotrypsin, lipase, and amylase.

The main function of the pancreas is to aid in food digestion and maintain a balance of glucose in the blood. Pancreatic enzymes remain inactive until they pass into the bowel, where they mix with bowel juices, become activated, and assist with digestion of carbohydrates, protein, and fats. Bile from the liver assists lipase in fat digestion by breaking the fat into tiny pieces. In pancreatitis, these powerful enzymes become activated prematurely and the pancreas begins digesting itself (autodigestion), resulting in bleeding. As the blood vessels are digested, they leak pancreatic chemicals into the abdominal cavity. When pancreatic blood vessels begin to erode, activated enzymes may gain access to the bloodstream, where they begin circulating throughout the body.

It is very easy to misdiagnose an acute case of pancreatitis because of vague patient complaints of fever, malaise, nausea, vomiting, and steady epigastric pain. However, one in four patients may have severe acute pancreatitis wherein the pain may become intense, radiating to the patient's back and flank, because the pancreas is located in the retroperitoneal space. The pain may lessen when the patient is sitting up and bending forward. Eating exacerbates the pain by stimulating secretion of prematurely activated enzymes that promote autodigestion of the gland. Pain is usually increased after vomiting, rather than decreased, because of an increase in intraductal pressure caused by retching that allows further obstruction of the outflow of pancreatic secretions, causing more damage to the organ.

One important note: No specific laboratory test is used to diagnose acute pancreatitis. Amylase, lipase, and trypsin serum levels may appear elevated early in the disease, only to return to normal values in cases of chronic pancreatitis.

Additional symptoms may include fever, tachycardia, low BP, and jaundice. Nausea, vomiting, and abdominal swelling are common symptoms as well. A rare sign found in pancreatic hemorrhage is the appearance of a reddish-purple or greenish-brown color located on the flank area (Turner's sign) or a bluish color around the navel (Cullen's sign), or both.

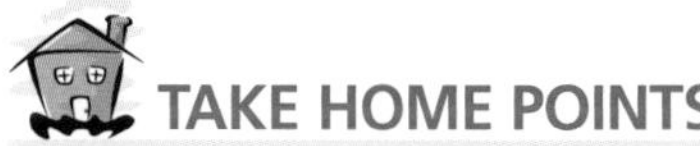

- A gland is any organ that produces chemicals for transport into the bloodstream or another organ.
- In pancreatitis, the pancreas autodigests itself.
- Pain is usually the main symptom in pancreatitis and is aggravated when lying down.

Turner's and Cullen's signs are evidence of necrotizing pancreatitis, in which death of pancreatic tissue causes bleeding into the abdomen.

Pancreatitis

Complication	Signs/Symptoms
Shock	Low blood pressure Increased heart rate Cold extremities Changes in mental status
Hypovolemia (secondary to internal and external bleeding and fluid loss)	Shock symptoms
Acute respiratory distress syndrome	Dyspnea Tachypnea Hypoxemia (Despite oxygen therapy)
Sepsis	Symptoms of shock with fever
Circulatory shock	Symptoms of shock
Pleural effusion	Respiratory distress Hypoxemia
Circulation of pancreatic enzymes throughout the body	Damage to kidneys, heart, liver, eyes, bone, skin, lining of gastrointestinal tract

A common cause of death in acute pancreatitis is secondary pancreatic infection. After the pancreatitis decreases, the pancreas becomes susceptible to infection because of extensive cell death caused by pancreatic necrosis. Prophylactic antibiotics are used to prevent potential septic complications. A pancreatic abscess can develop, causing a return of fever and pain, and is treated with broad-spectrum antibiotics.

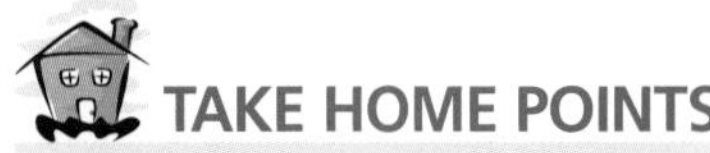

A pseudocyst, a severe complication of pancreatitis, is filled with pancreatic enzyme exudates.

A pancreatic pseudocyst is a severe complication of pancreatitis that can appear weeks after the illness begins. A pseudocyst is an encapsulated, saclike structure that forms on or around the pancreas and lacks the epithelial lining of a true cyst. The cyst may contain several liters of pancreatic enzyme exudates that may appear straw colored or dark brown. A pseudocyst may resolve spontaneously or may rupture, and death may occur if bleeding is a complication.

Loss of pancreatic function occurs in chronic pancreatitis as the gland begins to lose exocrine and endocrine functions. Although causes of chronic pancreatitis can rarely be identified, factors that produce the acute form can also cause the chronic form. In chronic pancreatitis, insulin-producing cells found in the islets of Langerhans that produce insulin to maintain proper glucose levels begin to malfunction and the patient may develop diabetes. As chronic pancreatitis continues and insulin levels drop, a patient may require insulin injections to be able to process sugars. A further complication of chronic pancreatitis is pancreatic insufficiency, which is caused by the malabsorption of nutrients in the small intestine because of the formation of fibrous tissue that replaces healthy acinar tissue. When acini are no longer able to produce necessary enzymes needed to digest proteins, carbohydrates, and fats, patients may complain of bulky, fatty, foul-smelling stool (steatorrhea), weight loss, fever, malaise, and nausea and vomiting. The inability to digest nutrients can also lead to muscle wasting, weakness, and malnutrition.

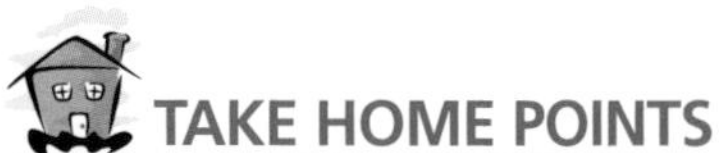

Transient rise in serum liver enzymes is common up to 24 hours after ERCP.

Several options are available to aid the physician in diagnosing pancreatitis. A contrast-enhanced CT scan provides the best image of the pancreas and surrounding structures. A CT scan of the abdomen can reveal fluid accumulation and noted inflammation of the pancreatic gland.

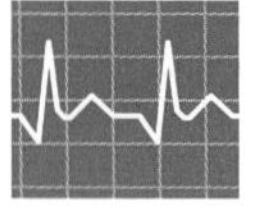

It is important to closely monitor blood glucose levels in patients with pancreatitis.

Endoscopic retrograde cholangiopancreatography (ERCP) allows the physician to view magnified images of the pancreas via a fiber-optic camera. ERCP is primarily indicated when patients have severe disease symptoms and are suspected to have biliary pancreatitis. During the ERCP procedure, the physician is able to remove impacted stones from the bile duct and drain cysts.

Ultrasonography is a noninvasive procedure acceptable for initial evaluation of the pancreas when biliary causes are suspected.

In pancreatitis, a malfunction of insulin production occurs; therefore, insulin needs to be administered.

Plain radiographic studies are helpful in revealing gallstones that may be blocking the pancreatic duct. Parts of the pancreas become calcified when previously healthy tissue is destroyed and is replaced by nonfunctioning scar tissue. These areas of calcification can be seen on radiographs.

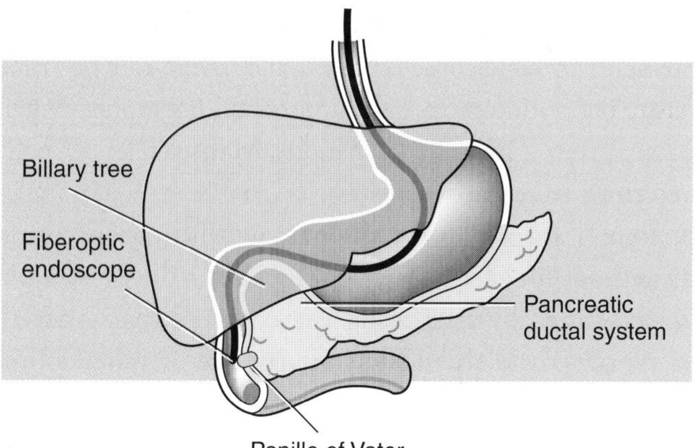

Endoscopic retrograde cholangiopancreatography diagnostic procedure.

What You DO

Management of the patient with pancreatitis focuses on the rest of the pancreas, supportive care, relief of symptoms, and management of complications. Treatment includes maintenance of circulatory volume, pain relief, and decreasing pancreatic secretions.

Vigorous IV replacement of electrolytes and proteins helps maintain circulatory volume and provides emergency treatment for shock. During IV rehydration, the nurse should pay close attention to BP and cardiac and pulmonary status. Nurses should monitor and report abnormalities in the patient's electrolyte profiles, including signs of tetany (a positive Trousseau's sign, carpopedal spasm, Chvostek's sign, and paresthesias of fingers and around the oral cavity). IV calcium gluconate should be readily available for the patient who experiences tetany.

Pain management is achieved by administering Demerol (meperidine), rather than morphine, because morphine can cause spasm of the sphincter of Oddi, which increases bile obstruction. Recently, fentanyl citrate (Sublimaze), also an opiate, has also been used to control the severe pain. The nurse should monitor for signs of analeptic activity (central nervous system [CNS] stimulation) caused by the metabolite of meperidine, normeperidine, with prolonged use of Demerol. The nurse should assess pain levels before and after the administration of analgesics.

Anticholinergics, such as atropine and propantheline (Propanthel), can be prescribed to decrease vagal stimulation, pancreatic secretion, and ampullary spasm. Cimetidine (Tagamet) and aluminum-magnesium can

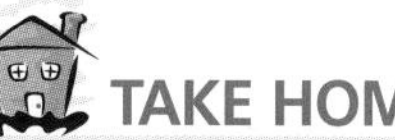

TAKE HOME POINTS

- Demerol is the drug of choice for managing the pain in pancreatitis, but fentanyl citrate (Sublimaze) has also been successful in controlling the pain.
- It may be necessary to replace the pancreatic enzymes to promote the GI digestion process in patients with pancreatitis.

Trousseau's sign of Tetany

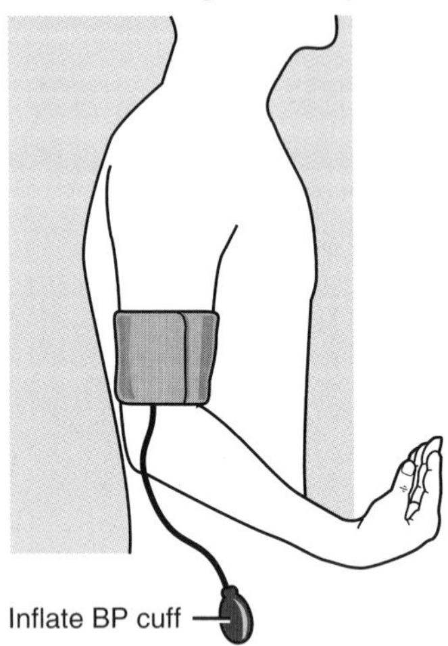

(From Bucher L, Melander S: Critical care nursing, *Philadelphia, 1999, WB Saunders.)*

Chvostek's sign of Tetany

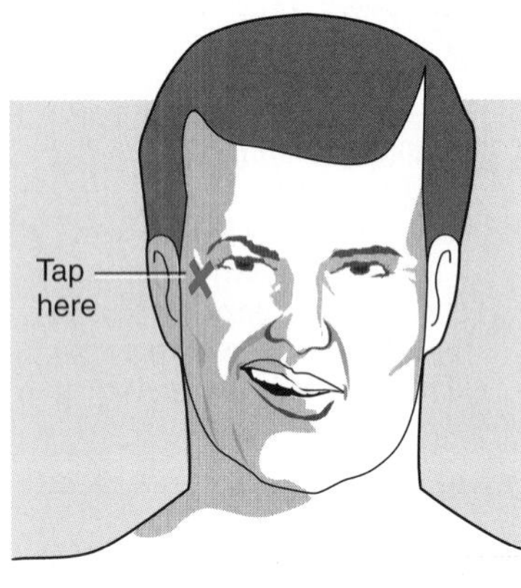

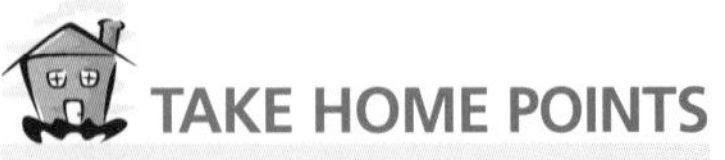

High-fat foods and alcohol should be avoided in patients with pancreatitis.

also be ordered to decrease hydrochloric acid production and further decrease pancreatic secretions. Acinar cell activity can be inhibited by administering octreotide acetate to suppress GI hormones that stimulate pancreatic secretions. In cases of pancreatic insufficiency, pancrelipase can be prescribed to replace enzymes.

NG suction is an option for the patient with consistent vomiting, gastric distention, or ileus. Suctioning also reduces stimulation of pancreatic secretions by decreasing the contents that enter the small intestines. Nursing care should include the use of water-soluble lubricant around the nares to prevent irritation. Good oral hygiene should promote clean mucous membranes and decrease irritation of the oropharynx and dryness. The patient should discontinue oral intake until symptoms subside. For those patients who do not recover quickly, or who have a complicated clinical course, total parenteral nutrition (TPN) therapy can be initiated to support nutritional status. Careful monitoring of laboratory studies will help prevent potential complications of hyperglycemia and hypoglycemia. Hyperglycemia will require an increase in IV insulin administration. In contrast, an IV bolus of dextrose 50% will reverse hypoglycemia.

Surgical intervention is usually a risky option because of the acutely ill presentation of the patient. A diagnostic laparotomy can be performed to débride a necrotic pancreas. Postoperative care includes management of several sump tubes that are placed to provide irrigation, air venting, and drainage. In severe cases, the surgical incision may remain open and be irrigated and repacked every 2 to 3 days to remove necrotic tissue. A cholecystectomy should be performed if gallstones or gallbladder disease are causative factors.

Patients who survive an episode of pancreatitis will be weak and debilitated for weeks or months after hospitalization. Because patients may not recall instructions during the acute phase, a home care referral would be appropriate, so the nurse can continue patient and family education. Written and verbal instructions should be included with dietary information, including the need to avoid high-fat foods, heavy meals, and alcohol. Information regarding resources and support groups are made available to the patient who is liable to return to previous alcoholic habits.

Nursing goals for the patient experiencing pancreatitis include pain relief, decreasing pancreatic stimulation, relieving discomfort associated with NG drainage, improving nutritional status, maintaining respiratory function, improving fluid and electrolyte status, and preventing shock.

Plate 1: Anaphylactic Shock Mediator Response and Clinical Manifestations

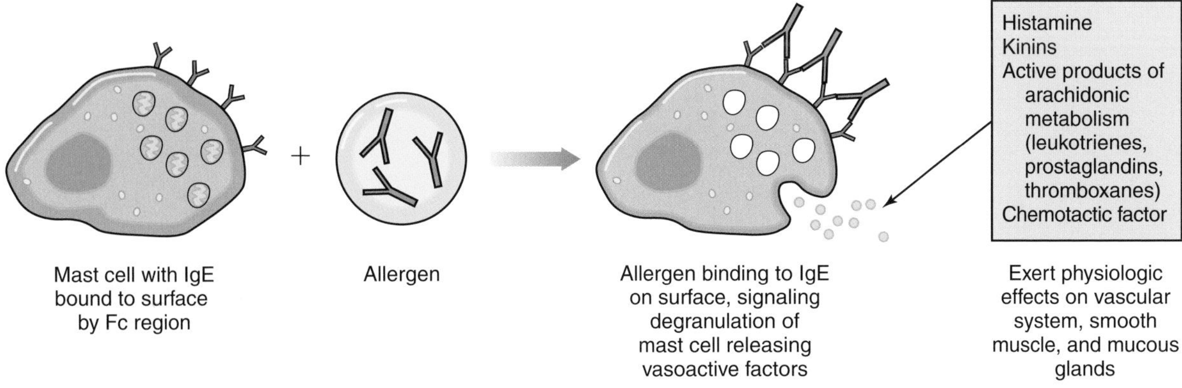

Clinical Manifestations of Type 1 Hypersensitivity Reactions

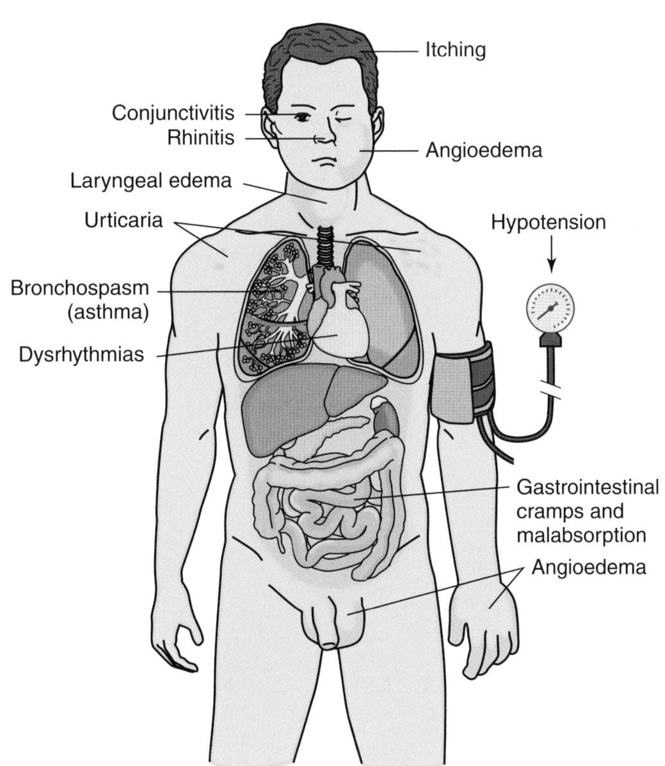

Reprinted with permission from Phipps W et al: Medical-surgical nursing: health and illness perspective, *ed 7, St Louis, 2003, Mosby (page 1635).*

Plate 2: Intraaortic Balloon Pump

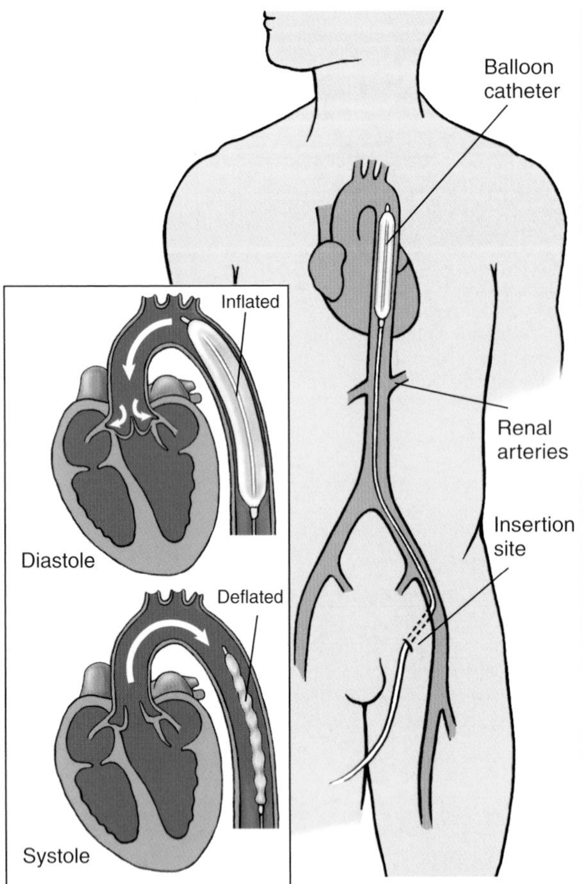

Plate 3: Application of Cricoid Pressure

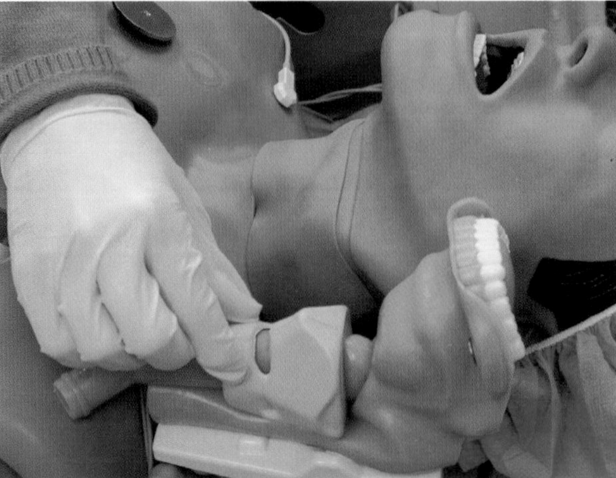

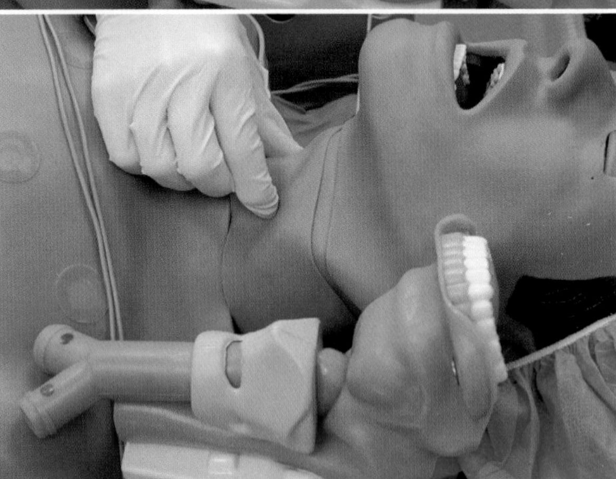

Plate 2: *Reprinted with permission from Phipps W et al:* Medical-surgical nursing: health and illness perspective, *ed 7, St Louis, 2003, Mosby (page 296).*
Plate 3: *Courtesy of Matthew W. Kervin, MN, CRNA.*

Plate 4: Coronary Arteries and Myocardial Infarction Localization

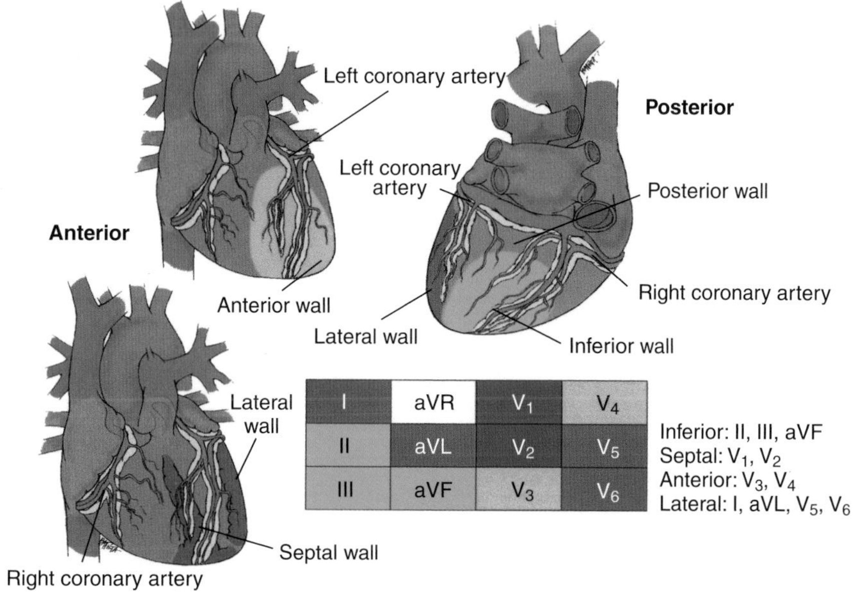

Plate 5: Blood Flow through the Heart

Plate 6: Osmosis and Diffusion

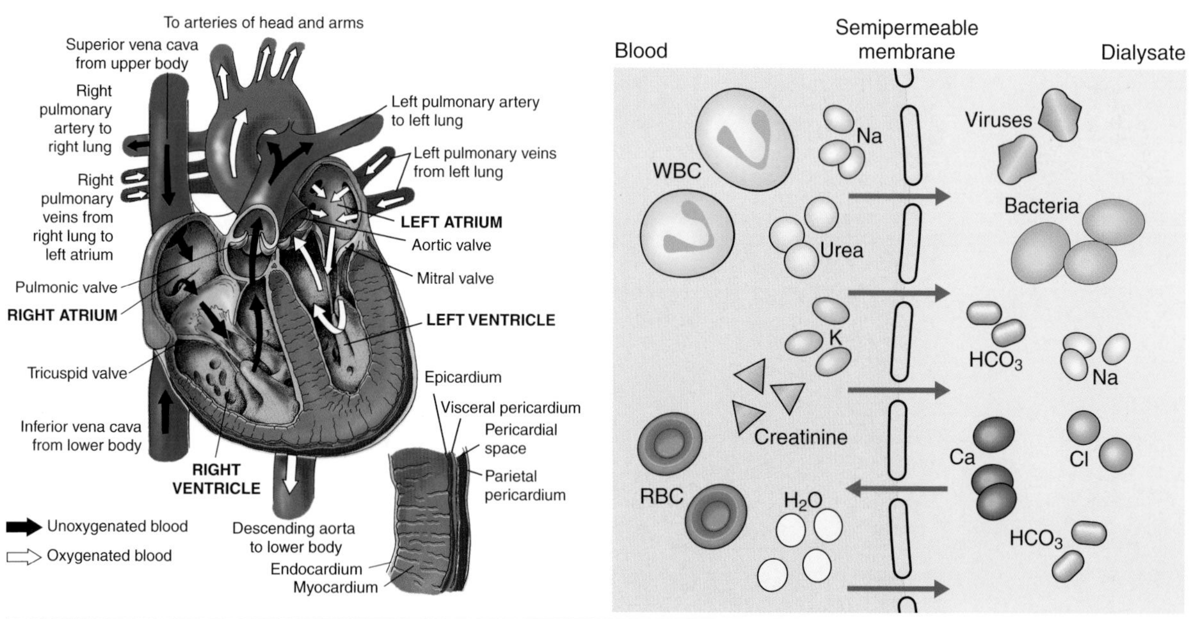

Plate 4: *Reprinted with permission from Aehlert B:* ECGs made easy, *ed 2, St Louis, 2002, Mosby (page 209).*
Plate 5: *Reprinted with permission from Ignatavicus, Workman:* Medical-surgical nursing: critical thinking for collaborative care, *ed 4, Philadelphia, 2002, WB Saunders (page 620).*
Plate 6: *Reprinted with permission from Lewis, Heitkemper, Dirksen:* Medical-surgical nursing: assessment and management of clinical problems, *ed 5 St Louis, 2000, Mosby (page 1321).*

Plate 7: Integumentary Problems

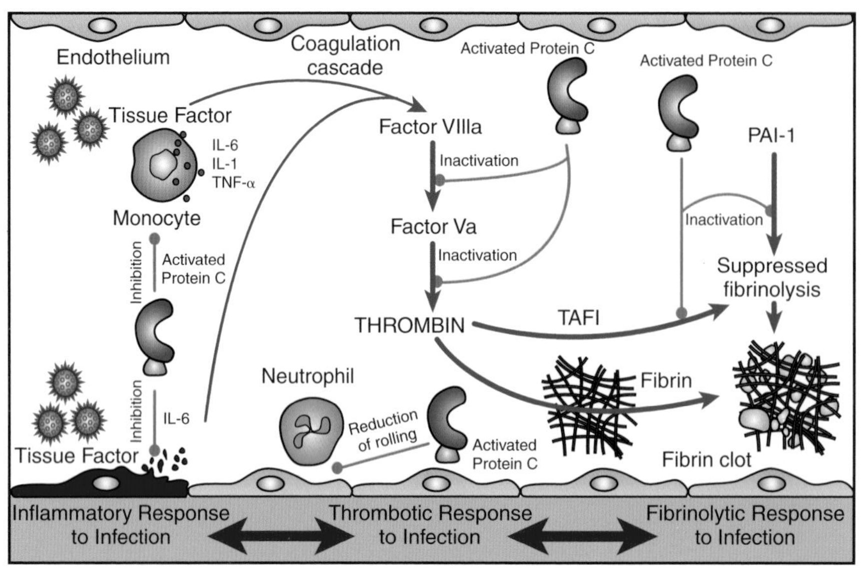

Plate 7: *Reprinted with permission from Lewis, Heitkemper, Dirksen:* Medical-surgical nursing: assessment and management of clinical problems, *ed 5, St Louis, 2000, Mosby (page 1321).*

Do You UNDERSTAND?

DIRECTIONS: **Complete the crossword puzzle on p. 240 using the clues listed below.**

Down

1. Endocrine cells that produce insulin, glucagon, and VIP are found in the islets of _____.
3. This drug can be prescribed to replace enzymes that are suppressed in cases of pancreatic insufficiency.
5. This takes place when pancreatic enzymes become prematurely activated while still inside the pancreas.
6. Pancreatic fluids enter the bowel from the head of the pancreas via the _____. (two words)
11. The trade name of the drug of choice for pain control.

Across

2. Chvostek's and Trousseau's signs indicate _____.
3. The main symptom in pancreatitis.
4. The abbreviation for therapy that supports nutritional status.
7. Pancreatic cells that produce exocrine secretions.
8. Describes the bulky, fatty, foul-smelling stool caused by the lack of enzymes needed to digest proteins, carbohydrates, and fats.
9. An anticholinergic used to decrease vagal stimulation, pancreatic secretion, and ampullary spasm.
10. Pancreatic _____ is caused by the malabsorption of nutrients in the small intestine.
12. Bleeding into the abdomen, caused by the death of pancreatic tissue, characterizes this type of pancreatitis.
13. A severe complication of pancreatitis that can appear weeks after the illness begins.
14. A common cause of death in acute pancreatitis.

Answers: *Down:* **1. Langerhans; 3. pancrelipase; 5. autodigestion; 6. pancreatic duct; 11. Demerol;** *Across:* **2. tetany; 3. pain; 4. TPN; 7. acini; 8. steatorrhea; 9. atropine; 10. insufficiency; 12. necrotizing; 13. pseudocyst; 14. infection.**

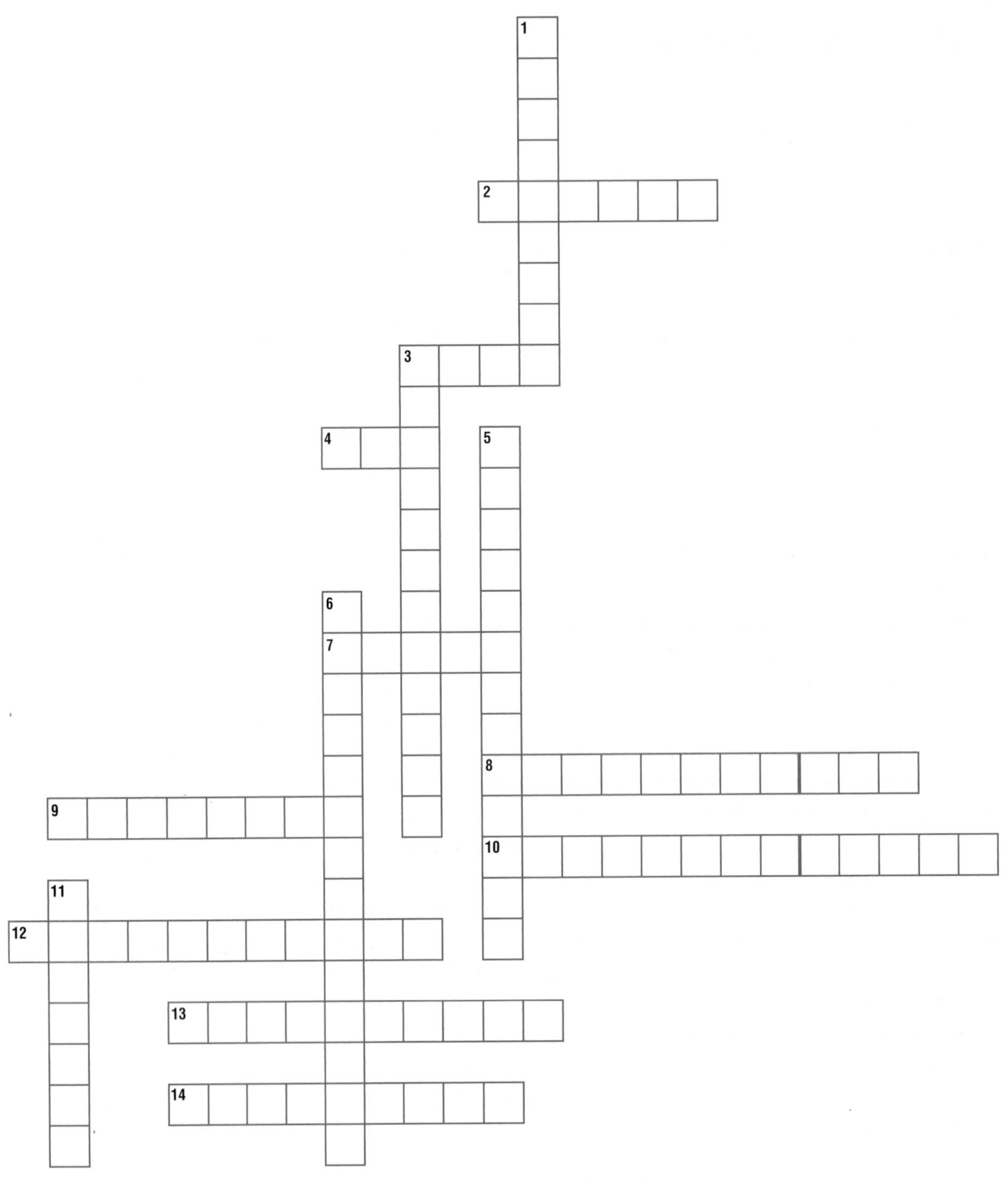
1
2
3
4
5
6
7
8
9
10
11
12
13
14

What IS Liver Failure?

Liver failure, also known as *hepatic failure,* is a condition in which the organ fails to fulfill its functions or is unable to meet the demands placed upon it. Acute diseases that cause sudden, massive hepatic destruction or chronic diseases that cause progressive hepatic damage can result in liver failure. Viral hepatitis, cirrhosis, benign or malignant neoplasms, biliary atresia, and primary or secondary cholangitis are examples of diseases that can lead to liver failure if their progression is not slowed or reversed. Liver failure can also be caused by the ingestion of toxic substances such as chemicals or overdoses of medications. Liver disease and subsequent liver failure can occur in any age group, from neonates to geriatric patients.

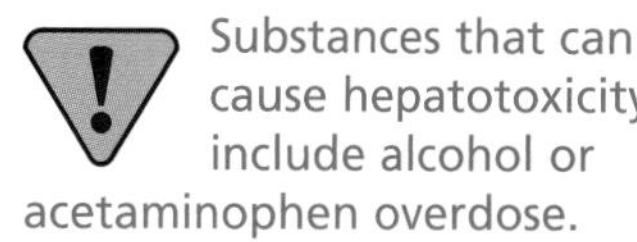
Substances that can cause hepatotoxicity include alcohol or acetaminophen overdose.

What You NEED TO KNOW

The first step in caring for a patient with liver disease is to understand the liver's functions. This foundational knowledge helps the nurse understand why clinical signs and symptoms occur and the rationale for treatment.

The liver is the largest solid organ in the body. The organ is located primarily in the right upper quadrant of the abdomen. A portion of the liver's left lobe extends into the left upper abdominal quadrant. The liver functions as a digestive, endocrine, hematologic, and excretory organ. The liver carries out more than 400 functions. Primary functions of the liver include storage and filtration of blood; bile production and metabolism; bilirubin elimination; carbohydrate, fat, and protein metabolism; storage of glycogen and fat; conversion of ammonia to urea; production of clotting factors and removal of activated clotting factors; metabolism of sex hormones; inactivation of aldosterone and antidiuretic hormones (ADHs); detoxification of drugs and foreign substances; and vitamin and mineral storage. The liver is composed of five parts: (1) the circulatory system, (2) the lobule and hepatocytes, (3) the reticuloendothelial system (RES), (4) the hepatobiliary system, and (5) the connective tissue structure.

The liver has a dual blood supply. Both the hepatic artery and portal vein supply the liver. Arterial flow enters the hepatic artery via the celiac trunk of the aorta. The portal vein carries blood, enriched with nutrients

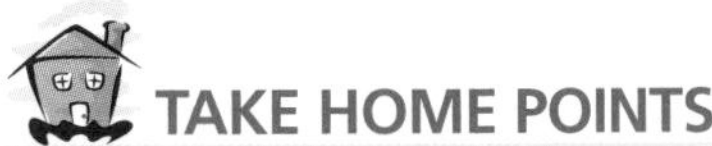

TAKE HOME POINTS

The key to the prevention of liver failure is early recognition and treatment of the underlying disease process.

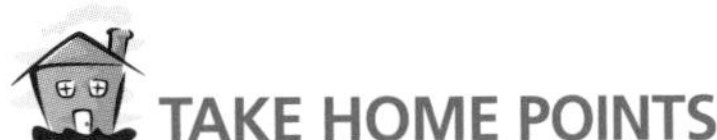

TAKE HOME POINTS

The most common cause of hepatitis is viral. Six types of viral hepatitis are A, B, C, D, E, and G.

and metabolic products, from capillaries in the stomach, small and large intestines, pancreas, and spleen to the liver. Blood is removed from the liver via the hepatic veins. The hepatic veins empty into the inferior vena cava. The liver is a highly vascular organ and contains about 25% of the body's total CO. Normal blood flow through the liver approximates 1500 mL/min.

The work of the liver is accomplished in the functional unit, the *lobule.* The lobule is composed of hepatocytes, arterioles and venules, sinusoids, Kupffer's cells, and bile canniculi. The liver's dual blood supply comes together in the sinusoid. Here the oxygenated arterial blood and the metabolic enriched venous blood are processed by the hepatocytes and the many functions of the liver are carried out. Kupffer's cells, which are a part of the reticuloendothelial system, line the walls of the sinusoids. The function of the Kupffer's cells is to phagocytize bacteria, foreign materials, and toxins. The bile canniculi are responsible for the transport of bile salts and pigments through the liver lobule to the gallbladder where the substances are stored.

The second step in caring for a patient with liver disease is to understand the diseases, both acute and chronic, that can lead to liver failure. Hepatitis is an inflammation of the liver cells caused by a viral or bacterial infection or toxic substances. If the inflammatory process is not reversed, liver cells are damaged and die. Hepatitis can be acute or chronic. Chronic hepatitis is an inflammation of the liver that lasts 6 months or longer. The mode of transmission, symptoms, and treatment differ among the many types of hepatitis.

Biliary diseases that can lead to liver failure include biliary atresia and sclerosing cholangitis. Biliary atresia is a pediatric disorder characterized by the congenital absence or underdevelopment of one or more of the biliary structures. As the condition progresses, jaundice, portal hypertension, biliary cirrhosis, and liver failure can result. Surgery is the recommended treatment for atresia. Sclerosing cholangitis is an inflammation of the bile ducts. The inflammation is brought about by a bacterial infection or an obstruction of the bile ducts from tumor or stones. If allowed to go untreated, the problem can lead to liver failure. Sclerosing cholangitis is treated with antibiotics and surgical intervention for obstruction.

Cirrhosis is a chronic, progressive, irreversible disease. The progression of cirrhosis can be slowed by treatment of the causative factors. Four classifications of cirrhosis based on the various causative agents are (1) alcoholic (Laennec's), (2) biliary, (3) cardiac, and (4) postnecrotic. A chronic inflammatory process causes disruption in the liver's blood and biliary flow, which results in hepatocyte damage and the formation of fibrotic tissue. The normal liver architecture is replaced with fibrotic, nodular scar tissue. The fibrosis and cellular damage of cirrhosis can lead to subsequent liver failure.

Other diseases that can lead to liver failure include Budd-Chiari syndrome, Crigler-Najjar syndrome, and cystic fibrosis. Budd-Chiari syndrome is characterized by obstruction of the hepatic vein, preventing outflow of blood from the liver. Cystic fibrosis is a genetic disease that can result in pancreatic fibrosis, biliary obstruction, hepatitis, and cirrhosis, all of which can lead to liver failure. Crigler-Najjar syndrome, a genetic disease characterized by severe unconjugated hyperbilirubinemia in the neonate, can lead to severe neurologic consequences and liver failure if not treated.

FIRST-LINE AND INITIAL TREATMENTS FOR LIVER DISEASE

- Understand the liver's functions.
- Understand the underlying diseases.
- Understand the clinical manifestations.

The third step in providing care for the liver failure patient is to understand the clinical manifestations of the liver failure. Initial symptoms of liver failure are vague; they include malaise, weakness, fatigue, exhaustion, loss of appetite, weight loss, abdominal discomfort, nausea, and vomiting. Progression of the disease brings about more severe, specific symptoms with systemic effects. These symptoms include jaundice, coagulopathies, fluid and electrolyte imbalances, nutritional deficiencies, portal hypertension, varices, ascites, hepatic encephalopathy, infections, and hepatorenal syndrome.

The pathway for the development of jaundice is complex. It begins when old or damaged RBCs are broken down by the reticuloendothelial system. Bilirubin is a product of hemoglobin breakdown. Bilirubin is released into the circulation and binds to albumin. In this form, bilirubin is called *unconjugated bilirubin.* Unconjugated bilirubin enters the liver via the general circulation. In the liver, bilirubin undergoes a process called *conjugation.* Conjugation changes bilirubin from a lipid-soluble product to a water-soluble product. In this form, bilirubin can be excreted. The liver then excretes conjugated bilirubin through the bile ducts. Bilirubin is moved through the biliary system as a component of

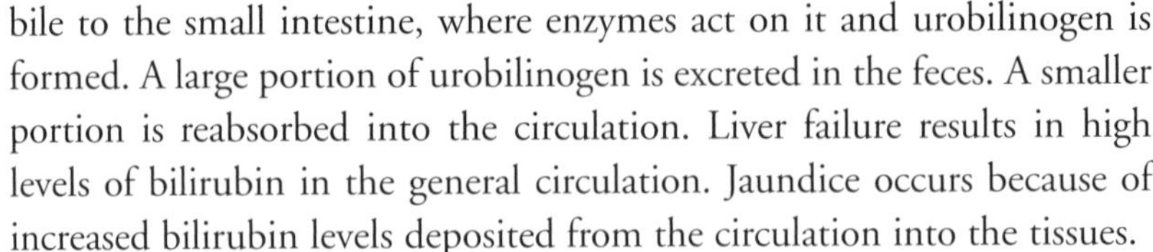

bile to the small intestine, where enzymes act on it and urobilinogen is formed. A large portion of urobilinogen is excreted in the feces. A smaller portion is reabsorbed into the circulation. Liver failure results in high levels of bilirubin in the general circulation. Jaundice occurs because of increased bilirubin levels deposited from the circulation into the tissues.

TAKE HOME POINTS

Signs and symptoms of liver failure are seen when the liver's functions cannot be carried out or are impaired.

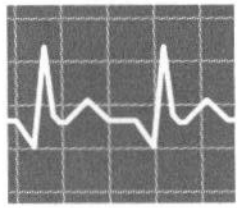

Bilirubin stains the tissues and causes a yellowish discoloration of the skin, mucous membranes, and sclera. Excess bilirubin in the general circulation is also filtered out by the kidneys and results in brownish, yellow-colored urine.

Acute renal failure can occur in association with liver failure. A decrease in renal blood flow and GFR and increased levels of aldosterone are thought to be the underlying causes. Hepatorenal syndrome is characterized by progressive azotemia, elevated serum creatinine levels, and oliguria. Treatment includes the administration of fluids and diuretics to improve renal blood flow, GFR, and urine output. Hemodialysis may be needed to support the kidneys while the underlying cause of the liver failure is treated.

TAKE HOME POINTS

Hepatorenal syndrome is renal failure that occurs in conjunction with liver failure.

Ascites is the accumulation of fluid within the peritoneal cavity. It is complicated by portal hypertension, hypoalbuminemia, and the inactivation of the hormones aldosterone and ADH. With liver failure, aldosterone and ADH are inactivated. The inactivation of aldosterone signals the kidneys, via the renin-angiotensin system, to hold on to sodium and water and excrete potassium. The inactivation of ADH results in additional fluid retention. The excess volume in the vascular space results in a hyperdynamic state. The excess volume cannot be maintained in the interstitial space because of the kidneys' inability to metabolize proteins. Albumin is responsible for maintaining colloid osmotic pressure in the vascular system. In the absence of albumin, fluids from the vascular system cross over into the interstitial space. The result is edema and ascites. With the loss of fluid from the vascular space, the kidneys sense a decreased blood volume and through the renin-angiotensin system signal the release of aldosterone. A problematic cycle is established through fluid retention in the vascular space (inactivation of aldosterone and ADH), loss of fluid into the interstitial space (inability of liver to metabolize protein resulting in hypoalbuminemia), fluid collection in the interstitial space (edema and ascites), and the body's own homeostatic mechanisms (renin-angiotensin system), which sense the loss of fluid from the vascular space and signal the kidneys to hold on to more sodium and water. Significant accumulation of ascitic fluids in the peritoneal cavity can cause abdominal organ compression and discomfort, respiratory compromise (because of pressure on the diaphragm), and impaired skin integrity. The treatment of ascites involves the restriction of sodium, bedrest, and pharmacologic therapy with diuretics. Abdominal paracentesis is another treatment modality.

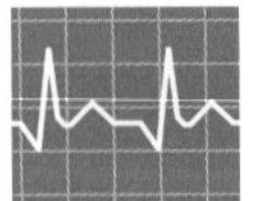

Monitoring of renal function via diagnostic tests and urine output is needed for persons in liver failure.

Paracentesis is accomplished by the insertion of a needle into the peritoneal cavity. Peritoneal (ascitic) fluid is then withdrawn. Abdominal paracentesis is used for the analysis of ascitic fluids and as a temporary relief measure for worsening or severe symptoms. LeVeen and Denver shunts have also been used for the treatment of ascites that has been refractory to medical management. The shunts use a pressure gradient or pump pressure to move ascitic fluid from the peritoneum into the general circulation. The excess fluid is then excreted via the kidneys.

Portal hypertension is a result of impaired blood flow caused by tissue damage and fibrosis. Increased pressure within the portal circulation; impaired blood flow to the liver; and slowed, congested circulation from the portal vein are the results. Splenomegaly can be a consequence of the increased pressure.

Esophageal, anterior stomach, and rectal veins are also affected. The veins become engorged, distended, and susceptible to hemorrhage as result of the increased pressure within the portal circulation. The distended veins are known as *varices.* Distended esophageal veins result in esophageal varices; distended rectal veins produce hemorrhoids. Rupture of the friable veins can result in life-threatening GI hemorrhage. Treatment of varices

Leveen shunt to treat ascites

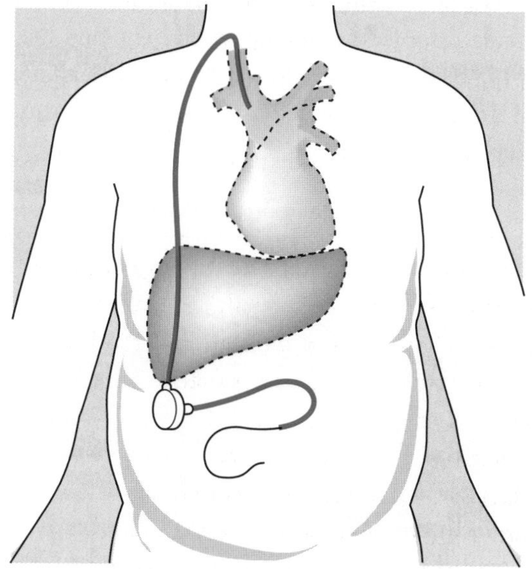

(From Sole ML, Lamborn ML, Hartshorn JC: Introduction to critical care nursing, *ed 3, Philadelphia, 2001, WB Saunders.)*

focuses on the reduction of portal pressures through the use of pharmacologic therapy, endoscopic procedures, and balloon tamponade.

If the treatment modalities do not effectively manage the esophageal varices, then radiographic or surgical intervention is considered. The radiographic procedure involves the placement of a stent that creates a portosystemic shunt. Surgical techniques to reduce portal hypertension include the placement of portacaval, mesocaval, or splenorenal shunts. The shunts divert blood flow and thus reduce portal pressures.

Hepatic *encephalopathy* is a term used for the CNS manifestations of liver failure. A range of symptoms from confusion to coma is seen. The cause of encephalopathy is not known. The cause is thought to be the inability of the liver to convert ammonia to urea. Protein is broken down in the GI tract. Ammonia is a product of protein metabolism. Ammonia ions diffuse from the GI tract into the circulation and are transported to the liver for conversion to urea. When the liver cells are unable to perform the conversion, ammonia levels build up. Elevated ammonia levels in the circulation have a neurotoxic effect on the CNS. The clinical signs of hepatic encephalopathy are defined in four progressively worsening stages.

Treatment of hepatic encephalopathy involves the reduction of ammonia levels. This is accomplished by dietary and pharmacologic means. Protein intake is reduced to 20 to 40 g per day. Neomycin and lactulose are used to reduce the breakdown of protein by bacteria. Neomycin reduces the normal bowel flora. Lactulose creates an acidic environment in the bowel that prevents ammonia from leaving the colon and entering the bloodstream. Lactulose also exhibits a laxative effect and eliminates ammonia from the GI tract, but it must be administered carefully because it can contribute to intravascular depletion.

Asterixis in hepatic encephalopathy

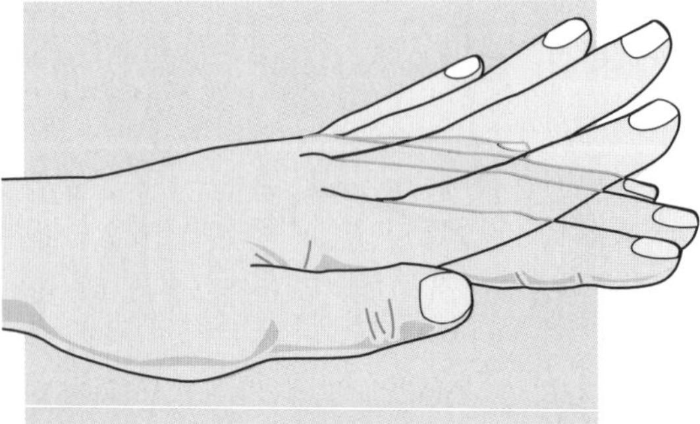

(From Ignatavicus DD, Workman ML: Medical-surgical nursing: critical thinking for collaborative care, *ed 4, Philadelphia, 2002, WB Saunders.)*

Stages of Hepatic Encephalopathy

Stage	Symptoms
Stage I	Tremors Slurred speech Impaired decision making
Stage II	Drowsiness Loss of sphincter control Asterixis
Stage III	Dramatic confusion Somnolence
Stage IV	Coma Unresponsiveness

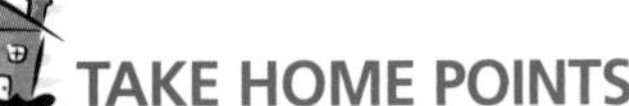

TAKE HOME POINTS

All treatment modalities for varices have side effects and potential complications that can worsen or complicate the liver failure condition.

Neomycin has a high risk of nephrotoxicity and is not specifically recommended.

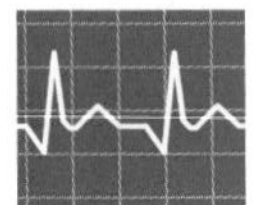

Asterixis is a hand-flapping tremor induced by extending the arm and dorsiflexing the wrist.

Carbohydrate, fat, and protein metabolism are affected by liver failure. When the blood glucose level exceeds the body's needs, excess glucose is converted to glycogen and stored in the liver. This is a process called *glycogenesis.* When the body needs glucose, glycogen is released from storage and used for energy. This is called *glycogenolysis.* If glycogen levels are used up, the liver uses amino acids and fats for energy via a process called *gluconeogenesis.* In liver failure, the organ is unable to effectively convert glucose to glycogen and use fats for gluconeogenesis. As a result, the body has no means for creating energy stores, and problems associated with meeting cellular energy needs develop. The clinical result is hypoglycemia, fatigue, weight loss, and malnutrition. The liver also metabolizes fats. The end results of fat digestion are fatty acids, glycerol, and cholesterol. In the liver, the metabolic substances are converted to the lipoproteins (LDL, HDL, and VLDL). When the process is interrupted, as with liver failure, fat accumulates in the liver, a condition known as *fatty liver.* The fat accumulation impairs the ability of the liver to carry out its functions. The liver produces three major plasma proteins: (1) albumin, (2) globulin, and (3) fibrinogen. Albumin maintains plasma oncotic pressure. Oncotic pressure helps hold fluids in the vascular space and prevents them from leaking out into the interstitial space, causing edema. Globulins promote cellular enzyme reactions, and fibrinogen plays an important role in coagulation and the establishment of hemostasis. Additional protein clotting factors II, V, VII, VIII, IX, and X are not synthesized by the failing liver. Liver failure patients who are unable to metabolize fibrinogen and synthesize clotting factors have a range of symptoms from petechiae, ecchymosis, bleeding from oral mucous, and nosebleeds to massive hemorrhage. Disseminated intravascular coagulation (DIC) can result from the inability of the liver to metabolize fibrinogen and other clotting factors. In the presence of liver failure, the lack of plasma protein production and metabolism can lead to edema, loss of certain cellular enzyme reactions, and coagulopathies.

Liver failure patients may exhibit problems with clotting abnormalities because the liver produces clotting factors.

Another problem with protein metabolism is the failed liver's inability to convert ammonia, an end product of protein metabolism, into urea. The increase in ammonia levels in turn affects the nervous system and skin (see the section on hepatic encephalopathy). A sign of abnormal protein metabolism is fetor hepaticus, which is characterized as a very sweet, acetone-like breath.

The liver also metabolizes and is a storage bank for vitamins A, B, D, K, and E. Vitamin K is necessary for the synthesis of clotting factors II,

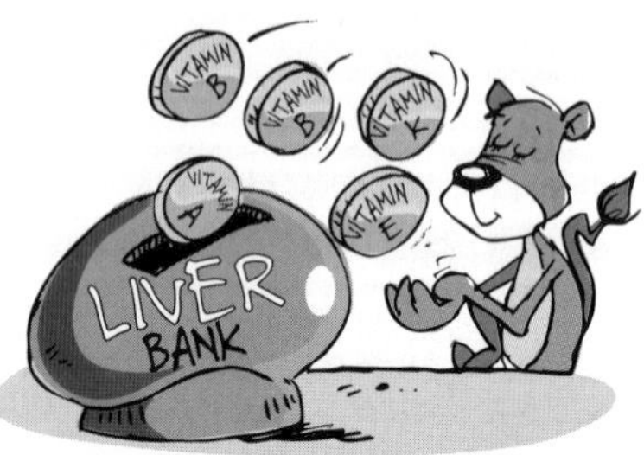

Vitamins are stored in the liver.

VII, VIII and X. Vitamin deficiencies and subsequent nutritional problems result from liver failure.

The liver plays a role in protecting the rest of the body from bacterial invasion, toxic substances, and poisons. Enzymes found in the liver metabolize a high percentage of drugs. Liver failure slows or stops the ability to filter medications from the blood and prolongs the duration of their action or their potentiated action. Kupffer's cells filter out bacteria. The loss of Kupffer's cell function can result in infection and sepsis.

The liver's inability to metabolize hormones can result in dermatologic lesions and changes in sexual characteristics or function. Dermatologic lesions such as vascular nevi (spiders), telangiectasias, and spider angiomas can be seen on the upper part of the body. Changes in male sexual characteristics such as testicular atrophy, gynecomastia, and decreased pubic or facial hair are seen. Sexual dysfunction in the form of impotence can also occur.

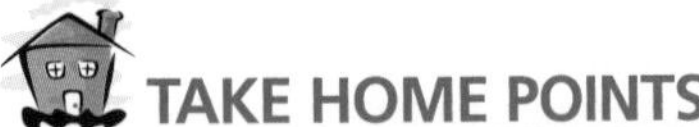

TAKE HOME POINTS

- Bile is a necessary component of fat digestion and absorption. The liver is responsible for bile synthesis. When the liver is unable to synthesize bile, fats are excreted and cannot be used as an energy source.
- The skin becomes itchy because of ammonia irritation of the skin cells.

The liver is a highly vascular organ and, as previously mentioned, the inactivation of aldosterone and ADH results in a hyperdynamic state because of an increased intravascular volume. Palmar erythema, redness of the palms of the hands, may be seen in association with a high CO and the hyperdynamic state. It is also thought to be associated with increased levels of circulating estrogens.

Diagnostic Tests

A number of diagnostic tests are used to determine the cause of liver disease, the range of complications, and the extent of organ damage. In liver failure, the liver enzymes, alkaline phosphatase, aspartate transaminase, and alanine transaminase, are elevated. Serum protein levels such as albumin are decreased. Clotting factors including prothrombin time (PT) and partial thromboplastin time (PTT) are elevated and prolonged. Serum ammonia, total bilirubin, and conjugated and unconjugated bilirubin levels are elevated. Urine bilirubin and urobilinogen elevations also occur. Electrolytes are monitored for alterations in serum glucose, sodium, and potassium. The CBC is assessed for anemia and infection. ABGs are obtained to assess the patient's acid-base status and for potential ventilatory problems. Stools and gastric samples should be assessed for the presence of blood (guaiac positive). Liver biopsy, ultrasound, CT scans, and MRI can be prescribed to determine the underlying cause of liver failure. A combination of history, clinical signs and symptoms, and diagnostic tools will help the medical team diagnose liver disease and determine whether the disease has progressed to the point of organ failure.

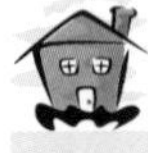

TAKE HOME POINTS

In patients with a high likelihood/suspicion of sepsis or systemic inflammatory response syndrome (SIRS) (temperature > 38° C or < 36° C, WBC > 12,000 or < 4000, HR > 90), prophylactic antibiotics also might be prescribed because these patients are already immunocompromised.

What You DO

The treatment of liver failure centers on the identification of the cause of liver disease, interventions to correct the cause or slow progression, and the provision of supportive therapy. Supportive therapy includes the correction of fluid and electrolyte abnormalities, nutritional support, elimination of hepatotoxins, and prevention and treatment of complications.

Patients with end-stage liver disease have few treatment options for cure. Transplantation is one possible option. Transplant criteria include the presence of an acute or chronic liver disease for which all forms of therapy have failed. Potential transplant candidates must undergo physiologic and psychologic evaluation to determine whether transplant is a viable treatment option. Survival rates are 85% at the end of 1 year and 70% at 5 years. Limitations of this treatment modality are the shortage of organs.

Clinical trials are in process to determine if extracorporeal liver assist devices can maintain a patient while the underlying cause of liver failure is treated, or whether the device can be used as a bridge to support the patient until a donor organ can be found.

The care of a patient with liver failure presents a clinical challenge for the nurse because of the complexity of liver functions and the systemic ramifications of liver failure. The nurse's role in the care of a patient with liver failure includes patient assessment, monitoring, documentation, reporting of patient responses to diagnostic and treatment plans, observation for complications, supportive care, and patient and family teaching. Consistent systems assessments; monitoring of vital signs, intake, and output; measurement of hemodynamic parameters; and documentation of findings to identify complications or a worsening condition are the foundations of care. Laboratory values are obtained, assessed, and monitored. Nutritional assessment and support is necessary. Dermatologic assessment should include observing for bruising, petechiae, itching, spider angiomas, edema, and pressure ulcer formations. Pressure reduction measures should be prophylactically established. For patients with ascites, the head of the bed should be elevated to reduce fluid pressure exerted on the diaphragm and to promote lung expansion. The patient should be assessed for any signs and symptoms of pleural effusions and monitored for signs of inadequate hemostasis. Testing of stool and gastric contents by guaiac should occur. Bleeding precautions should be implemented because of the coagulopathies associated with liver failure. Neurologic assessments are needed to identify hepatic encephalopathy and whether the condition had progressed. Medications that are metabolized by the liver should be minimized. If these medications

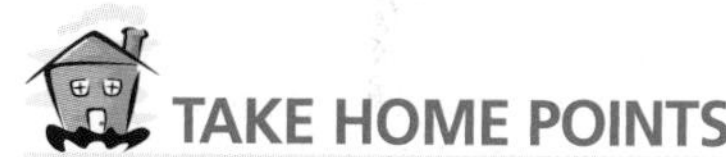

Signs and symptoms of pleural effusion include cough, dysphea, and pleuritic chest pain.

cannot be eliminated and are necessary for the patient, the multidisciplinary team should be consulted for dose review and adjustment. Discussion with the patient, family, or both on the treatment plan and options for treatment is required. The establishment of advanced directives should be accomplished and possible end-of-life decisions discussed.

Do You UNDERSTAND?

DIRECTIONS: Match the descriptions in Column A with appropriate symptoms of liver failure in Column B.

Column A

_____1. Progressive azotemia, elevated serum creatinine levels, and oliguria

_____2. A yellowish discoloration of the skin, mucous membranes, and sclera

_____3. Fluid accumulated within the peritoneal cavity

_____4. Engorged, distended veins caused by increased pressure within the portal circulation

_____5. Coma caused by inability of liver to convert ammonia to urea

Column B

a. Hepatorenal syndrome
b. Ascites
c. Jaundice
d. Varices
e. Hepatic encephalopathy

DIRECTIONS: Identify the following statements as *true* (T) or *false* (F).

_____ 6. Cirrhosis is a reversible disease process.

_____ 7. Stage IV of hepatic encephalopathy is characterized by coma and unresponsiveness.

_____ 8. The functional unit of the liver is the hepatocyte.

_____ 9. Alcohol and acetaminophen are substances that can cause hepatotoxicity.

_____10. In a patient with hepatic encephalopathy, the nurse would expect to find an elevated serum ammonia level.

_____11. Liver transplant survival rates are 50% or less at the end of 1 year.

Answers: 1. a; 2. c; 3. b; 4. d; 5. e; 6. F; 7. T; 8. F; 9. T; 10. T; 11. F

References

Alspach JG: *American Association of Critical Care Nurses core curriculum for critical care nursing,* ed 6, St Louis, Saunders/Elsevier, 2006.

Barada K, Karrowni W, Abdallah M, Shamseddeen W, Sharara AI, Dakik HA: Upper gastrointestinal bleeding in patients with acute coronary syndromes clinical predictors and prophylactic role of proton pump inhibitors, *Journal of Clinical Gastroenterology,* 42(4):368-372, 2008.

Burke M: Acute intestinal obstruction: diagnosis and management, *Hospital Medicine,* 63(2):104, 2002.

Burkill G, Bell J, Healy J: Small bowel obstruction: the role of computed tomography in its diagnosis and management with reference to other imaging modalities, *European Radiology,* 11(8):1405, 2001.

Chulay M, Burns SM: *American Association of Critical Care Nurses essentials of critical care nursing,* New York, 2006, *McGraw Hill.*

Dauphne CE, et al: Placement of self-expanding metal stents for acute malignant large-bowel obstruction: a collective review, *Annals of Surgical Oncology,* 9(6):74, 2002.

Davis MP, Nouneh C: Modern management of cancer-related intestinal obstruction, *Current Pain and Headache Reports,* 5(3):257, 2001.

De Giorgio R, et al: Review article: the pharmacologic treatment of acute colonic pseudo-obstruction, *Alimentary Pharmacology & Therapeutics,* 15(11):1717, 2001.

Diaz JJ, Bokhari F, Mowery NT, Acosta JA, Block EF, Bromberg WJ, et al: Guidelines for management of small bowel obstruction, *The Journal of Trauma Injury, Infection and Critical Care,* 64(6):1651-1664, 2008.

Edlich RE, Woods JA: Wangensteen's transformation of the treatment of intestinal obstruction from empiric craft to scientific discipline, *Journal of Emergency Medicine,* 15(2):235, 1997.

Fischer CP, Doherty D: Laparoscopic approach to small bowel obstruction, *Seminars in Laparoscopic Surgery,* 9(1):40, 2002.

Fleshner PR, et al: A prospective, randomized trial of short versus long tubes in adhesive small-bowel obstruction, *American Journal of Surgery,* 170(4):366, 1995.

Frager D: Intestinal obstruction role of CT, *Gastroenterology Clinics of North America,* 31(3):777, 2002.

Furukawa A, et al: Helical CT in the diagnosis of small bowel obstruction, *Radiographics,* 21(2):341, 2001.

Morton PG, Fontaine DK, Hudak CM, Gallo BM: *Critical care nursing: a holistic approach,* ed 8, Philadelphia, Lippincott Williams & Wilkins, 2004.

Onoue S, et al: The value of contrast radiology for postoperative adhesive bowel obstruction, *Hepatogastroenterology,* 49(48):1576, 2002.

Platt V: Malignant bowel obstruction: so much more than symptom control, *International Journal of Palliative Nursing,* 7(11):547, 2001.

Ripamonti C, Bruera E: Palliative management of malignant bowel obstruction, *International Journal of Gynecological Cancer,* 12:135, 2002.

Sharma PK, Madan K, Garg PK: Hemorrhage in acute pancreatitis: should gastrointestinal bleeding be considered an organ failure? *Pancreas,* 36(2), 141-145, 2008.

Singh S, Gagneja HK: Stents in the small intestine, *Current Gastroenterology Reports,* 4(5):383, 2002.

Siow E: Enteral versus parenteral nutrition for acute pancreatitis. *Critical Care Nurse,* 28(4),19-31, 2008.

Sole ML, Klein DG, Moseley MJ: *Introduction to critical care nursing,* ed 4, St Louis, 2005, Elsevier, Saunders.

Stravitz RT, Kramer AH, Davern T, Shaikh OS, Caldwell SH, Mehta RL, et al: Intensive care patients with acute liver failure: recommendations of the U.S. Acute Liver Failure Study Group, *Critical Care Medicine,* 35(11):2498-2508, 2007.

Taourel P, et al: Non-traumatic abdominal emergencies: imaging of acute intestinal obstruction, *European Radiology,* 12(9):2151, 2002.

Urden LD, Stacy KM, Lough ME: Thelan's critical care nursing diagnosis and management, ed 5, St Louis, Elsevier, 2006.

NCLEX® Review

1. A patient is admitted to the hospital with the diagnosis of peptic ulcer disease. The patient develops a sudden, sharp pain in the midepigastric region of the abdomen. The abdomen is rigid and boardlike. The clinical manifestations most likely indicates:
   1 The ulcer has perforated.
   2 Additional ulcers have formed.
   3 The patient has hemorrhagic shock.
   4 An intestinal obstruction has developed.

2. A patient has been diagnosed with chronic gastritis caused by *Helicobacter pylori.* The nurse anticipates that the patient will be administered which medications?
   1 Antacids.
   2 Mucosal protectant agents.
   3 Histamine 2–receptor antagonists.
   4 Antibiotic combinations.

3. Which diagnostic tool is used in patients with peptic ulcer disease and provides direct visualization of the gastrointestinal tract and the bleeding site?
   1 Endoscopy.
   2 Angiography.
   3 Radionuclide scanning.
   4 Barium enema.

4. The patient arrives at the emergency department with nausea and bloody vomitus that has occurred for the past 48 hours. Which acid-base imbalance would you expect to find when laboratory results return?
   1 Respiratory acidosis.
   2 Respiratory alkalosis.
   3 Metabolic acidosis.
   4 Metabolic alkalosis.

5. The nurse is completing dietary teaching for the patient recovering from an episode of gastrointestinal bleeding. The nurse explains to the patient that he or she will be able to eat:
   1 High-protein, low-fat foods.
   2 Any foods that are tolerated.
   3 Low-calorie, low-fat foods.
   4 High-fiber foods.

6. The nurse is caring for a patient who was admitted with massive gastrointestinal bleeding. The nurse assesses the patient and notes the following: tachycardia, decrease in urine output to less than 30 mL/hr, skin cool to the touch, and pallor. The nurse believes these symptoms are associated with:
   1 Cardiogenic shock.
   2 Neurogenic shock.
   3 Distributive shock.
   4 Hemorrhagic shock.

7. The endocrine cells reside in the:
   1 Acini cells.
   2 Islets of Langerhans.
   3 Duodenum.
   4 Liver.

8. The main symptom of acute pancreatitis is:
   1 Nausea and vomiting.
   2 Severe pain.
   3 Elevated lipase and amylase serum levels.
   4 Hypocalcemia or hypercalcemia.

9. Which of the following is a nursing diagnosis for the patient with pancreatitis?
   1 Imbalanced nutrition: more than body requirements.
   2 Excess fluid volume.
   3 Ineffective tissue perfusion: peripheral.
   4 Potential for hemorrhage.

10. In chronic pancreatitis, diabetes may develop as a result of:
    1 Shock.
    2 Effects of the disease on the islets of Langerhans.
    3 Secondary infection.
    4 The formation of fibrous tissue that replaces healthy acini tissue.

NCLEX® Review Answers

1.1 Complications of peptic ulcer disease include hemorrhagic shock, perforation, and obstruction. Perforation occurs when an erosion of all the layers of the gastrointestinal (GI) wall occurs and the contents of the GI tract spill into the peritoneum. The result is an inflammatory process known as peritonitis. Sudden onset of abdominal pain; a rigid, boardlike abdomen; nausea and vomiting; fever; tachycardia; hypotension; and paralytic ileus can result. No signs of hemorrhage or bleeding are observed to indicate hemorrhagic shock. An obstruction has no bowel sounds.

2.4 Patients with *Helicobacter pylori* infection are treated with antibiotics. Antibiotics are used in combination to minimize the potential for bacterial resistance. Antacids, mucosal protectant agents, and histamine 2–receptor antagonists are used in the pharmacologic management of peptic ulcer disease. However, when *H. pylori* is identified as the cause of the ulcer, antibiotics are the most appropriate therapy.

3.1 Endoscopy is the diagnostic tool that provides direct visualization of the gastrointestinal (GI) tract and bleeding site. Radiographic studies such as barium enemas do not allow for direct visualization of the GI tract. Angiography and radionuclide scanning are used to identify the site of a bleeding vessel.

4.4 Metabolic alkalosis results from the loss of hydrogen ions when vomiting. Metabolic acidosis, respiratory acidosis, and respiratory alkalosis are not associated with vomiting and the loss of hydrogen ions.

5.2 When a patient is recovering from a gastrointestinal (GI) bleeding episode, the diet is prescribed as tolerated. No specific diet prescriptions are recommended for patients who are recovering from GI bleeding. The diet is geared to the treatment of the underlying cause of the bleeding.

6.4 The symptoms of tachycardia—decrease in urine output to less than 30 mL/hr, skin cool to the touch, confusion, and pallor—are indicative of hemorrhagic shock. Hemorrhagic shock is characterized by a decrease in preload to the heart (as a result of massive blood loss) and an associated reduction in CO. Hemorrhagic shock results in the inability of the body to meet cellular needs. The body responds by increasing the heart rate (tachycardia), shunting blood to the cerebral and cardiovascular systems (and away from the integumentary system), cooling the skin, producing a pallor to the skin, and decreasing urine output. Cardiogenic shock is caused by direct pump failure, neurogenic shock is paralysis and bradycardia, and distributive shock occurs with sympathetic stimulation causing vasodilation.

7.2 Endocrine cells, found in the islets of Langerhans, produce several hormones that pass directly into the bloodstream. Exocrine secretions are produced by the acini cells, which are then received by the duodenum. The liver drains bile into the bowel.

8.2 The main symptom is found in one of four patients with acute pancreatitis. Nausea and vomiting are specific to many gastrointestinal disorders. Normal levels of lipase and amylase serum appear in chronic cases of pancreatitis; consequently, elevated lipase and amylase serum levels are not specific for diagnosis. Hypocalcemia and hypercalcemia are found in chronic pancreatitis when islets of Langerhans cells malfunction and glucose levels are unable to be maintained.

9.4 As the pancreas digests itself, bleeding results and the patient has the potential to exhibit signs and symptoms of hypovolemic shock. Nutrition at a level less than the body requires occurs as a result of enzymatic dysfunction. No hypervolemia occurs as a result of hemorrhage. No peripheral tissue perfusion is found in the patient with pancreatitis.

10.2 Diabetes develops when the islets of Langerhans are no longer able to produce hormones necessary to maintain proper glucose levels. Shock occurs when circulating blood volume is low. Because of a susceptibility of infection as a result of pancreatic necrosis, secondary infection may appear after the acute attack subsides. The formation of fibrous tissues that replaces healthy acini tissue refers to the formation of pseudocyst structures.

Chapter 8 Renal System

What You WILL LEARN

After reading this chapter, you will know how to do the following:

- ✔ Differentiate between the various pathologic processes of acute tubular necrosis and chronic renal failure.
- ✔ Describe the physical manifestations associated with the various types of renal failure.
- ✔ Compare and contrast the various types of renal failure.
- ✔ Discuss the complications of renal failure.
- ✔ Identify appropriate nursing interventions for caring for a patient with renal failure and a patient receiving continuous renal replacement therapy.
- ✔ Describe prevention approaches that can be instituted in the critical care environment.
- ✔ Describe relevant patient education topics.

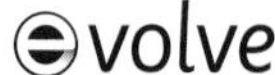

See http://evolve.elsevier.com/Schumacher/criticalcare for additional NCLEX® review questions.

What IS Acute Tubular Necrosis?

Acute tubular necrosis (ATN) is a term used to describe a form of acute renal failure (ARF) caused by ischemic (loss of blood supply) or nephrotoxic (chemical) injury. Although "necrosis" is part of the term, a more accurate wording would be acute tubular injury because cell death is not always a feature of the condition. Any hypotensive event can lead to ATN, with sepsis being the leading cause. Pathologic changes causing death of the tubular endothelium lead to obstructive sloughing by the dead cells, blocking the flow of filtrate. However, necrosis is not always present in ATN, and current research focuses on the roles of the inflammatory response, free radical production, retrograde blood flow, back leak, and apoptosis on tubule function. In fact, even in severe organ dysfunction, histologic changes can be minimal.

The cause of ATN varies because of the types of insults that lead to renal tubule injury. Recovery follows a predictable sequence of events, although prognoses vary. As a form of ARF, ATN can also be classified as prerenal (before the kidney), intrarenal (inside the kidney), and postrenal failure (after the kidney). Another way to classify ATN is by identifying whether the cause was ischemic or nephrotoxic.

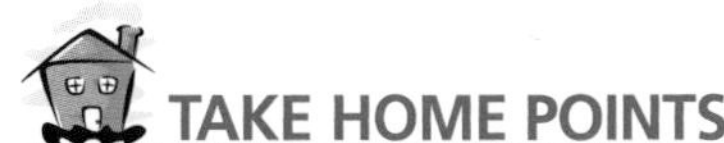

ATN is a type of ARF that follows a sequence of events.

What You NEED TO KNOW

ATN usually occurs after an acute ischemic or toxic event such as untreated prerenal failure (hypoperfusion) or the use of nephrotoxic medications (aminoglycosides) or contrast agents. ATN unfolds as a well-defined sequence of events that starts with an acute decrease in glomerular filtration rate (GFR). GFR is the amount of ultrafiltrate that passes through the glomerulus into the renal tubules. It is regulated by the amount of blood that circulates through the kidney, and is the key component of urine production. Normal GFR for the average adult is 125 mL/min. In the initial phase of ATN, the GFR drops to low levels, which leads to a decline in urine production, below 400 mL in 24 hours. As a result, sudden increases in serum creatinine and blood urea nitrogen (BUN) concentrations occur. The presence of abnormal levels of creatinine and BUN, nitrogenous byproducts of protein breakdown, is referred to as *azotemia.* The second phase, maintenance, is characterized by reduction and stabilization of GFR for a variable length of time but usually approximately 1 to 2 weeks. The BUN and creatinine continue to rise as a result of the sustained decreased GFR; however, there may be a slight improvement in urinary output. Recovery, the final phase in which tubular function and GFR are restored, is characterized by an increase in urine volume and gradual decrease in BUN and serum creatinine to preinjury levels. The following table summarizes the GFR, BUN, and creatinine levels occurring in each phase.

Summary of the Stages of Acute Tubular Necrosis

Initial Phase	Maintenance Phase	Recovery Phase
Hours to Days	*1 to 2 Weeks*	*Several Months to a Year*
• From acute insult to signs of injury	• Glomerular filtration rate (GFR) continues to decrease/stabilize	• Tubular function and GFR begin restoration
• Acute decreased GFR	• Increased blood urea nitrogen (BUN) and creatinine continue	• Increased urine production
• Urine production < 400 mL per 24 hours	• Increased urine production	• Gradual decrease in BUN and creatinine
• Increased BUN and creatinine		• Full recovery/renal insufficiency/dialysis

Ischemic Acute Tubular Necrosis

Ischemic ATN can result from prerenal and intrarenal blood flow problems. Risk factors for developing ATN include:

- Systemic vasodilation—sepsis, anaphylaxis, anesthesia, antihypertensives.
- Hypovolemia—dehydration, hemorrhage, burns, gastrointestinal (GI) and renal losses, dialysis, fluid questration (third spacing), surgery, trauma.
- Low cardiac output—heart failure, tamponade, mitral valve dysfunction, dysrhythmias.
- Renal vasoconstriction/hypoperfusion—abdominal compartment syndrome, hypercalcemia, hypertension, amphotericin B, cocaine, cyclosporine.
- Toxic injury—contrast media, rhabdomyolysis.
- Tubule obstruction—disseminated intravascular coagulation (DIC), transfusion reaction.

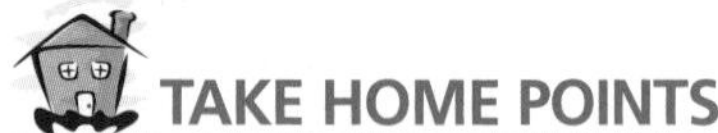

Any event or disease process that contributes to a decrease in renal blood flow can result in ischemic ATN.

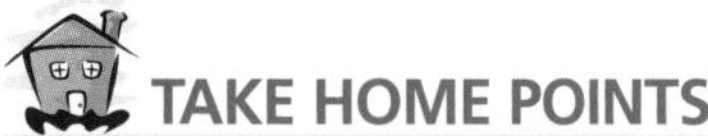

Due to the age-induced decreased GFR in the elderly, doses of medication for these patients may be lowered and/or infusion times prolonged.

The preexisting ability of the kidney to filter and clear toxins directly affects the chances of developing ATN.

Nephrotoxic Acute Tubular Necrosis

The kidney has a rich blood supply, receiving 25% of cardiac output, which makes it easily accessible to toxins. In addition, the kidney concentrates and clears toxins from the body. Toxins may be exogenous or endogenous.

Exogenous Nephrotoxins

Exogenous nephrotoxins originate from outside the body, often in the form of medications. The most common hospital nephrotoxins are aminoglycosides, amphotericin B, and contrast media. ATN occurs in up to 20% of patients receiving aminoglycosides, even at therapeutic dosages. Nonoliguric renal failure ensues within 5 to 10 days and recovery is delayed by persistence of aminoglycosides in renal tissue for up to a month. Peak and trough levels are monitored for renal toxicity, although trough levels are more predictive. Risk factors for the development of aminoglycoside-induced ATN include preexisting renal disease, concomitant use of other nephrotoxins (e.g., vancomycin, intravenous acyclovir, and cephalosporins), and age. Aminoglycosides are saturable in the proximal tubule; therefore, once daily dosing may be renal-protective because aminoglycoside uptake is reduced.

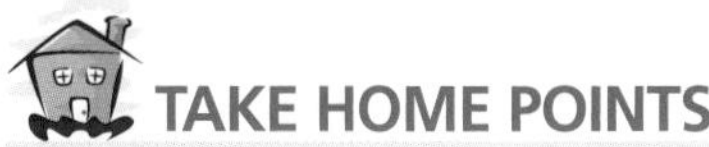

TAKE HOME POINTS

Exogenous nephrotoxins are external substances taken in by the patient.

Risk of ATN from amphotericin B is dose related. It occurs in up to one-third of patients receiving amphotericin B, with likelihood of ATN at cumulative dosages greater than 2 to 3 g. Injury is a result of distal tubule vasoconstriction leading to nonoliguric failure from nephrogenic diabetes insipidus. Lipid formulations of amphotericin B are less nephrotoxic than standard formulations.

Contrast-induced nephrotoxicity (CIN) is a preventable form of ATN. Unfortunately, CIN has become more frequent because of increased use of radiocontrast media for diagnostic and therapeutic purposes. Chronic kidney disease (CKD) and diabetes mellitus (DM) are major risk factors for development of CIN. Increased incidence of CKD and DM therefore contributes to CIN. Other risk factors include preexisting renal insufficiency, diabetes, volume depletion, large contrast load, malnourishment, and advanced age. Iodinated contrast media cause vasoconstriction and also have a direct toxic effect on tubular cells through hypoperfusion and osmotic stress.

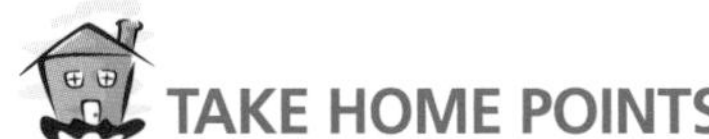

TAKE HOME POINTS

Power injections of contrast should be implemented through a power-PICC, not a regular PICC catheter, which can rupture.

Actions to prevent CIN are aimed at identifying patients at risk and reducing nephrotoxicity. Research suggests the use of iso-osmotic low dose contrast media reduces the likelihood of clinical nephrotoxicity. Isotonic infusions of saline or bicarbonate solutions 12 hours before and after (1 mL/kg/hr for 24 h) may also minimize nephrotoxicity, especially when pretreatment and posttreatment are given with the oral medication N-acetylcysteine (Mucomyst), which acts as an antioxidant. Other renal protective agents under investigation are theophylline and ascorbic acid. Studies suggest that normal saline is more effective than other saline solutions, and the intravenous route superior to the oral route.

Combinations of insults are even more deleterious to kidney function. Aminoglycosides administered to septic patients, radiocontrast agents in conjunction with angiotensin-converting enzyme (ACE) inhibitors (which decrease GFR), and nonsteroidal antiinflammatory agents (NSAIDs) (directly nephrotoxic) given to heart failure patients predisposes patients to ATN. Use of diuretics during contrast administration also has prenephrotoxic effects.

Other nephrotoxic substances include:

- Cyclosporine (dose dependent) and tacrolimus: induce renal vasoconstriction.
- Sulfonamides, acyclovir, and methotrexate: crystal formation blocks tubular flow.
- Cisplatin and foscarnet: directly toxic.
- Heavy metals: cadmium, mercury, arsenic: direct toxic effect, tubular necrosis.

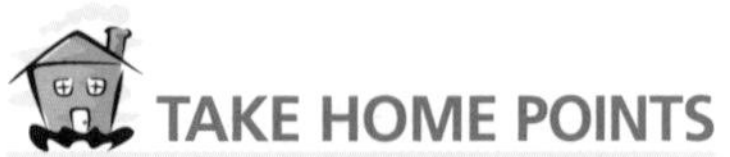

Endogenous nephrotoxins are internally occurring substances.

Endogenous Nephrotoxins

Endogenous nephrotoxins are produced within the body system. Myoglobinemia, hemoglobinemia, urinary crystal formation, and myeloma are examples of endogenous nephrotoxins. Myoglobin is the oxygen-storing component of skeletal muscles, and functions similarly to hemoglobin and is not normally present in blood. The breakdown of muscle (i.e., rhabdomyolysis) leads to myoglobinemia. Myoglobinemia is induced by any mechanical injury to skeletal muscle, such as crush injuries, severe exercise, seizures, and nonmechanical injury, including viral illness, excessive heat, multiple wasp/bee stings, and medications. Alcohol and coma are risk factors due to unrelieved muscle pressure caused by immobility.

Hemoglobinuria occurs from massive destruction of red blood cells (RBCs) as a result of a hemolytic transfusion reaction or hemolytic anemias. Transfusion reaction from ABO incompatibility occurs in less than 4 per million transfusions, usually due to human error. Pathologically, renal effects from hemoglobinuria are similar to myoglobinuria. In both myoglobinuria and hemoglobinuria, ATN occurs through obstruction of the renal tubule by pigments as well as direct toxicity.

Crystal formation in the renal tubule is caused by conditions such as dehydration and by crystal-forming substances. Crystals may be directly cytotoxic or cause tubule obstruction. Medications such as sulfonamides, methotrexate, and acyclovir can cause crystal precipitation in renal tubules as can certain toxic substances such as ethylene glycol, which forms calcium oxalate crystals.

Multiple myeloma, a cancer of the bone marrow, may cause ATN by several means. Hypercalcemia from bone destruction, intratubular light chain proteins, uric acid crystal precipitation, and antineoplastic drug toxicity may all play a role in ATN from myeloma.

TAKE HOME POINTS

The exact mechanisms of ATN are not always clearly understood. Theories include intrarenal ischemia, direct toxic injury, and mechanical tubular obstruction.

Diagnostics

No single test can diagnose ATN. Patient history, clinical findings, and laboratory studies are interpreted jointly. Radiologic studies and renal biopsy are reserved for differentiation of ATN from primary renal disease. Unfortunately, biopsy may not be conclusive, especially in ATN, where minor histologic changes belie major organ dysfunction.

Laboratory values are especially useful in distinguishing prerenal azotemia from ATN.

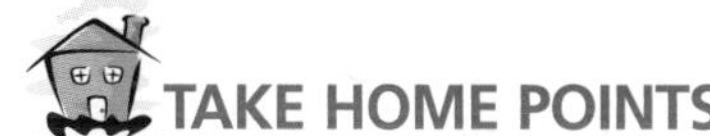

TAKE HOME POINTS

- Urine casts, characteristic of ATN, may not always be present.
- Anemia, due to diminished production of erythropoietin, and bleeding due to uremia-induced platelet dysfunction may occur.
- Hypercalcemia and hyperuricemia (tumor lysis syndrome) may suggest a malignant cause of ATN.
- Urine electrolytes may help differentiate ATN from prerenal azotemia.

Acute Tubular Necrosis Laboratory Values

Laboratory Study	Characteristics
Serum chemistries	• BUN increased • Creatinine increased • Hyponatremia • Hyperkalemia • Hypermagnesemia • Hypocalcemia • Hyperphosphatemia • Metabolic acidosis
CBC	• Anemia
Urinalysis	• Sediment: muddy brown granular casts
Urine Na, mEq/L	• >40
Urine osmolality, mOsm/kg H_2O	• <400

BUN, Blood urea nitrogen; *CBC*, complete blood count.

Prognosis

The mortality rate of ATN is between 37.1% and 78.6%. Higher mortality is associated with intensive care unit admission, which may point to the severity of underlying disease as a risk factor. For example, the mortality rate in patients with ATN after sepsis or severe trauma is much higher (about 60%) than the mortality rate in patients with ATN that is nephrotoxin related (about 30%). However, the nurse should remember the following points:

- Nonoliguric ATN has a worse prognosis than oliguric ATN, probably related to the magnitude of renal insult. Transforming oliguric ATN to a nonoliguric state with diuretics or dopamine improves urine output but has no effect on long-term outcomes.

- Of the survivors of ATN, approximately 60% have full recovery of renal function. Another 5% to 11% never recover kidney function and require dialysis. The remainder experience varying levels of renal insufficiency.

What You DO

Nursing Care

- Assessment (history): During history-taking, pay close attention for events that may lead to ischemic or toxic kidney insult, such as an episode of sustained hypotension or administration of contrast media for whole body imaging posttrauma. In addition, review patient medication type and dosages, including over-the-counter (OTC) medications. A renal history should include usual voiding pattern, amount and difficulty, and estimated output. Changes in weight should also be evaluated daily and accurate intake and output maintained.
- Assessment (physical examination): Physical assessment parameters focus on fluid volume status related to decreased output. Nurses should assess for high blood pressure, increased pulse, basilar lung crackles, jugular vein distention, hepatomegaly, peripheral edema, and weight gain. If the patient is in the diuretic phase, signs of dehydration may be present, such as dry mucous membranes, poor skin turgor, flat neck veins, orthostatic hypotension, and weight loss. Observe for weakness and fatigue, nausea and vomiting, and pruritus for patients in renal failure.
- Assessment (psychological): Accumulation of metabolic wastes may cause patients to be drowsy, confused, irritable, or even combative. Anxiety may be a problem because patients are unsure of the outcome.
- Interpretation of laboratory data: Expect serial examinations of blood and urine chemistries to be prescribed, as well as a CBC to rule out infectious causes and to monitor for anemia and bleeding. During renal failure, potassium levels may rise drastically, and metabolic acidosis can occur.
- Nursing interventions: The nurse has an important role in preventing and mitigating ATN. Most important is recognizing at-risk patients and early onset of renal dysfunction. Treat hypotensive events aggressively. Closely monitor serum creatinine and BUN when administering nephrotoxic agents. At-risk patients should receive adequate hydration before and after iso-osmotic low-dose contrast media, and

possibly N-acetylcysteine or other protective agents before and after the examination. If the cause of ATN was a nephrotoxic medication, eliminate or change dosing. Collaborate with physicians to discuss possible daily dosing of aminoglycosides and use of lipid-based amphotericin B. Continue assessments throughout the course of ATN and support the patient and family. Explain fluid and dietary restrictions, and prepare to administer erythropoietin and phosphate binders. If appropriate, prepare the patient for dialysis. Monitor laboratory results and assess for hyperkalemia, hypermagnesemia, hyperphosphatemia, and acidosis. Monitor serum sodium, which may be high or low depending on fluid balance. Sudden shifts in sodium balance can affect cerebral function. In addition, monitor RBCs for anemia, platelets for bleeding, and white blood cell count (WBC) for infection because renal failure alters function of the immune system. Promote healthy skin as a barrier to infection and treat dry skin and pruritus.

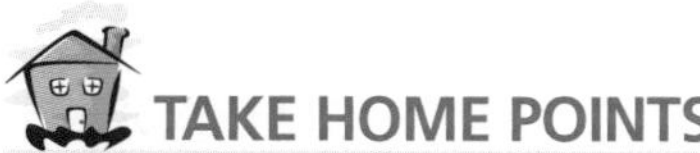

Usually, patients who experience ATN are previously healthy and may have developed renal failure as a result of an iatrogenic problem.

If the cause of ATN is a nephrotoxic agent, preventing further exposure to the agent should be a primary nursing goal.

FIRST-LINE AND INITIAL TREATMENTS FOR ACUTE TUBULAR NECROSIS

- Assess and recognize at-risk patients and the signs of ATN.
- Assess fluid volume status.
- Monitor for hyper/hypotension.
- Weigh daily, report weight gains or losses.
- Monitor urine output, report output less than 30 mL/hr.
- Restrict fluids.
- Restrict intake of sodium, phosphorous, potassium, magnesium, and protein; consult dietician.
- Monitor serum electrolyte laboratory values.
- Avoid catabolic/high-energy states (e.g., fever; increased nitrogenous wastes).
- Administer prescribed medications, adjust dosages for nephrotoxic agents.
- Prevent infection.

The following formula should be used to calculate the fluid intake for the next 24 hours:

Urinary output (previous day or nondialysis day if on dialysis)
− 500 to 800 (insensible water loss) = Amount of intake next 24 hours

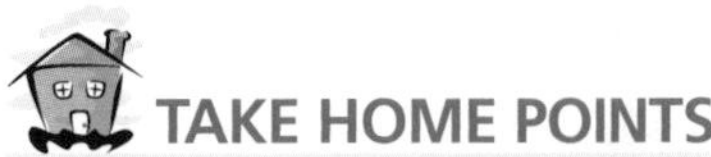

TAKE HOME POINTS

Prevention of infection is crucial in preventing further complications in patients with ATN.

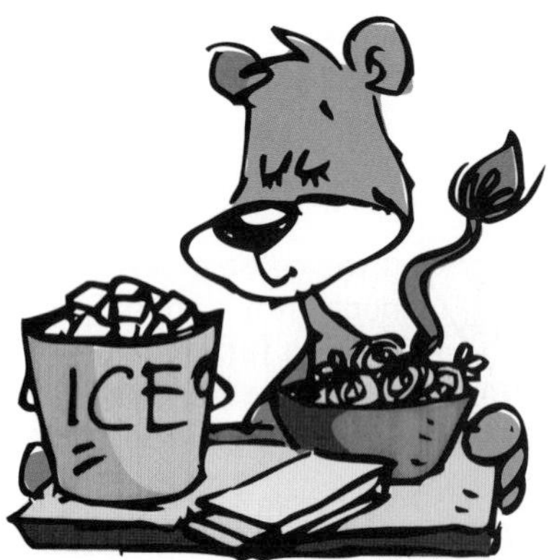

Fluid restriction interventions: ice chips, gum, hard candy

Treatment for ATN means correcting underlying pathologies that contributed to ARF. For example, hypotension due to shock or trauma, and diminished cardiac output in heart failure must be improved. Nurses should be aware that common OTC medications such as NSAIDs may contribute to ATN and combinations of events and medications may contribute to the development of renal failure or prevent exacerbation of existing renal compromise.

Discharge and Home Health Guidelines

All patients who experience ATN should be discharged with an understanding of ATN, signs and symptoms of impending renal failure, and how to monitor basic renal function. OTC medications need to be discussed with the nephrologist. Daily weight checks and daily rest periods to prevent overexertion should be encouraged. The nurse should explain dietary and fluid restrictions, emphasizing the importance of follow-up and compliance to recovery in renal failure. Continued follow-up with the nephrologist during the recovery phase and inclusion of the social worker and spiritual advisor are important to promoting wellness.

Do You UNDERSTAND?

DIRECTIONS: **Identify the following statements as *true* (T) or *false* (F).**

_____1. The BUN and creatinine should decrease in the initial phase of ATN.

_____2. A normal adult's GFR is approximately 125 mL/hr.

_____3. In ATN, one of the first signs is a decrease in urine production below 400 mL/24 hr.

_____4. Fluid volume excess is an important focus of the nurse's assessment and physical examination when caring for patients at risk for ATN.

_____5. When caring for patients with ATN, the nurse needs to use the following formula to calculate fluid allotment: Urinary output (previous day/nondialysis day if on dialysis) – 500 mL to 800 mL (insensible water loss) = Intake in next 24 hours.

DIRECTIONS: Match the following incident with the appropriate cause of ARF (each can be used more than once).

Column A	Column B
______ 6. Patient overdoses on a nephrotoxic drug	a. Prerenal
______ 7. Patient has hypertension	b. Intrarenal
______ 8. Patient develops ATN because of enlarged prostate	c. Postrenal
______ 9. Patient experienced a hypotension episode	
______ 10. Patient is diagnosed with renal artery stenosis	

What IS Chronic Renal Failure?

Chronic renal failure (CRF) is a slow, progressive, irreversible loss of renal function and reduction in the GFR. It is a form of chronic kidney disease (CKD), which is incompatible with life and requires renal replacement through dialysis or transplantation. Without kidney function, death ensues in 3 to 4 weeks.

As the GFR approaches zero, the patient enters the last phase of CKD—called CRF, end-stage renal disease (ESRD), or stage 5 CKD. Homeostatic regulation of water and electrolytes no longer occurs, and metabolic wastes accumulate within the body, resulting in the development of the clinical syndrome called *uremia. Uremia* is the term used to describe the clinical effects of *azotemia* (elevated serum BUN and creatinine). Every organ system is affected by retention of nitrogenous wastes and loss of fluid and electrolyte regulation. Cyanate, polyamines, and guanidine—other toxic metabolites of protein breakdown—may also contribute to uremia. Signs and symptoms of ESRD include fluid and electrolyte disturbances, acid-base imbalances, anemia, fatigue, anorexia, nausea, vomiting, pruritus, and cardiovascular, neurologic, GI, and skeletal manifestations.

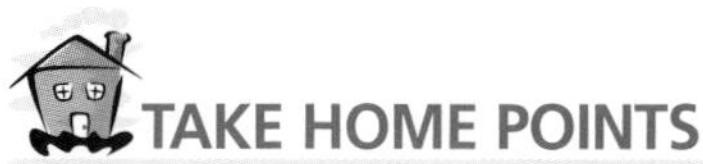

- *Azotemia* refers to elevation of BUN and creatinine levels with decreased GFR.
- Before a change in BUN is detected, up to 60% to 70% of renal function is already permanently lost.

Answer: 1. F; 2. F; 3. T; 4. T; 5. T; 6. b; 7. a; 8. c; 9. a; 10. a.

Pathogenesis

DM and hypertension are responsible for 69% of ESRD, although the pathogenesis can be multifactorial and includes atherosclerosis, bacterial infection, lupus, obstruction, cancer, and polycystic kidney disease (PKD). ESRD is the end result of all chronic renal disorders and is often related to repeated insult as is seen with chronic glomerulonephritis, use of nephrotoxic drugs, and ureteral and prostate obstruction. Even though there is progressive loss of nephrons, renal adaptation maintains function for a time. The intact nephron hypothesis suggests that, as total nephrons are lost, remaining nephrons hypertrophy and hyperfunction to adjust to the increased load. Other theories suggest that hyperfiltration caused by shunting of renal blood flow to functioning nephrons causes capillary hypertension, which further speeds nephron loss. Lastly, the location of kidney damage, cortical, medullar, or vascular, affects kidney function. The kidneys are able to compensate until the GFR (most frequently measured by urine creatinine clearance) drops to less than 10 mL/min (normal 125 mL/min). More than 90% of functioning nephrons are lost at this point. The pattern of progression from normal renal function to ESRD involves four stages: (1) reduced renal reserve, (2) renal insufficiency, (3) renal disease, and (4) ESRD.

Pattern of Progression of Renal Disease

Disease Stages	Characteristics
Reduced renal reserve	• GFR is reduced to 50% of normal. • BUN slightly elevated. • No clinical symptoms.
Renal insufficiency	• GFR is reduced to 75% of normal. • Azotemia (elevated serum BUN and creatinine). • Mild anemia and hypertension. • Nocturia (frequent voiding at night).
Renal disease	• Reduction in GFR to less than 20% of normal. • Azotemia, acidosis, severe anemia, impaired urine dilution, fluid and electrolyte imbalances • Patient may exhibit overt uremia with cardiovascular, gastrointestinal, and neurologic complications.
End-stage renal disease	• Reduction in GFR to less than 10% of normal. • Represents the terminal stage of uremia.

BUN, Blood urea nitrogen; *GFR*, glomerular filtration rate;

The National Kidney Foundation classifies CKD in five stages according to GFR function:

Stages of Chronic Kidney Disease

Stage	Description	GFR mL/min/1.73 m^3
1	Kidney damage: no symptoms	normal to ≥ 90
2	Mild: no or rare symptoms	60-89
3	Moderate: clinical and laboratory signs	30-59
4	Severe: prominent signs	15-29
5	Kidney failure: uremic syndrome	<15 or on dialysis

From Eknoyan G, Levin A, Levin NW: Bone metabolism and disease in chronic kidney disease, *American Journal of Kidney Diseases,* 42(3 suppl):1-201, 2003.

At-Risk Populations

Diabetic nephropathy is the leading cause (42.8%) of CRF in the United States, followed by hypertension (25.9%), glomerulonephritis (9.0%), cystic kidney disease (2.3%), and other causes (20%). At-risk populations include African ancestry; those older than 65 years of age (47.9% of all cases); or persons with autoimmune disease, a family history of renal disease, a previous episode of acute renal failure, the presence of proteinuria, abnormal urinary sediment, or structural abnormalities of the urinary tract. A potentially undiagnosed cause of renal failure is atheroembolic disease found particularly in white men older than 60 years with a history of DM, hypertension, or smoking.

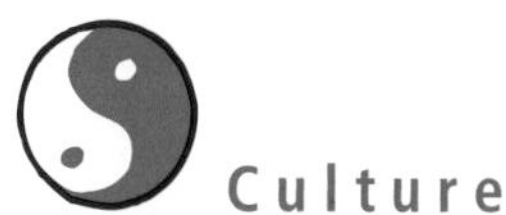

Culture

African-American men experience a higher incidence of renal dysfunction as a result of hypertension than white men for reasons that are unclear.

What You NEED TO KNOW

Signs and symptoms of CRF occur late in the course of the disease after significant damage has occurred. Progression of CKD may be subtle so that the presenting symptom is CRF (ESRD stage 5 CKD). The delay between the occurrence of damage to the nephrons and the onset of symptoms is due to the ability of the kidney to compensate until approximately 90% of renal function is lost.

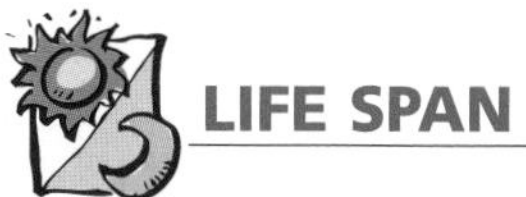

LIFE SPAN

Older adults are at increased risk for CRF because of the annual decline in GFR, which is more pronounced in women than men. A woman in her 80s with a normal serum creatinine may have a GFR of just 50 mL/min/1.73 m^3.

Clinical Manifestations of Chronic Renal Failure

Fluid and electrolyte imbalances	• Edema • Weight gain (fluid) • Hyperkalemia
Acid-base imbalance	• Metabolic acidosis
Abnormalities of calcium, phosphate, and bone metabolism	• Hyperphosphatemia • Hypocalcemia • Hyperparathyroidism • Renal osteodystrophy
Cardiovascular disease	• Hypertension • Dysrhythmias • Uremic pericarditis • Heart failure
Hematopoietic disorders	• Anemia • Bleeding tendencies
Gastrointestinal effects	• Anorexia • Nausea and vomiting • Diarrhea or constipation • Weight loss (nutritional) • Gastrointestinal bleeding • Uremic esophagitis • Uremic gastritis • Uremic colitis • Uremic fetor (breath)
Integumentary manifestations	• Sallow/gray complexion • Pruritus • Uremic frost
Neuromuscular complications	• Headache • Altered mental status • Peripheral neuropathy • Restless leg syndrome • Encephalopathy • Myopathy • Seizures • Coma

The rate of progression in CKD varies among individuals. If left untreated, fluid and electrolyte imbalance, acidosis, and accumulation of toxic metabolites eventually lead to cardiac dysrhythmias, pulmonary edema, cerebral edema, and death. Renal replacement therapy (RRT) and renal transplant provide the only means of prolonging life once the patient has reached end-stage renal failure.

What You DO

Treatment of CKD includes interventions aimed at slowing the progression of the disease, managing symptoms, and providing renal replacement for CRF.

- Management of fluid balance includes daily fluid restriction and/or diuretics and monitoring daily weight. Earlier stages of CKD may not limit fluids.
- Management of electrolyte balance consists of dietary modifications, which may limit sodium, potassium, and phosphorus. Potassium balance is of particular concern in CRF due to cardiac effects. Oral phosphate binders may be taken to remove phosphorus. Calcium and phosphorus have an inverse relationship; high levels of phosphorus cause serum calcium to fall. Low calcium leads to demineralization of bones, resulting in osteodystrophy. Supplemental vitamin D (Calcitrol) and calcium may be needed to enhance dietary calcium absorption and prevent broken bones.
- A true renal diet is a very restricted diet. Consult a dietician.
- Management of metabolic wastes includes limiting dietary protein. Protein metabolism produces BUN and creatinine, which when abnormally retained, cause uremic syndrome.
- Management of weakness and fatigue by providing iron and folic acid to enhance RBC production, and administer erythropoietin (Epoetin alfa, Epogen, or Procrit) in CRF. Monitor serum albumin and calorie intake to ensure adequate nutrition and immune function.
- Manage symptoms such as bleeding, hyperlipidemia, nausea and vomiting, and pruritus. In later stages of CKD, platelet dysfunction prolongs bleeding time.
- Monitor cardiovascular, neurologic, and endocrine effects of uremia, such as pericarditis, encephalopathy, muscular cramping, and hyperinsulinemia.
- Management of psychosocial functioning by addressing fear, anxiety, and powerlessness.

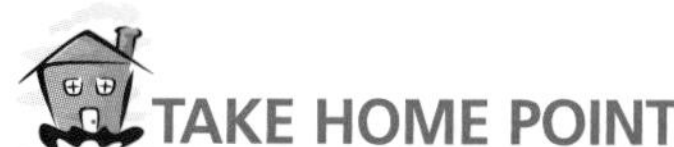

CKD is progressive and irreversible.

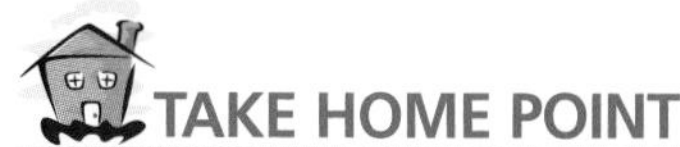

Fluid management and dietary control can be used to slow the progression of CKD for several years.

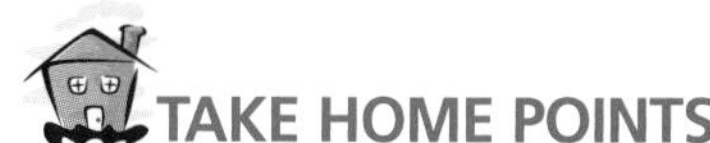

The cost of erythropoietin is about $5oo per injection.

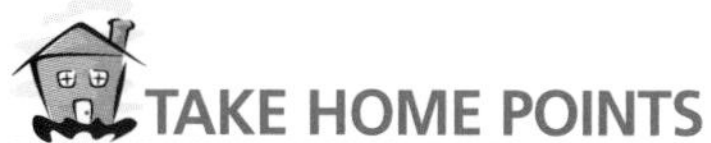

Renal diets are low in sodium, potassium, and phosphorus. Do NOT eat processed or seasoned foods, most canned foods, salted foods, and pickled products. You can eat grits, toast, lettuce, fish, fresh peaches, and 2 oz. chicken breasts, for example.

FIRST-LINE AND INITIAL TREATMENTS FOR CHRONIC RENAL FAILURE

- Dialysis to treat: severe hyperkalemia, volume overload, acidosis, or uremia.
- Management of cardiovascular effects begins with the treatment of hypertension as a result of salt and water retention. Administration of angiotensin-converting enzyme (ACE) inhibitors and angiotensin receptor–blocking (ARB) agents are effective in conjunction with non–potassium-sparing diuretics. Failure to regulate fluid balance may lead to overload with development of heart failure and pulmonary edema. Dialysis may help treat both effects.
- Treat metabolic acidosis resulting from retained organic acids and hyperkalemia. Hyperkalemia moves hydrogen ions out of the cell and into the blood, causing acidosis. Acidosis can be managed with sodium bicarbonate supplements and dialysis. Potassium excess can also be managed with sodium polystyrene sulfonate (Kayexalate), glucose and insulin, or IV calcium.
- Monitor for adequate nutrition and complications such as anemia, infection, bleeding, hyperlipidemia, and electrolyte imbalances such as hyperkalemia (loss of regulation) or hypokalemia (diuretic administration), hyperphosphatemia, and hypocalcemia.

The only effective treatments for ESRD are RRT and renal transplant. *RRT* is a term that describes modalities that act as an artificial kidney to remove excess fluid, electrolytes, and metabolic waste products when the kidneys are no longer able. RRT is divided into intermittent and continuous therapies. Intermittent therapy includes traditional hemodialysis (IHD) and peritoneal dialysis (PD). IHD is usually performed three times per week in a dialysis center for 3 to 4 hours at a time. PD is performed at home four to five times a day, with exchanges taking about 30 minutes. Continuous renal replacement therapy (CRRT) is performed continuously in a hospital setting. Each technique involves filtering blood across a semipermeable membrane that causes water and solute molecules to move across a gradient from higher to lower concentration for elimination from the body. In IHD and CRRT, the semipermeable membrane is artificial, but in PD, the peritoneum serves as the semipermeable membrane.

IHD is accomplished using a machine to pump blood from the patient to a dialyzer filter. The filter has two compartments, one for the patient's blood and the other with a dialysate solution. The compartments are separated only by a semipermeable membrane. What type, how much, and how fast fluids and solutes move from the patient's blood into the dialysate fluid is a function of the osmolality, chemistry, and hydrostatic pressure of the dialysate. The membrane allows water, urea, creatinine, potassium, magnesium, chloride, and other electrolytes to move from the patient's blood into the dialysate fluid. The membrane is too fine to allow large molecules such as RBCs or albumin to pass. After dialyzing, the dialysate fluid contains waste products that would normally be filtered by healthy kidneys. Blood leaves the patient and returns via an arteriovenous (AV) fistula or graft. An AV fistula is a permanent surgical connection made between a vein and an artery, usually in the arm. Grafting uses a synthetic tube between the vessels. If permanent access is not available, intravenous access with a specialized catheter (e.g., Vas-Cath) allows temporary access.

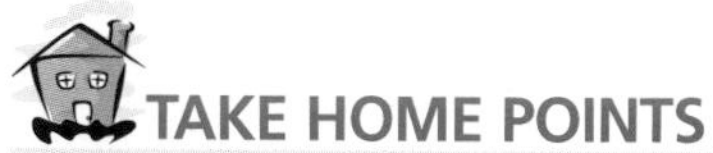

RRT involves an exchange or movement of molecules in and out of the blood across a semipermeable membrane.

A major concern is the loss of vascular access because of clot formation, infection, or inadequate blood flow. An anticoagulant given during dialysis prevents clotting during treatment; however, the access site must be regularly assessed for the presence of a bruit and thrill. A bruit is the noise heard with a stethoscope over the graft as blood flows quickly from the arterial to venous circulation. A thrill is the vibration felt over the graft caused by movement of blood. The nurse also avoids compression or restriction of blood flow to the site, and any invasive procedures near the site. If the access becomes occluded, immediate intervention such as embolectomy, angioplasty, or thrombolysis may be needed to restore patency.

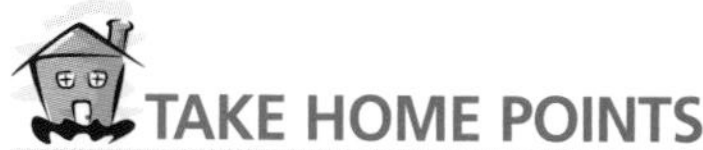

Hemodialysis requires the removal of blood through vascular access.

Instead of vascular access, PD requires a catheter (e.g., Tenckhoff) placed in the abdomen to access the peritoneal cavity. PD uses the same principles of osmosis, diffusion, and filtration as hemodialysis. The patient's peritoneum serves as a natural semipermeable membrane separating the patient's blood in the mesenteric vasculature from the dialysate, which is instilled into the peritoneum via the catheter. In a cycle of fill, dwell, and drain, the peritoneum continuously filters blood. In *continuous ambulatory peritoneal dialysis* (CAPD), the patient drains dialysate that has stayed in the abdominal cavity for 5 to 6 hours, and then refills the cavity with fresh dialysate and leaves it to dwell. While the dialysate dwells in the abdomen, the catheter is capped and the patient goes about daily activities. The cycle of drain

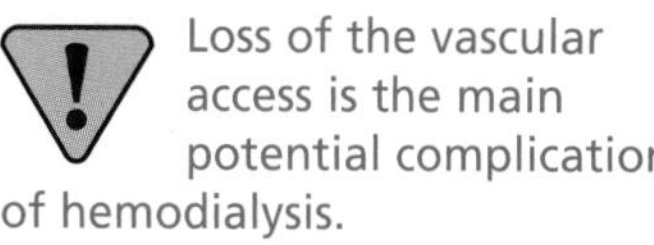

Loss of the vascular access is the main potential complication of hemodialysis.

Hemodialysis circuit

(From Ignatavicus DD, Workman ML: Medical-surgical nursing: critical thinking for collaborative care, *ed 4, Philadelphia, 2002, WB Saunders.)*

and fill takes about 30 minutes, but dwelling occurs over hours. During dwell time, water and solutes move into the dialysate, which are drained out of the body with each drain cycle. A programmable cycler provides automated multiple overnight exchanges as an alternative form of CAPD. Complications of PD include infection at the catheter insertion site, peritonitis, occlusion of the catheter, and failure of the peritoneum to function as an adequate dialyzing membrane. Protein loss through the peritoneum and absorption of glucose from the dialysate may also pose endocrine and nutritional problems. Nonglucose starch and protein-based dialysates are available. Sterile technique using masks, sterile gloves, and supplies must be observed when performing PD. The catheter insertion site should be carefully assessed and drained dialysate inspected for color, clarity, and amount. The patient's output is calculated as the difference between the volume of dialysate instilled and the amount that empties into the collection bag during the next drain. The output should be a positive number.

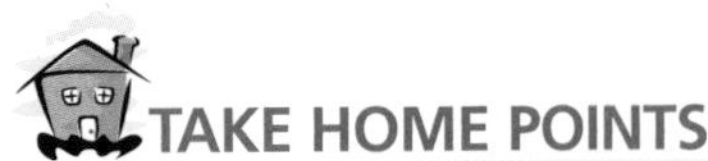

PD removes fluid and waste products from the body using the peritoneal cavity as the dialysate membrane.

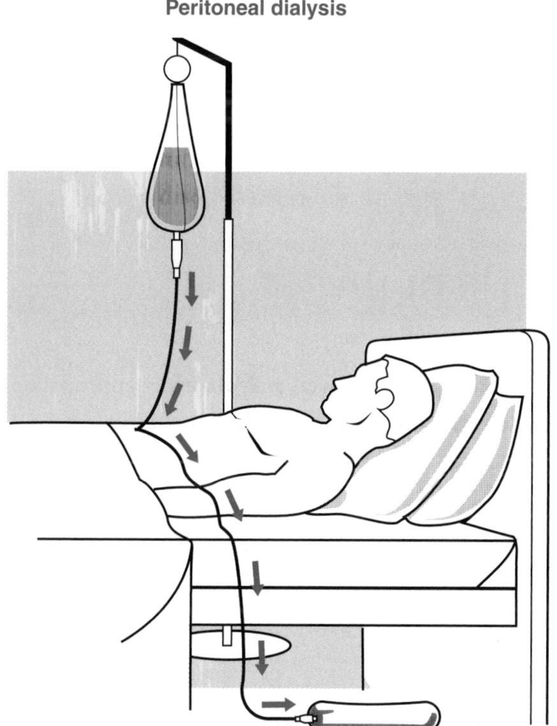

(From Ignatavicus DD, Workman ML: Medical-surgical nursing: critical thinking for collaborative care, *ed 4, Philadelphia, 2002, WB Saunders.)*

TAKE HOME POINTS

One pound of weight gain represents approximately 500 mL of fluid retention.

Nursing Responsibilities

- Keep accurate records of intake and output, including net output from RRT, and daily weight.
- Ensure patient understanding of fluid and diet restrictions.
- Monitor serum electrolytes, BUN, creatinine, and albumin.
- Monitor RBCs, hemoglobin, hematocrit, and WBC count.
- Know which medications are dialyzed out and which are not affected.
- Assess for signs and symptoms of uremia.
- Report signs of infection, such as fever or productive cough.
- Instruct patients experiencing pruritus to avoid strong soap, rinse thoroughly, and shower rather than bathe when possible.
- Provide psychosocial support for the patient and family. Educate patients about dietary changes, renal replacement therapies, kidney transplant, and right to refuse or withdraw from treatment.
- Assess and protect the vascular access site for HD. Assess for bruit and thrill.

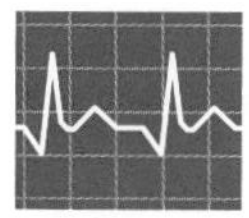

The nurse should assess for the presence of a thrill and bruit every 4 to 6 hours in the patient with an arteriovenous (AV) fistula or graft.

- The nurse should never compromise the vascular access—it is the patient's lifeline.
- The nurse should never perform venipuncture, administer an injection, or inflate a blood pressure cuff on the extremity where the fistula or graft is located.

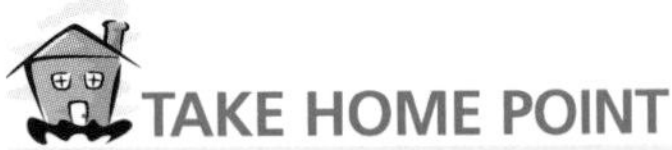

TAKE HOME POINT

The nurse should instruct the person with CRF to avoid tight or restrictive clothing around the affected arm and to not rest the head on the affected arm while sleeping.

- Assess and protect the peritoneal catheter for PD. Assess for signs and symptoms of peritonitis such as cloudy dialysate, abdominal pain, rebound tenderness, and fever. Monitor protein levels, appetite, and blood glucose for patients on PD.
- Use strict sterile technique when accessing the patient for RRT.

Do You UNDERSTAND?

DIRECTIONS: **Select the best answer, and place the appropriate letter in the space provided.**

_____ 1. Compensatory mechanisms that allow normal renal function to be maintained for long periods of time despite renal injury include:
1. Hyperfiltration.
2. Vasodilation.
3. Atrophy.
4. Homeostasis.

_____ 2. ESRD is said to have occurred when kidney function is reduced to:
1. 10%.
2. 50%.
3. 75%.
4. 90%.

_____ 3. The potential life-threatening electrolyte imbalance most common in the patient with ESRD is:
1. Hyponatremia.
2. Hypercalcemia.
3. Hypophosphatemia.
4. Hyperkalemia.

_____ 4. For each pound a patient gains, the nurse can estimate the patient is retaining fluid of approximately:
1. 100 mL.
2. 250 mL.
3. 500 mL.
4. 1000 mL.

Answers: 1. 1; 2. 1; 3. 4; 4. 3.

What IS Continuous Renal Replacement Therapy?

CRRT is a slow continuous form of hemodialysis often used as emergency treatment for patients with ARF, fluid overload, BUN greater than 100 mg/dL, symptomatic uremia (encephalopathy, bleeding, pericarditis), hyperkalemia (>6.5 mEq/L), dialyzable toxins, or metabolic or hemodynamic instability. CRRT continuously operates during 24 hours over one to several days and is most commonly used in the intensive care unit. In addition to slow removal of toxins and wastes, CRRT may remove inflammatory mediators from the blood. There are two CRRT options: venous only and arteriovenous.

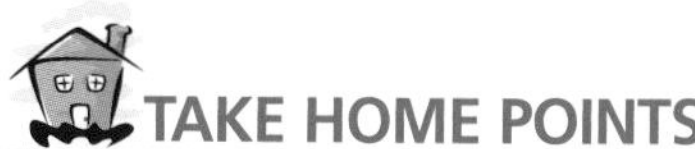

CRRT provides a means of dialyzing a critical care patient who is hemodynamically unstable.

What You NEED TO KNOW

CRRT relies on the principles governing fluid and solute transport across a semipermeable membrane. These include diffusion, convection, and ultrafiltration. Diffusion describes the movement of solutes across a semipermeable membrane from an area of higher concentration to one of lower concentration. In convection, a solvent carries solutes along with it, called *solvent drag*, by the force of water through a semipermeable membrane. Ultrafiltration describes the process in which plasma water and crystalloids are separated from whole blood across a semipermeable membrane in response to a transmembrane pressure gradient, the same

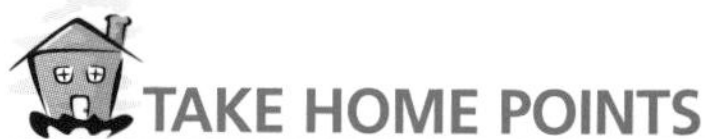

Diffusion is the process of solutes moving across a semipermeable membrane from an area of higher concentration to one of lower concentration.

Diffusion

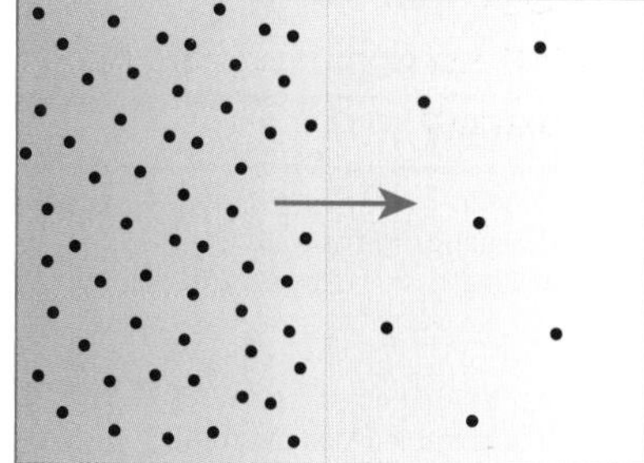

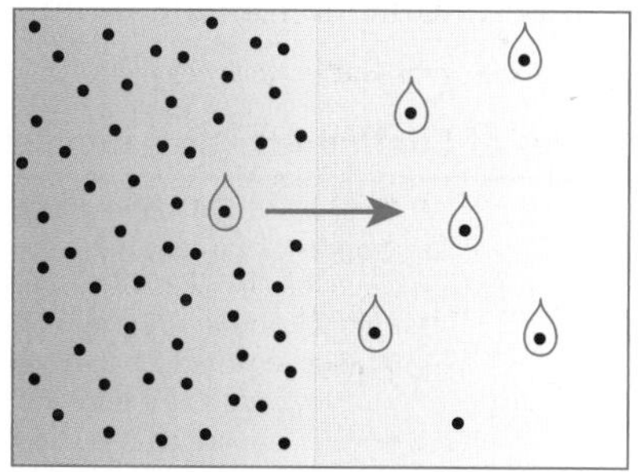

Passage of solutes from area of higher to lower concentration.

process that normally occurs in the nephron at the glomerulus. Higher pressure and faster flow rates increase the rate of ultrafiltration.

Modes of Continuous Renal Replacement Therapy

The most common form of CRRT is venous. Arteriovenous modes require accessing both an artery and a vein. No blood pump is needed because the force of the arteriovenous pressure gradient moves blood through the circuit. However, this requires the patient to have a high enough mean arterial pressure (MAP) to create an effective gradient between arterial and venous pressures. Aside from the difficulty for patients in ICU maintaining an effective MAP, there is increased risk of blood clotting.

In contrast, venovenous modes require only venous access. Vascular access is most commonly achieved by inserting a double lumen catheter into a central vein. One lumen functions as an arterial (or outflow) line and the other as the venous (or inflow) line. Blood is circulated through this system by use of a pump, which decreases the likelihood of clot formation. Placement of the CRRT catheter must be considered because if it is inadvertently located near other vascular devices blood will be drawn into the circuit and all dialyzable substances will be removed.

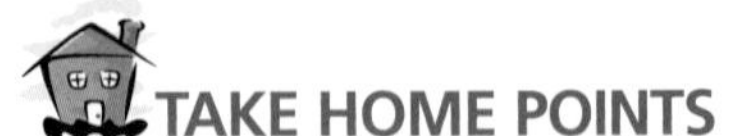

To operate, CRRT needs a vascular outflow and an inflow line. Most current CRRT modes are venous.

Modes of CRRT include continuous arteriovenous hemofiltration (CAVH), continuous arteriovenous hemodialysis (CAVHD), continuous venovenous hemofiltration (CVVH), continuous venovenous hemodialysis (CVVHD), continuous venovenous hemodiafiltration (CVVHDF), slow continuous ultrafiltration (SCUF), and slow extended daily dialysis (SLEDD). Venovenous modes have almost completely replaced arteriovenous modes of CRRT. Replacement fluids are used in some modes to replace volume of ultrafiltrate for hemodynamic stability and to increase flow against the filter's semipermeable membrane to improve convection.

Modes of Continuous Renal Replacement Therapy

CAVH	• Original and simplest form of CRRT.
	• Requires cannulation of both an artery and vein (usually femoral).
	• Blood flow through the system depends on a mean arterial pressure (MAP).
	• Advantage: relatively simple to use.
	• Disadvantages include the following:
	  • Arterial bleeding if disconnections or leaks in circuit occur
	  • Poor clearance rates in patients with low or unstable blood pressure
	  • Risk of clot formation in extracorporeal circuit as a result of low blood flow

Modes of Continuous Renal Replacement Therapy—cont'd

CAVHD	• Used when CAVH cannot provide adequate waste removal. • Uses the principle of diffusion. • Dialysate delivered to an extracorporeal compartment removes solutes, resulting in more rapid reduction in BUN and creatinine. • Similar to CAVH, MAP must be maintained to ensure proper blood flow through the system. • Decreases blood flow, resulting in the same disadvantages as CAVH.
CVVH	• Relies on the principle of convection. • Ultrafiltration rate is high. Replacement fluid is added to the extracorporeal circuit to enhance convective transport and maintain hemodynamic stability. No dialysate is required. • Does not require arterial access. CVVH relies on a pump to control blood flow rather than arterial pressure. • Venovenous modes incorporate safety devices to detect low pressures and presence of air in circuit.
CVVHD	• Works by diffusion and can be understood as simply a slow form of dialysis. • Use of dialysate increases the clearance rate of small solutes. Countercurrent dialysate (dialysate and blood move in opposite directions across the semipermeable membrane) increases waste removal. • No replacement fluid is used.
CVVHDF	• Uses convection and diffusion to remove water, wastes, and toxins. • Diffusion occurs as dialysate is run counter to the blood. • Convection occurs as an electrolyte replacement fluid is pumped into the blood.
SCUF	• Form of CRRT used to treat refractory fluid overload. • Slow form of CVVH. Works by ultrafiltration. No dialysate is used. • Fluid replacement is unnecessary because of the slow rate of fluid removal. Not effective for removing wastes. Up to 2 L of water is removed in 24 hours.
SLEDD	• Intermittent form of CRRT completed over 8 to 12 hours to allow freedom for tests, rehabilitation, or ventilator weaning. • Higher blood flow rates, fluid flow rates, and volume of hourly fluid removed.

BUN, Blood urea nitrogen; *CAVH,* continuous arteriovenous hemofiltration; *CAVHD,* continuous arteriovenous hemodialysis; *CRRT,* continuous renal replacement therapy; *CVVH,* continuous venovenous hemofiltration; *CVVHD,* continuous venovenous hemodialysis; *CVVHDF,* continuous venovenous hemodiafiltration; *SCUF,* slow continuous ultrafiltration, *SLEDD,* slow extended daily dialysis.

CRRT provides a slow, gentle method of fluid and solute removal that helps maintain hemodynamic stability and prevent complications in critically ill patients. PD can be limited by insufficient solute clearance, inability to correct hyperkalemia quickly, a high risk of peritonitis, hyperglycemia, poor fluid removal, and respiratory difficulty because of large volumes of fluid instilled in the peritoneal cavity. In addition, because it requires an intact peritoneal membrane, it is contraindicated for patients with abdominal wounds, infections, or adhesions. These limitations prevent the use of PD in the management of most ARF patients.

The most commonly used RRT is IHD. The usefulness of IHD is limited, however, in the unstable or critically ill patient because it may result in severe hemodynamic instability that causes therapy to be discontinued. The most significant complication is hypotension, especially

IHD (intermittent hemodialysis) can cause an increase in intracranial pressure from the rapid solute movement and can contribute to the development of massive cerebral edema causing herniation and death.

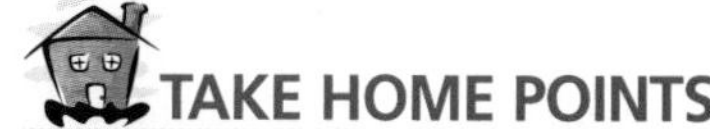

TAKE HOME POINTS

Dialysis disequilibrium syndrome occurs when hemodialysis causes a rapid decrease in BUN, which results in the development of cerebral edema.

in the critically ill patient with multiorgan dysfunction. Other complications of IHD include dysrhythmias, hypoxemia, hemorrhage, infection, dialysis disequilibrium syndrome, and seizures. Despite the need for specialized dialysis staff, the cost of IHD is lower than CRRT.

CRRT provides better, more natural, fluid control than IHD, enhancing fluid volume removal without compromising intravascular volume. CRRT also improves both electrolyte balance and nutritional support because parenteral nutrition can be given with less risk of fluid overload. Patients with heart failure resistant to diuretics are able to maintain hemodynamic stability. CRRT is also the treatment of choice in patients with, or at risk for, cerebral edema. Unlike IHD, where rapid solute removal from the blood shifts water into the cell, causing increased intracranial pressure, seizures, and possible death (dialysis disequilibrium syndrome), CRRT does not induce increased intracranial pressure.

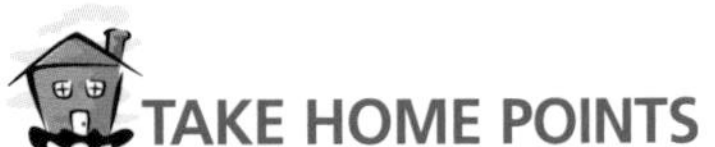

CRRT assists in maintaining hemodynamic stability during fluid removal process.

What You DO

CRRT is usually performed in the critical care unit by the nurse who is responsible for caring for the patient. Before beginning CRRT, the nurse should know the patient's diagnosis, past medical history, allergies, and current medications. Baseline vital signs, temperature, SpO_2, cardiac rhythm, hemodynamic parameters (if available), and current weight and laboratory values should be assessed. The nurse should check the physician's CRRT prescriptions to determine mode, type of replacement fluids, and dialysate (if used); the flow rates for blood, fluids, and medications; and parameters for the amount of fluid to be removed. The CRRT machine should be set up according to the manufacturer's directions. This includes hanging fluids, priming the tubing, and adding an anticoagulant to the system if prescribed (usually heparin or trisodium citrate). The patient should be connected to the machine via the established vascular access.

The physician may or may not order anticoagulation to maintain blood flow during CRRT. Citrate, an excellent anticoagulant, binds with calcium to interrupt the clotting cascade. As a result, however, calcium levels may fall during CRRT when citrate is used. Therefore, ionized, or free calcium, is routinely monitored. If levels are low, calcium may need to be replaced postfilter.

Nursing Responsibilities

The nurse should do the following:

- Prepare for CRRT by collecting patient data and baseline assessments, including vital signs, SpO_2, hemodynamic status, and cardiac rhythm.
- Monitor hourly output from CRRT and assess fluid volume status, including vital signs, central venous pressure (CVP), pulmonary artery pressure (PAP) and pulmonary artery occlusion pressure (PAOP) (if available), breath sounds, SpO_2, skin turgor, edema, and weight (especially important if using SLEDD). Note the color of the ultrafiltrate.
- Measure hourly and cumulative intake and output. The nurse should include all forms of intake, such as medications, blood products, and enteral or parenteral feedings, as well as output such as chest tube or nasogastric (NG) drainage.
- Administer correct fluid replacement based on hourly fluid balance goal as determined by the physician. Replace dialysate, if prescribed, with correct fluid as indicated.
- Assess for neurologic changes. Confusion or altered mentation could signal fluid shifts or build up of nitrogenous wastes.
- Assess electrolyte and acid-base balance routinely.
- Assess for bleeding. The entire circuit should always be visible, connections secure, and the patient positioned to avoid disconnection. Sedation may be needed for agitated or restless patients.
- Assess temperature. During CRRT, 110 to 200 mL blood is in the circuit at any one time. Cooling effects on the extracorporeal circulation plus room temperature replacement fluids and dialysate may induce hypothermia. Euthermia can be achieved with an in-line warmer or warming blankets. Blankets should be used with care to avoid concealing the blood circuit.
- Assess for infection. Monitor for fever and elevated WBC count and assess catheter insertion site. Use sterile technique when accessing lines and sterile dressing changes according to institution policy. Be aware that cooling effects of CRRT may mask fever.
- Assess coagulation status. Monitor catheter patency and coagulation laboratory studies.
- Assess and maintain patency of the circuit. The nurse should flush the system with saline or heparin according to policy.
- Assess the system for air and blood leakage. Loose connections can lead to hemorrhage or introduce air into the vascular space. The

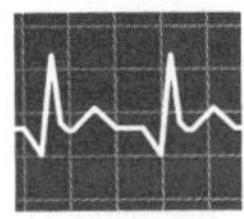

Once CRRT has begun, the nurse must monitor the patient and assess for any complications. Complications may include hypotension, hemorrhage, hypothermia, infection, and air embolism.

system should be monitored for air bubbles and blood loss, and all alarms investigated. When discontinuing, blood from the circuit tubing should be returned to the patient before removal.

- Give patient support. Patients are immobile during CRRT and need to be repositioned frequently. Educational support should be provided for patients and families.

Do You UNDERSTAND?

DIRECTIONS: **Select the best answer, and place the appropriate letter in the space provided.**

_____ 1. Principles governing fluid and solute transport across a semipermeable membrane in CRRT include diffusion and:
1. Conversion.
2. Convection.
3. Active transport.
4. Capillary membrane permeability.

_____ 2. The type of vascular access required for a patient undergoing CVVHDF is:
1. Arterial.
2. Venous.
3. Arteriovenous.
4. Venovenous.

_____ 3. SCUF is a form of CRRT used to treat:
1. Azotemia.
2. Dehydration.
3. Fluid overload.
4. Uremia.

_____ 4. IHD may be unsuitable for the critically ill patient because it can result in:
1. Fluid overload.
2. Hypertension.
3. Multiorgan failure.
4. Severe hemodynamic instability.

Answers: 1. 2; 2. 4; 3. 3; 4. 4.

References

Aghasadeghi K, Akbari V: Comparison of *N*-acetylcysteine and ascorbic acid in prevention of renal dysfunction after coronary angioplasty, *Journal of Renovascular Disease* 6:1-5, 2008.

Bednarski D, Castner D, Douglas C: Managing acute tubular necrosis, *Nursing,* 38(6):56hn1-2, 56hn4, 56hn6, 2008.

Bhatta N, Singh R, Sharma S, Sinnha A, Raja S: Acute renal failure following multiple wasp stings, *Pediatric Nephrology,* 20:1809-1810, 2005.

Broscious SK, Castagnola J: Chronic kidney disease, *Critical Care Nurse,* 26(4):17-27, 2006.

Chungang G, Cenac TA, Li Y, McMartin E: Calcium oxalate, and not other metabolites, is responsible for the renal toxicity of ethylene glycol, *Toxicology Letters* 173:8-16, 2007.

Crawford-Bonadio TL, Diaz-Buxo JA: Comparison of peritoneal dialysis solutions, *Nephrology Nursing Journal,* 31:500-507, 520, 2004.

Devarajan P: Cellular and molecular derangements in acute tubular necrosis, *Current Opinion in Pediatrics* 17(2):193-199, 2005.

Dirkes S, Hodge K: Continuous renal replacement therapy in the adult intensive care unit: history and current trends, *Critical Care Nurse Supplement,* 8-27, 2008.

Doherty RA: Continuous peritoneal dialysis, *Nursing Standard,* 19:55-65, 2005.

Gill N, Nalley JV, Fatica RA: Renal failure secondary to acute tubular necrosis: epidemiology, diagnosis, and management, *Chest,* 128:2847-2863, 2005.

Hoffman RS, Nelson LS, Howland MA, Lewin NA, Flomenbaum NE, Goldfrank LR: *Goldfranks's manual of toxicologic emergencies,* 2007, New York: McGraw-Hill.

Lamiere N, Biesen WV, Vanholder R: Acute renal failure, *Lancet,* 365:417-430, 2005.

McCance KL, Huether SE: *Pathophysiology: the biologic basis for disease in adults and children,* ed 5, St Louis, 2006, Elsevier Mosby.

McLaren BK, Zhang PL, Guillermo HA: P53 protein is a reliable marker in identification of renal tubular injury, *Applied Immunohistochemistry & Molecular Morphology,* 12:225-229, 2004.

Mitra A, Zolty E, Wang W, Schrier RW: Clinical acute renal failure: diagnosis and management, *Comprehensive Therapy,* 31:262-269, 2005.

Morton PG, Fontaine DK, Hudak CM, Gallo BM: *Critical care nursing: a holistic approach,* ed 8, Philadelphia, 2005, Lippincott.

National Kidney Foundation: Nutrition and chronic kidney disease, 2006, from www.kidney.org/atoz/pdf/nutri_chronic.pdf.

Piraino B, Bailie GR, Bernardini J, Boeschoten E, Gupta A, Holmes C, et al: International Society for Peritoneal Dialysis guidelines/recommendations, *Peritoneal Dialysis International,* 25,107-131, 2005.

Rosen S, Stillman, I: Acute tubular necrosis is a syndrome of physiologic and pathologic dissociation, *Journal of the American Society of Nephrology,* 19:871-875, 2008.

Russell TA: Acute renal failure related to rhabdomyolysis: pathophysiology, diagnosis, and collaborative management, *Nephrology Nursing Journal,* 32:409-417, 2005.

Tintinalli JE, Kelen GD, Stapczynski S: *Tintinalli's emergency medicine: a comprehensive study guide,* ed 6, The American College of Emergency Physicians, New York: McGraw-Hill, 2004.

Tomlins MJ: Practice change in peritoneal dialysis exit site care, *Renal Society of Australasia Journal,* 4:26-29, 2008.

Weisbord SD, Palevsky PM: Radiocontrast-induced acute renal failure, *Journal of Intensive Care Medicine,* 20:63-75, 2005.

West B, Picken M, Leehey D: Albuminuria in acute tubular necrosis, *Nephrology, Dialysis, Transplantation* 21:2953-2956, 2006.

Venkataraman R, Kellum JA: Prevention of acute renal failure, *Chest,* 131:300-308, 2007.

NCLEX® Review

1. The earliest sign of acute tubular necrosis (ATN) is:
   1 Decreased urinary output.
   2 Uremic frost.
   3 Chills and fever.
   4 Cardiac friction rub.

2. Which of the following urine patterns is seen in the recovery phase of ATN?
   1 Anuria.
   2 Polyuria.
   3 Oliguria.
   4 Hypovolemia.

3. As a nurse caring for a patient in acute renal failure, you are observing your patient's heart rate. Which electrolyte would you be concerned about?
   1 Sodium.
   2 Potassium.
   3 Chloride.
   4 Phosphorous.

4. Which of the following should the nurse expect to find when assessing an arteriovenous fistula?
   1 Redness.
   2 Pulselessness.
   3 Presence of thrill and bruit.
   4 Mottled skin distal to site.

5. The nurse is teaching a patient about the classic signs and symptoms of renal failure. The nurse realizes the patient needs additional instruction when he includes which of the following?
   1 Loss of appetite.
   2 Fatigue.
   3 Hair loss.
   4 Fluid retention.

6. Which of the following patients does the nurse recognize as being at greatest risk for the development of renal disease?
   1 A 72-year-old African-American woman with osteoporosis.
   2 A 55-year-old African-American man with hypertension.
   3 A 32-year-old obese white woman.
   4 A 15-year-old white adolescent with cerebral palsy.

7. The use of which medication would the nurse most likely question when caring for a patient with a diagnosis of CKD stage 4?
   1 Ibuprofen.
   2 Epogen.
   3 Calcium carbonate.
   4 Phos-Lo.

8. Which of the following medications may be prescribed to prevent clot formation in the extracorporeal circuit?
   1 Vitamin K.
   2 Warfarin (Coumadin).
   3 Trisodium citrate.
   4 Protamine sulfate.

9. A patient is scheduled for multiple tests using iodinated contrast media. Which interventions below may be helpful in preventing ATN?
   1 Restrict fluids for 8 to 12 hours before the test.
   2 Administer acetaminophen 625 mg before and after the test.
   3 Force fluids orally for 24 hours after the test.
   4 Start isotonic IV fluids 12 hours before and run for 12 hours after the test.

10. The patient receiving CRRT has a temperature of 96.2° F. The nurse knows this is best treated by:
    1 Using an in-line fluid warmer to warm the blood returning to the patient.
    2 Ensuring that the patient is fully covered with a warming blanket.
    3 Applying warm compresses to the vascular access site.
    4 Encouraging a family member to bring a pair of warm flannel pajamas for the patient.

NCLEX® Review Answers

1.1 Urinary output is dependent on glomerular filtration rate (GFR). The GFR decreases in ATN, which causes a decrease in urinary output. In renal failure, uremia takes time to develop, and uremic frost is a late sign. Chills and fever should not be present unless the patient has an infection or is septic. Cardiac friction rub could be heard as a result of uremic pericarditis but would be a late sign.

2.2 GFR increases in the recovery phase and BUN and creatinine levels slowly decrease. The concentrating ability of the nephron is weak, resulting in polyuria, and there is poor filtration of wastes, so BUN and creatinine fall slowly.

3.2 An increased serum potassium level can contribute to irritability of the heart and should be monitored closely. Although sodium, chloride, and phosphorus are important electrolytes, they are not the most important for heart conduction (dysrhythmias) problems.

4.3 A bruit and thrill indicate adequate blood flow through a fistula. Redness is not an expected finding, and no skin discoloration at the site should be found. A loss of pulse is indicative of circulatory compromise and needs to be reported to the physician immediately.

5.3 Anorexia from retained nitrogenous wastes, fatigue from anemia and loss of nutrition, and fluid retention are all signs of renal failure. Hair loss is not associated with kidney function.

6.2 African-American men with hypertension are among the populations most likely to develop renal disease. Osteoporosis is not a risk factor for renal disease. Age may contribute to the development of renal disease but not to the extent of hypertension. Obesity is a risk factor for hypertension but not necessarily renal disease. Cerebral palsy is not a risk for renal disease.

7.1 The use of nonsteroidal antiinflammatory drugs (NSAIDs) such as ibuprofen are contraindicated in the patient with renal disease (CKD stage 4 has severe loss of GFR). Epogen (erythropoietin alfa) is commonly used to treat anemia; calcium carbonate is commonly used to treat hypocalcemia; Phos-Lo is commonly used to reduce hyperphosphatemia in a patient with end-stage renal disease (ESRD).

8.3 Trisodium citrate may be used to prevent clot formation in the extracorporeal circuit. Vitamin K is an antagonist of Coumadin. Coumadin, although an anticoagulant, is not indicated to prevent clot formation during CRRT. Protamine sulfate is an antagonist for heparin.

9.4 IV administration of isotonic fluid for 12 hours before and after contrast media may be effective in decreasing the risk of nephrotoxic ATN. Tylenol is not appropriate and can even be nephrotoxic under certain circumstances. IV hydration is believed more effective than oral but must begin before the examination. Restricting fluids would concentrate the contrast media, possibly increasing toxicity.

10.1 An in-line fluid warmer helps control hypothermia. The complete circuit, including the access site, must remain visible. Do not cover the access site with a blanket or pajamas. The use of warm compresses at the vascular access site is not appropriate.

Endocrine System

What You WILL LEARN

After reading this chapter, you will know how to do the following:

- ✔ Compare and contrast the various types of alterations in glucose metabolism: diabetic ketoacidosis, hyperglycemic hyperosmolar state, hypoglycemia.
- ✔ Describe the pathophysiologic process associated with each alteration in glucose metabolism and the effect on the critical care patient.
- ✔ Identify appropriate nursing interventions for caring for a patient with altered glucose metabolism.
- ✔ Discuss the pathophysiologic processes associated with pituitary disorders.
- ✔ Differentiate between the various endocrine pituitary disorders: syndrome of inappropriate antidiuretic hormone and diabetes insipidus.
- ✔ Explain the nursing management for the care of a patient with pituitary disorders.
- ✔ Describe prevention approaches that can be instituted in the critical care environment.
- ✔ Describe relevant patient education topics.

evolve
See http://evolve.elsevier.com/Schumacher/criticalcare for additional NCLEX® review questions.

What IS Diabetes Mellitus?

Diabetes mellitus is a disorder of the endocrine system that causes alterations in glucose metabolism. Two primary classifications of diabetes exist: type 1 and type 2. Both classifications of diabetes result from dysfunctional pancreatic cells.

What You NEED TO KNOW

Pancreas

The pancreas is an organ with both endocrine and exocrine functions. The exocrine function is to release a juice full of enzymes and other components that helps with the process of digestion. One of the functions of this juice is to adjust the pH of the contents of the duodenum, so the pancreatic enzymes can work efficiently. Pancreatic enzymes include proteases, amylases, and lipases to facilitate the breakdown of proteins, starches, and fats. Tissue in the pancreas is called the *islets of Langerhans*. This tissue contains the primary endocrine cells referred to as *alpha, beta,* and *delta* cells.

Alpha, Beta, and Delta Cells

- Alpha cells produce glucagon, which helps maintain normal blood sugar levels through the breakdown of glycogen (glycogenolysis) and the formation of glycogen from fats and proteins (gluconeogenesis). Hypoglycemia stimulates the release of glucagon, and hyperglycemia inhibits glucagon release.
- Beta cells produce insulin, which is the key that allows cells to be permeable to glucose along with amino acids, potassium, magnesium, and phosphate. Insulin assists in carbohydrate, protein, and fat metabolism and in the formation of new proteins. Patients who are insulin deficient have depleted protein and decreased glucose in muscle cells. An abnormal release of stored body fat occurs because of a shift from carbohydrate to fat metabolism. Ketone formation results from the metabolism of fats; if left untreated, it results in ketoacidosis and coma.
- Delta cells secrete somatostatin, which inhibits growth hormone, thyroid-stimulating hormone, insulin, glucagon, and other gastrointestinal (GI) hormones.

Pancreatic tissue.

TAKE HOME POINTS

In Type 1 Diabetes:

There is typically an autoimmune process that causes islet cell antibodies. Most frequently it is associated with an absolute lack of insulin and typical onset is before the age of 30. People with type 1 diabetes are often at their expected ideal body weight or below. These patients require exogenous administration of insulin.

In Type 2 Diabetes:

There is a relative insulin deficiency and absence of circulating islet cell antibodies. It typically occurs in obese people older than 40 years of age. A proper diet and exercise, as well as oral hypoglycemic agents, may be used to manage the condition early on. After 5 or more years, insulin therapy may be required.

Multiple factors including genetics, diseases or trauma of the pancreas, infections, and drugs can contribute to both types of diabetes.

Prevalence

- Diabetes has been diagnosed in more than 16 million Americans.
- An additional 6 million Americans are estimated to have undiagnosed diabetes.
- Ninety percent to 95% of cases are type 2.

Complications

Many acute and chronic complications are associated with type 1 and type 2 diabetes. Other complications often are a result of chronic hyperglycemia and alterations in metabolism. Serious complications result from vascular and neuropathic alterations. Diabetes is the leading cause of end-stage renal failure and new blindness in adults.

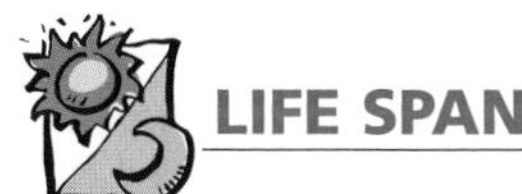

LIFE SPAN

Approximately 15% of type 1 diabetic patients die by the age of 40 years.

What IS Diabetic Ketoacidosis?

Diabetic ketoacidosis (DKA) is one of the more serious metabolic crises that can result from hyperglycemia in patients with uncontrolled diabetes mellitus. The incidence of DKA occurs most frequently in adolescents and older adults with type 1 diabetes; however, several recent studies have identified DKA in patients with type 2 diabetes. DKA results from a deficiency of insulin, which leads to four life-threatening metabolic derangements. First, because the beta cells in the pancreas are unable to produce insulin, the ensuing hyperglycemia causes a hyperosmolar state. This hyperosmolarity results in fluid shifting from inside the cell to the serum; eventually, this fluid is lost in the urine, causing electrolyte shifts and total body dehydration. Other metabolic derangements occur because no insulin exists to allow glucose to enter the cells; therefore, cells begin to break down fats and proteins to use for fuel. This process causes the formation of ketones. Ketones decrease the blood pH and the bicarbonate concentration, causing a ketoacidosis.

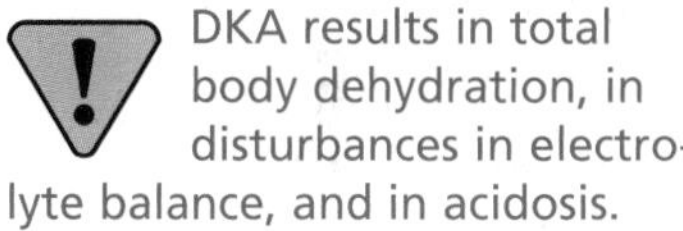

DKA results in total body dehydration, in disturbances in electrolyte balance, and in acidosis.

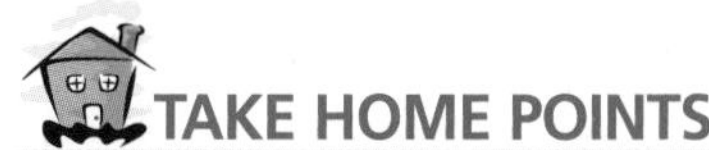

TAKE HOME POINTS

In type 2 diabetes, insulin deficiency can contribute to the development of DKA, along with insulin resistance at the cellular level.

What You NEED TO KNOW

Clinical Manifestations

The definition of DKA includes plasma glucose level greater than 250 mg/dL, blood pH less than 7.35, bicarbonate less than 15 mEq/L, and a significant anion gap. DKA can occur in type 2 diabetes; however, most frequently it is the initial presentation of undiagnosed type 1 diabetes or can appear when patients have missed or reduced insulin doses. Glucoregulatory hormone excess at levels sufficient to promote hyperglycemia occurs with illness, stress, growth spurts, and pregnancy. Medications that interfere with insulin secretion or action include thiazide diuretics, Dilantin, sympathomimetics, and glucocorticoids. The result of excess glucose (hyperglycemia) and insufficient insulin can lead to DKA.

The hallmark symptoms of DKA include dehydration, ketosis, metabolic acidosis, and ketonuria. The patient may also exhibit weakness, anorexia, vomiting, abdominal pain, altered mental status, tachycardia, orthostatic hypotension, poor skin turgor, dry mucous membranes, and Kussmaul respirations (the attempt of the body to eliminate ketones through respirations, giving the breath a fruity, sweet odor).

In DKA, diagnostic findings may include serum glucose levels of greater than 250, often more than 500 mg/dL, glycosuria, increased serum osmolarity, serum acidosis, elevated blood urea nitrogen (BUN), and initially a hyperkalemia.

Serum Osmolality

Serum osmolality is the concentration of solute particles in the blood. Serum osmolality can be calculated by using the serum measurements of sodium, glucose, and BUN. Serum osmolality is increased in patients with acidosis, DKA, hyperglycemia, hyperglycemic hyperosmolar nonketotic coma, hypernatremia, methanol poisoning, and nephrogenic diabetes insipidus. The serum osmolality formula is the following:

$$\text{Serum osmolatily} = (2 \times \text{Serum sodium}) + \frac{\text{Serum glucose}}{18} + \frac{\text{BUN}}{2.8}$$

Anion Gap

The anion gap is a calculation of the difference between the major positively charged electrolytes (cations) and the major negatively charged electrolytes (anions) in the serum. It helps determine the cause of metabolic acidosis. The anion gap formula is the following:

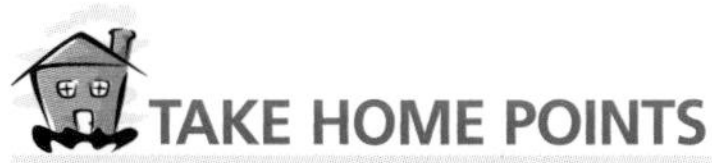

TAKE HOME POINTS

Normal serum osmolality: 280 to 300 mOsm/kg. Normal anion gap: 8 to 20 mEg/L.

$$\text{Anion gap} = \frac{(\text{Serum sodium } [Na^{+}] + \text{Serum potassium } [K^{+}])\ -}{(\text{Serum chloride } [Cl] + \text{Serum bicarbonate } [HCO_3])}$$

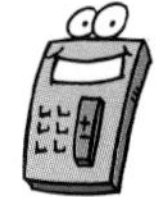

Causes of DKA:

- Initial presentation in undiagnosed type 1 diabetes
- Missed or reduced insulin doses
- Illness, particularly infection and stress hormone excess, that increases blood sugar levels
- Stress
- Growth spurts
- Pregnancy

Medications that interfere with insulin secretion or action include glucocorticoids (hydrocortisone, prednisone, dexamethasone), phenytoin (Dilantin), thiazide diuretics (hydrochlorothiazide), sympathomimetics (albuterol, dobutamine, dopamine, epinephrine, norepinephrine, phenylephrine).

DKA laboratory values:

- Serum glucose levels elevated (usually >250 mg/dL)
- Elevated BUN
- Glucosuria
- Elevated serum osmolality (usually >300 mOsm/L)
- Arterial pH: <7.35
- Hyperkalemia (often, initially): >5.4 mEq/L
- Anion gap: >20 mEq/L

What You DO

Goals of treatment include correction of the acidosis, correction of the electrolyte and fluid disturbances, insulin to lower serum glucose levels, prevention of ketosis, and prevention of complications. When treating patients with DKA, the medical team should do the following:

FIRST-LINE AND INITIAL TREATMENTS FOR DKA

- Closely monitor blood glucose levels and acidosis (arterial blood gasses [ABGs]).
- Administer insulin.
- Replace fluids and electrolytes.
- Monitor cardiac, pulmonary, and neurologic systems.
- Identify and correct precipitating event.
- Educate the patient and the patient's family.

Medical Interventions and Nursing Responsibilities

When treating patients with DKA, the medical team should do the following:

- Monitor serum glucose levels at least every 2 hours. Serum glucose levels should be monitored every 1 to 2 hours while the patient is receiving a continuous insulin infusion.
- Administer rapid-acting insulin. Administration of regular intravenous (IV) insulin at a rate of 0.1 to 0.2 U/kg/hr is recommended via continuous infusion to accomplish a gradual decrease in serum glucose.
- Replace life-threatening fluid and electrolyte deficits. The fluid of choice is usually 0.9% normal saline (NS), which allows for replacement of extracellular fluid (ECF) volume deficits. Initial replacement is usually rapid; then, when the patient's blood pressure (BP) is normal, hypotonic saline (0.45% NS) can be used.
- Monitor acidosis by assessing arterial blood gases (ABGs). Correction of fluid and electrolyte imbalance will allow the kidneys to conserve bicarbonate and restore acid-base balance. Acidosis is usually treated with bicarbonate when the serum pH is 7.10 or less. In this setting, bicarbonate is added to hypotonic NS and replaced slowly.
- Monitor cardiac, pulmonary, and neurologic status.
- Monitor and correct electrolyte imbalances. IV replacement of potassium, chloride, phosphate, and magnesium may be required. Osmotic diuresis can result in a major potassium deficit. If no contraindication such as renal disease exists, potassium replacement usually begins with fluid therapy but should be based on serum and urine laboratory values. Phosphate depletion can result in impaired cardiac and respiratory function. Follow hospital treatment protocol/policies during potassium replacement.
- Monitoring of potassium during treatment is mandatory.

Lowering glucose levels too rapidly can cause cerebral edema, resulting in seizures, coma, or both. *Any* change in level of consciousness in a patient on an insulin drip should include the intervention of seizure precautions and an immediate assessment of blood glucose level.

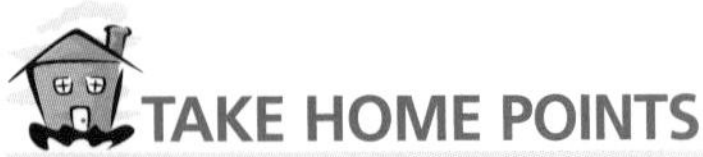

Total body water deficit may be 3 to 4 L in hyperglycemia.

- Observe for potential electrocardiogram (ECG) abnormalities, including ST depression (sign of hypokalemia) or widened QRS and tall, peaked T waves (sign of hyperkalemia). Refer to *Saunders Nursing Survival Guide: ECGs & the Heart,* 2nd ed.
- Correct sodium levels with volume replacement of normal saline. To calculate for corrected sodium in hyperglycemia, add 1.6 mEq to measured sodium for each 100 mg/dL of glucose above a serum glucose level of 100 mg/dL.
- Correct underlying, precipitating events (usually infection). With infections, WBCs (white blood cell count) may be greater than 25,000 with more than 10% neutrophils.
- Provide patient and family support and education. Education is essential in prevention of further episodes of diabetic crisis. Emphasis should be placed on glucose monitoring and regulation, eating schedules, diet, exercise, and rest.
- Avoid complications of therapy.

The most common complications are a result of treatment and include the following:

- Hypoglycemia due to overaggressive treatment with insulin
- Hyperglycemia due to interruption of IV insulin with other coverage
- Hypokalemia resulting from insulin administration and from the treatment of acidosis with sodium bicarbonate

Rapid correction of acidosis can result in severe hypoxemia at the cellular level.

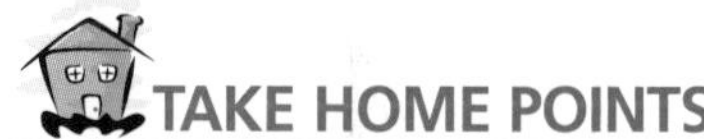

- The goal of treating hyperglycemia is to prevent complications of excess insulin administration and to restore normal uptake of glucose by the cells.
- Potassium phosphate can be used to treat a potassium deficit in hyperglycemia.

Do You UNDERSTAND?

DIRECTIONS: **After reviewing the following results of a patient's physical examination, calculate serum osmolarity and anion gap.**

A 34-year-old woman has a 4-year history of insulin-dependent diabetes. A recent episode of influenza has led to her admission to the intensive care unit (ICU). A physical examination reveals the following:

Respiratory rate: 40 (respirations deep and rapid)
Heart rate (HR): 118 bpm
BP: 88/50 mm Hg
Temperature: 101.8° F, rectally
Skin: Dry, with poor turgor (patient is lethargic but responsive to simple commands)

Admission laboratory data:

- Serum glucose: 540 mg/dL
- BUN: 70
- Hemoglobin (Hgb): 14 g/dL
- Hematocrit (HCT): 48%
- Serum sodium: 129 mEq/L
- Serum potassium: 5 mEq/L
- Serum chloride: 94 mEq/L
- pH: 7.23
- Partial pressure of carbon dioxide (pCO_2): 22
- HCO_3: 8

1. Calculate the serum osmolarity.

    ____

2. Calculate the anion gap.

    ____

What IS Hyperglycemic Hyperosmolar State?

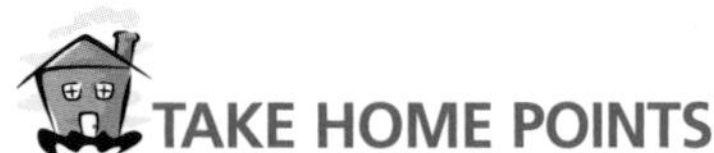

HHS occurs in type 2 diabetes and results in total body dehydration and disturbances in electrolyte balance, without acidosis.

Hyperglycemic hyperosmolar state (HHS) is also a serious metabolic complication of diabetes, but it is usually seen in patients with type 2 diabetes. Because type 2 diabetes is a problem of relative insulin deficiency rather than an absolute deficiency, the cells are able to use some glucose. However, not enough glucose is available for cellular metabolism because of the insulin deficiency, so hyperglycemia develops. This promotes cellular dehydration, osmotic diuresis, and fluid and electrolyte disturbances, but ketosis and acidosis are minimal or absent. These patients are profoundly dehydrated with blood glucose levels typically exceeding 600 mg/dL or greater. Marked hyperosmolarity and elevated BUN levels also exist.

Answers: **1.** Serum osmolarity = 313 mOsm/L = (2 × 129) + (540 ÷ 18) + (70 ÷ 2.8);
2. Anion gap = 32 mEq/L = (129 + 5) − (94 + 8).

What You NEED TO KNOW

HHS usually occurs in individuals with type 2 diabetes who have omitted or reduced their hypoglycemic agent. Other precipitating causes include drugs, enteral feedings, hyperalimentation, and peritoneal dialysis.

Clinical manifestations include:

- Profound dehydration
- Hypotension
- Tachycardia
- Diminished central venous pressure (CVP)
- Dry mucous membranes
- Poor skin turgor
- Neurologic impairments including confusion, seizures, and coma

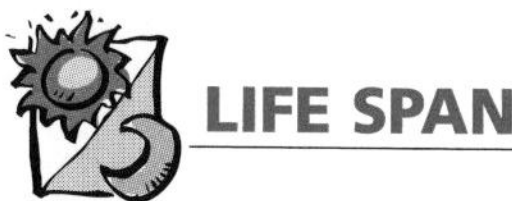

LIFE SPAN

The older adult population is predisposed to HHS, and a concurrent illness or underlying cause usually exists.

What You DO

The treatment goals for HHS are similar to the interventions for DKA. Rapid replacement of fluids to correct dehydration is one of the most important interventions. Often, physicians use isotonic fluids to replace half of the estimated fluid deficit within the first 12 hours and the remainder within 24 hours.

A fast-acting form of insulin is typically administered by IV infusion to closely control blood glucose levels. When the blood glucose level approaches 300 mg/dL, addition of dextrose into the IV infusion should be considered, because the blood glucose level can precipitously drop and the patient can become hypoglycemic. The patient's cardiovascular and neurologic status should be monitored, along with monitoring for embolic complications. The nurse should remember that HHS and DKA are precipitated by underlying problems, often infection, so it is essential to treat the underlying problem. In addition, to prevent future recurrences, patient and family education should be reinforced.

When treating DKA or HHS patients, the nurse should closely monitor serum potassium levels! Because patients with DKA or HHS are hyperosmolar, dehydrated, and depleted of potassium intracellularly, rehydration by replacement fluids alone can decrease serum potassium levels. In addition, insulin therapy causes potassium to move into the cell along with glucose, further decreasing serum potassium levels.

Do You UNDERSTAND?

DIRECTIONS: **After reviewing a patient's history and results of laboratory studies, provide short answers to the two following questions.**

RK is a 76-year-old woman who lives alone. Her medical history includes twice daily diuretics for the treatment of hypertension and a recent complaint of thirst and urination over the past month. Her daughter took her to the emergency department because she was lethargic and difficult to arouse. Her skin and mucous membranes appeared dry. She was in a sinus tachycardia. Laboratory studies disclosed the following values:

Blood glucose level: 1230 mg/dL
Serum sodium: 144 mEq/L
Serum potassium: 5.5 mEq/L
BUN: 79 mg/dL
Creatinine: 2.8 mg/dL
Serum osmolarity: 361 mOsm/kg
pH: 7. 35
HCO3: 18 mEq/L
Urine: Positive for glucose
Serum and urine ketones: Negative

1. Is patient RK more likely to have DKA or HHS? Why?

____
____
____
____

2. What are some important nursing and medical interventions for patient RK?

____
____
____
____

Answers: **1. RK is more likely to have HHS. RK's laboratory values reflect a glucose level of >1000, no acidosis, and no urine and serum ketones;** 2. RK's serum osmolarity and BUN reflect dehydration. RK needs IV replacement of fluids and rapid-acting insulin to reduce the glucose levels (usually in an insulin drip, so glucose levels can be closely controlled and monitored). RK also needs close monitoring of serum electrolyte levels. RK should be frequently assessed for changes in heart rhythms, respiratory rate and rhythms, and alterations in levels of consciousness.

What IS Hypoglycemia?

Acute hypoglycemia occurs when the blood sugar (glucose) levels drop rapidly. Without enough glucose, brain cells cannot use adenosine triphosphate (ATP) for energy, and this causes cerebral dysfunction. This process causes sympathetic nervous system (SNS) stimulation and increased levels of epinephrine, glucagons, growth hormone, cortisol, and adrenocorticotrophic hormone. These hormones suppress the secretion of insulin and act to increase blood sugar levels by gluconeogenesis and glycogenolysis. Epinephrine and cortisol also inhibit glucose use in muscles. Causes of hypoglycemia include adrenal insufficiency, alcohol ingestion, oral antihyperglycemic agents, and insulin.

What You NEED TO KNOW

The following are clinical manifestations of hypoglycemia:

- Sweating, tremors
- Blurred vision, hunger, weakness
- Behavior changes and confusion
- Anxiety, paresthesias, and poor coordination
- Slurred speech, headache
- Palpitations, nausea
- Seizures, stupor, coma

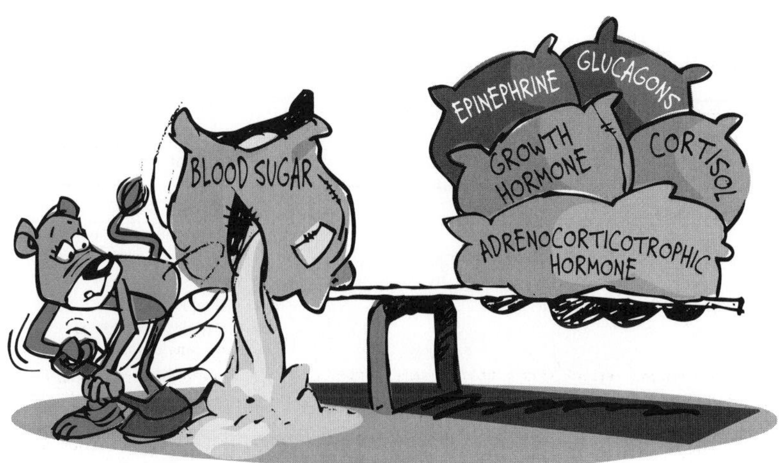

Hypoglycemia causes increases in hormones and other substances.

What You DO

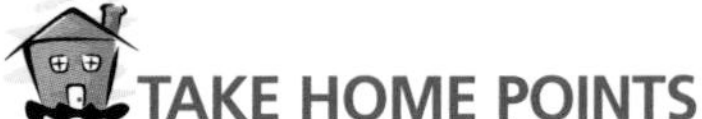

TAKE HOME POINTS

- Nocturnal hypoglycemia may present as night sweats, nightmares, and a morning headache.
- It is important to do a complete assessment and history of the hypoglycemic patient, because the hypoglycemia might be a symptom of another health problem such as myxedema coma (complication of hypothyroidism).

Severe, prolonged hypoglycemia can cause brain damage. Any abnormal behavior in a patient taking insulin should be considered a hypoglycemic reaction until proven otherwise.

It is essential to identify patients at risk for hypoglycemic episodes and monitor these patients for manifestations of hypoglycemia. If the patient has a blood glucose level above 80 mg/dL with symptoms, fast-acting carbohydrates (FACs) are typically not administered. A diet drink should be administered, and the blood glucose level rechecked in 15 minutes. If the patient's blood glucose level has dropped below 80 mg/dL at recheck, the nurse should assess the patient's ability to swallow and administer FACs.

FACs include **ANY ONE** of the following:

- 4 oz (½ cup) of apple juice
- 4 oz of orange juice
- 4 oz of cranberry juice
- 4 oz of cola
- 8 oz of skim milk

If the patient has a blood glucose level of less than 60 mg/dL, the nurse should assess the patient's ability to swallow and immediately administer FACs. The patient and blood glucose level should be assessed every 15 minutes until the blood glucose level is greater than 70 mg/dL. If the patient has not been placed on nothing by mouth (NPO) status, a complex carbohydrate snack may be given. If the patient is unable to swallow, is NPO, or is unresponsive, glucagon can be given intramuscularly or subcutaneously or dextrose 50 (D50) can be given through an established IV site.

Differences Among Diabetic Ketoacidosis, Hyperglycemic Hyperosmolar State, Hypoglycemia

	DKA	HHS	Hypoglycemia
Symptoms			
	• Confusion, lethargy • Warm, dry, flushed skin • Weakness • Anorexia, nausea • Abdominal pain • Tachycardia • Fruity, acetone breath • Deep, rapid respirations • Thirst	• Confusion, lethargy • Warm, dry flushed skin • Weakness • Tachycardia • Rapid respirations • Acetone breath absent • Thirst	• Cold, clammy skin • Pallor • Profuse sweating • Normal mucous membranes • Irritability, tremors • Poor concentration • Tachycardia • Bradycardia (in coma) • Normal-to-rapid respirations • Acetone breath absent • Hunger

Differences Among Diabetic Ketoacidosis, Hyperglycemic Hyperosmolar State, Hypoglycemia—cont'd

	DKA	HHS	Hypoglycemia
Laboratory Values			
Blood glucose	300-800 mg/dL	Significantly elevated (600-2000 mg/dL)	Below normal
Serum sodium	Normal to decreased	Variable	Normal
Serum potassium	Variable (or low)	Variable (or elevated)	Normal
Serum osmolarity	Elevated but usually <330 mOsm/L	Significantly elevated >350 mOsm/L	Normal
Arterial blood gases	Decreased pH Metabolic acidosis with compensatory respiratory alkalosis	Normal-to-mild acidosis	Normal-to-slight respiratory acidosis
Serum ketones	Positive	Negative	Negative
Urine	Positive for glucose or ketones	Negative for glucose or ketones	Negative for glucose or ketones
Interventions			
	Insulin, fluid, and electrolyte replacement	Insulin, fluid, and electrolyte replacement	Glucose, glucagon

DKA, Diabetic ketoacidosis; *HHNK,* hyperglycemic hyperosmolar state.

Do You UNDERSTAND?

DIRECTIONS: **Identify the following statements as *true* (T) or *false* (F).**

_____1. The key to identifying hypoglycemia is the presence of acidosis.

_____2. Any abnormal behavior in patients taking insulin should be considered a hypoglycemic reaction until proven otherwise.

_____3. A hypoglycemic patient will have positive serum ketones.

What IS Syndrome of Inappropriate Antidiuretic Hormone?

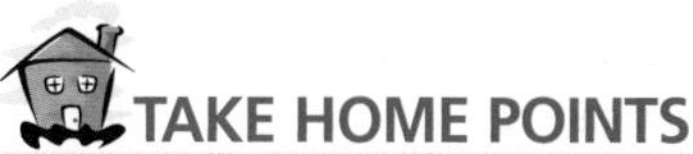

In SIADH, an excessive amount of ADH is released, resulting in water being reabsorbed, which contributes to fluid and electrolyte imbalances.

Syndrome of inappropriate antidiuretic hormone (SIADH) is caused by excessive release of antidiuretic hormone (ADH). The syndrome is characterized by increased water reabsorption in the kidneys, serum sodium

Answers: 1. F; 2. T; 3. F.

dilution (hyponatremia), and elevated serum levels of ADH. Symptoms associated with SIADH-related hyponatremia include lethargy, confusion, and in extreme cases, coma and death. SIADH is strongly associated with neoplasm, particularly small-cell carcinoma of the lung. Nursing care focuses on improving fluid and electrolyte balance and neurologic status.

What You NEED TO KNOW

Under normal conditions, ADH, also called *vasopressin,* is secreted by the posterior pituitary gland in response to increased osmolarity. ADH regulates osmolarity by increasing the permeability of distal tubules and collecting ducts in the kidney to water. Large amounts of water are reabsorbed, diluting solutes, lowering serum osmolarity, and concentrating urine.

In SIADH, ADH levels are increased several-fold, causing an excessive increase in water reabsorption. An increase of water in the ECF dilutes sodium. As water is reabsorbed, small increases in BP cause loss of sodium from the ECF in the urine through pressure natriuresis.

The following place a person at high risk for developing SIADH:

- Neoplasm—specifically small-cell lung cancer and lymphoma
- Central nervous system (CNS) disorders—head trauma, stroke, tumor, meningitis
- Postoperative patients—especially after pituitary surgery
- Antineoplastic agents—cisplatin, vincristine, cyclophosphamide, vinblastine
- Nicotine use
- Medications—tranquilizers, barbiturates, anesthetics, thiazide diuretics

The symptoms depend on the severity of the hyponatremia and the length of time the patient has been hyponatremic.

Clinical Manifestations Associated with Hyponatremia

Serum Sodium Levels	Associated Symptoms
120-135 mEq/L	None
110-120 mEq/L	Headache, apathy, disoriented, weakness, fatigue, thirst, anorexia, possible seizures
100-110 mEq/L	Confusion, severe gastrointestinal symptoms including nausea or vomiting and abdominal cramps, muscle twitching
<100 mEq/L	Convulsions, coma, areflexia, death

Other syndromes can be associated with hyponatremia and increased urine sodium levels; these include hypothyroidism, adrenal insufficiency, metabolic acidosis associated with vomiting, osmotic diuresis, diuretics, and renal failure. In addition, during pregnancy, women may develop hyponatremia as low as 130 mEq/L because of the release of the hormone relaxin. This is a normal change. A thorough history of illness and medication use is instrumental in diagnosis.

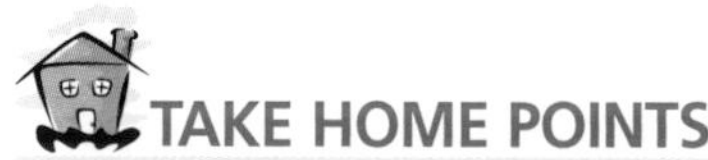

Symptoms of SIADH may be the presenting symptom in patients with small-cell lung cancer.

Comparison of Laboratory Values: Normal vs SIADH

Normal Laboratory Values of Adults	SIADH Diagnostic Evaluation
Serum sodium (137-145 mEq/L)	Serum hyponatremia (<130 mEq/L)
Urine sodium (40-220 mEq/L/day)	Urine hypernatremia (>40 mEq/L)
Serum osmolality (280-300 mOsm/kg)	Serum osmolality (<275 mOsm/kg)
Urine osmolality (50-1200 mOsm/kg)	Urine hyperosmolarity (>100 mOsm/kg)
Uric acid (2-7 mg/dL)	Low uric acid concentration (<4 mg/dL)
Serum potassium (3.5-5.0 mEq/L)	Normal serum potassium
pH (7.35-7.45)	Normal pH
Urine specific gravity (1.002-1.028)	Elevated urine specific gravity
ADH level (0-4.7 pg/mL)	Elevated ADH level

ADH, Antidiuretic hormone; *SIADH,* syndrome of inappropriate antidiuretic hormone.

Prognosis

The prognosis of SIADH depends on the cause. In ectopic ADH secretion, SIADH normally resolves with tumor regression. Any neurologic deficit is usually reversible. In transient SIADH after surgery, ADH levels gradually return to normal within 5 to 7 days.

What You DO

Treatment for SIADH is primarily focused on elimination of the cause. Water restriction (500 to 1000 mL/day) is instituted. The patient may be placed on a high-salt, high-protein diet, and any medications that might potentiate ADH are discontinued. In severe hyponatremia, IV hypertonic saline is administered and may be given with diuretics such as furosemide (Lasix) or mannitol (Osmitrol). Medications that interfere with the action of ADH on the kidney may be initiated, including lithium carbonate

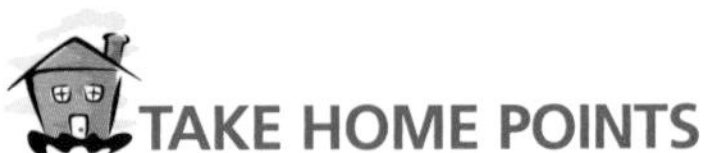

TAKE HOME POINTS

Infusion of hypertonic saline must be implemented slowly, at a rate of ≤ 0.05 mL/kg/min, so as to not cause heart failure due to rapid fluid shifts.

Serum sodium levels must be continuously monitored every 2 hours and the infusion discontinued once the serum sodium level has increased by 12 or reaches 130 mEq/L.

Hyponatremic patients are at risk for seizures and falls.

(Lithobid, Lithonate) or demeclocycline (Declomycin). No drug therapy is available to suppress ectopic release of ADH.

If the cause is unknown, the medical history may provide clues. A history of stroke, cancer, pulmonary disease, or head injury should be considered as significant in the diagnosis of SIADH.

The patient should be assessed for symptoms of hyponatremia, including neurologic status. The level of consciousness should be determined, and any change should be noted. The patient's safety should be protected at all times, and the nurse should assist with ambulation. Fall precautions and seizure precautions should be initiated as appropriate. Frequent neurologic assessments should be performed and daily electrolyte laboratory results monitored.

Fluid restrictions should be maintained and input and output documented. The patient should be weighed daily, and comfort measures for thirst should be provided, such as lozenges, swabs, or ice chips. Water or ice chips should not be kept at the bedside. The nurse should help the patient and family understand the importance of fluid restriction and monitoring daily weights. In addition, the signs and symptoms of hyponatremia should be taught.

FIRST-LINE AND INITIAL TREATMENTS FOR SIADH

- Monitor electrolyte laboratory values.
- Restrict fluids.
- Infuse hypertonic saline.
- Administer prescribed medications, such as furosemide, mannitol, lithium carbonate, and demeclocycline.
- Protect the patient from possible injury (seizures).
- Ensure accurate intake and output.
- Weigh the patient each day.

Do You UNDERSTAND?

DIRECTIONS: **Select the best answer, and place the appropriate letter in the space provided.**

_____1. SIADH is most strongly associated with:

a. Small-cell lung cancer.

b. Pregnancy.

c. Breast cancer.
d. Surgery.

_____2. The symptoms of SIADH are most strongly associated with:
a. Hypernatremia.
b. Hyponatremia.
c. Water intoxication.
d. Urine hyperosmolarity.

_____3. The following are appropriate nursing actions associated with SIADH ***EXCEPT***:
a. Monitor strict intake and output.
b. Institute safety procedures.
c. Keep water and ice chips at bedside.
d. Weigh the patient each day.

What IS Diabetes Insipidus?

Diabetes insipidus (DI) is caused by a deficiency in the production or release of ADH by the posterior pituitary gland. The insufficient amount of circulating ADH results in the renal tubules being unable to conserve free water, which is clinically seen as polyuria.

What You NEED TO KNOW

Normally, ADH is secreted by the posterior pituitary gland and regulates water balance and serum osmolality. In DI, interference with the production, transport, or release of ADH causes excessive water loss and the inability to dilute serum solutes. The following are common categories of DI:

Neurogenic

- Posterior pituitary region lesion (hypothalamus, pituitary, craniopharyngioma)
- Congenital defect

Answers: 1. a; 2. b; 3. c.

- Severe head trauma
- Intracranial surgery (especially region of pituitary)
- Increased intracranial pressure (ICP)
- CNS infections (meningitis, encephalitis)
- Metastatic malignancies
- Autoimmune response
- Granulomatous disease (tuberculosis [TB], sarcoidosis)
- Idiopathic diseases and conditions

Nephrogenic

- Renal disease (pyelonephritis, polycystic disease, obstructive uropathy)
- Decrease or absence of ADH receptors
- Cellular damage to loop of Henle nephrons
- Drugs (lithium, ethanol, amphotericin, demeclocycline, phenytoin)
- Hypokalemia
- Hypercalcemia

Psychogenic

- Water intoxication
- Excessive IV fluid administration
- Drugs (anticholinergics, tricyclic antidepressants)

Clinical Manifestations

- Polyuria (30 to 40 L/24 hr)
- Polydipsia
- Hypotension (systolic blood pressure [SBP] in adult < 90 mm Hg)
- Tachycardia (HR >100 beats per minute)
- Weight loss
- Dehydration (decreased skin turgor, dry mucous membranes)
- Mental status changes (confusion, restlessness, irritability, lethargy, coma)
- Seizures
- Constipation
- Diagnostic evaluation includes serum and urine laboratory tests

Serum Findings

- Serum sodium > 145 mEq/L
- Serum osmolality > 300 mOsm/kg
- Serum ADH decreased in neurogenic DI, may be normal with nephrogenic or psychogenic diabetes insipidus

Urine

- Urine specific gravity (USG) < 1.005
- Urine osmolality < 300 mOsm/kg

What You DO

Treatment for DI is focused on correcting the underlying cause, as well as restoring and maintaining fluid volume. To restore and maintain fluid volume, the patient requires volume replacement. Depending on the patient's mental status and ability to ingest fluid, the patient should be able to drink enough water to maintain fluid volume. Patients who are unable to orally take in adequate amounts of fluid will most likely require IV administration of fluids. In either case, it is important that the patient be adequately hydrated; otherwise, he or she will exhibit signs and symptoms of fluid volume loss (hypotension, tachycardia). If the DI is psychogenic, then the management is to remove the causative agent, which in this case would be by restricting fluid intake.

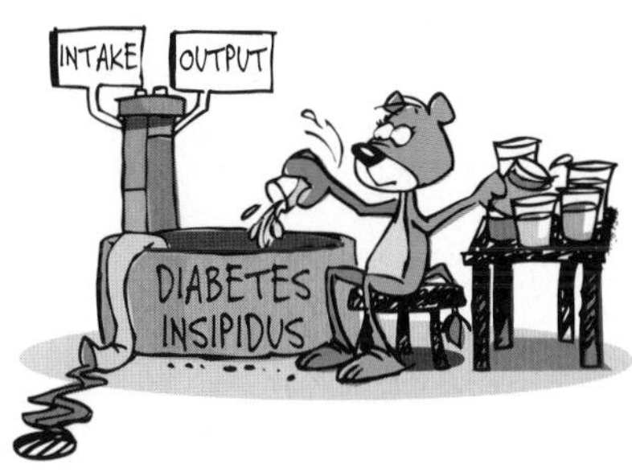

Assessing fluid intake and output is imperative in patients with DI.

Medications Used to Treat Diabetes Insipidus

Drug	Dose	Limitations	Side Effects
Desmopressin acetate	**Intranasally** 10-40 mcg (micrograms) at bedtime or in divided doses **Parenteral** 2-4 mg twice daily	High cost ($2000/yr)	Nasal congestion Headache Flushing Hyponatremia (overtreatment)
Vasopressin (Pitressin)	**Intramuscularly or subcutaneously** 5-10 units every 6 to 12 hours	Very short duration (1-2 hours)	Sweating Tremor
	Intravenously 0.2-0.4 units/min up to 0.9 units/min		Pounding in head Abdominal cramps Nausea Angina Increased blood pressure Water intoxication

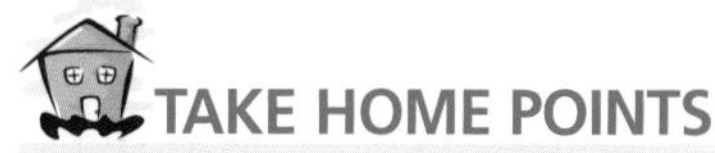

TAKE HOME POINTS

Overmedication with an exogenous ADH medication can cause water overload resulting in third spacing, pulmonary congestion, and weight gain.

Medications that are used in the management of DI include an exogenous hormone supplement to replace the ADH. For the initial management of the patient in DI, the medication of choice is vasopressin

(Pitressin); for the patient with a chronic neurogenic DI, the medication of choice is desmopressin acetate (DDAVP).

Nursing management of the patient with DI includes astute assessment skills of fluid volume and neurologic status. Monitoring the patient's intake and output, weight, vital signs, laboratory values, and treatment outcomes is crucial in effectively managing the patient with DI. In addition, patient and family education is important in assisting the patient and family to understand the DI disease process, the importance of drinking fluid, and the importance of the medication regimen prescribed.

Do You UNDERSTAND?

DIRECTIONS: **Select the best answer, and place the appropriate number in the space provided.**

_____1. In which cause of DI would you implement fluid restriction?
1. Neurogenic
2. Psychogenic
3. Anatomic
4. Pleurogenic

_____2. Overmedication with an exogenous ADH medication in a person with DI can cause:
1. Constipation.
2. GI hemorrhage.
3. Third spacing.
4. Dehydration.

DIRECTIONS: **Unscramble the italicized letters to complete each of the following statements.**

3. The _____________________ gland is responsible for the production and release of ADH. *(ripseoort; rtiuyaipt)*
4. To maintain fluid volume, the patient will require _____________________ replacement. *(elvmuo)*
5. A medication given intranasally that is the exogenous replacement of ADH is _____________________. *(sopsienemdsr)*

Answers: 1. 2; 2. 3; 3. posterior pituitary; 4. volume; 5. desmopressin.

References

American Association of Critical Care Nurses: *Core curriculum for critical care nursing,* JG Alspach (Ed), ed 6, St Louis, 2006, Saunders/Elsevier.

Barker E: *Neuroscience nursing: a spectrum of care,* ed 3. St Louis, 2008, Mosby.

Chernecky CC, Berger BJ: *Laboratory tests and diagnostic procedures,* St Louis, 2008, Elsevier.

Chih-hung C, Jui-Jung L, Chang C, Lee C: Recurrent hyponatremia after traumatic brain injury. *American Journal Medical Science,* 335(5):390-393, 2008.

Chulay M, Burns SM: *American Association of Critical Care Nurses essentials of critical care nursing,* New York, 2006, McGraw Hill.

Guerrero R, Pumar A, Soto A, et al: Early hyponatraemia after pituitary surgery: cerebral salt-wasting syndrome, *European Journal of Endocrinology,* 156:611-616, 2007.

Morton PG, Fontaine DK, Hudak CM, Gallo BM: *Critical care nursing: a holistic approach,* ed 8, Philadelphia, 2004, Lippincott Williams & Wilkins.

Urden LD, Stacy KM, Lough ME: *Thelan's critical care nursing,* ed 5, St Louis, 2006, Elsevier.

NCLEX® Review

1. Which of the following is caused by a total lack of endogenous insulin?
   1 Metabolic alkalosis.
   2 Hypotension.
   3 Hyperglycemic hyperosmolar state (HHS).
   4 Diabetic ketoacidosis (DKA).
2. Severe hyperosmolarity, dehydration, and blood glucose levels above 1000 mg/dL are most likely associated with:
   1 Metabolic alkalosis.
   2 Hyperglycemic hyperosmolar state.
   3 Diabetic ketoacidosis.
   4 Adrenal insufficiency.
3. A patient is admitted to the intensive care unit with a decreased level of consciousness. She has a 4-year history of type 1 diabetes. Her skin is dry with poor turgor. A physical examination reveals the following:
   RR: 40, deep and rapid
   HR: 118 bpm, weak pulse
   PB: 100/58 mm Hg
   Temperature: 101.8° F, rectally
   Serum glucose level: 510 mg/dL
   Serum osmolarity: 315 mOsm/L
   HGB: 14 g/dL
   Hematocrit (HCT): 48%
   Na^+: 130 mEq/L
   K^+: 5 mEq/L
   pH: 7.23
   Which would be the primary cause of the patient's dehydration and increased serum osmolarity?
   1 Hyponatremia.
   2 Hyperthermia.
   3 Ketosis.
   4 Osmotic diuresis.
4. The primary goal during initial treatment of a patient who has a hyperglycemic hyperosmolar state is to:
   1 Lower serum glucose levels as quickly as possible.
   2 Correct the patient's dehydrated state.
   3 Restore normal serum potassium levels.
   4 Identify the precipitating problem.
5. A primary danger of insulin shock is:
   1 Increased uptake of glucose.
   2 Severe dehydration and hypovolemia.
   3 Increased alertness.
   4 Irreversible brain damage.
6. Which of the following is true concerning syndrome of inappropriate antidiuretic hormone secretion (SIADH)?
   1 Antidiuretic hormone (ADH) levels are increased; serum sodium levels are increased; urine specific gravity is increased.
   2 ADH levels are increased; serum sodium levels are decreased; urine-specific gravity is increased.
   3 ADH levels are decreased; serum sodium levels are decreased; urine-specific gravity is decreased.
   4 ADH levels are decreased; serum sodium are increased; urine-specific gravity is unchanged.
7. SIADH is suspected in which of the following patients?
   1 An older patient with a recent stroke who is confused and on diuretics.
   2 A patient recovering from surgery with a serum sodium level of 150 mEq/L and increased urine sodium level.
   3 A pregnant woman with serum sodium level of 130 mEq/L.
   4 A patient with small-cell carcinoma of the lung who is complaining of muscle cramps, whose urine-specific gravity is 1.030, and whose serum sodium is 120 mEq/L.
8. Which vital signs indicate the possibility of diabetes insipidus?
   1 BP 210/140 mm Hg, temperature 97.8° F.
   2 HR 66 bpm, temperature 102° F.
   3 RR 28 breaths/minute, HR 40.
   4 BP 70/40 mm Hg, HR 124.

9. What clinical manifestation occurs in the gastrointestinal tract as a result of polyuria associated with DI?
   1 Diarrhea.
   2 Constipation.
   3 Hemorrhage.
   4 Ulcerative colitis.

10. What two main areas of nursing assessment are crucial in monitoring the patient with DI?
   1 Cardiac rate and psychologic status.
   2 Airway and GI loss.
   3 Fluid volume and neurologic status.
   4 Pain and pulmonary status.

NCLEX® Review Answers

1.4 DKA occurs in patients with type 1 diabetes who lack any production of endogenous insulin. Lack of endogenous insulin leads to hyperglycemia; if left untreated, it can lead to DKA, which results in metabolic acidosis. Hypotension is not a direct result of a lack of endogenous insulin. HHS is commonly associated with type 2 diabetes, in which there is a relative but not total lack of insulin.

2.2 HHS coma is usually accompanied by blood glucose levels greater than 1000 mg/dL and severe dehydration that is the result of hyperosmolarity and osmotic diuresis. Causes of metabolic alkalosis include loop diuretics, antacids, hypokalemia, blood products, lactate administration, nasogastric suction, and H_2-blockers. DKA is commonly associated with blood glucose levels greater than 250 mg/dL but usually less than 1000 mg/dL, as well as dehydration, hyperosmolarity, and acidosis. Adrenal insufficiency from glucocorticoid insufficiency results in fever, nausea and vomiting, abdominal pain, hypotension, and altered mental status. Adrenal insufficiency caused by mineralocorticoid insufficiency results in hyponatremia and hypokalemia.

3.4 The primary cause of dehydration in patients with DKA and HHS is osmotic diuresis. Because the serum is hyperosmolar, water is pulled from the cells into the serum and then eliminated through the kidneys as urine. Normal serum levels are 136 to 145 mEq/L. Although this value represents hyponatremia, it is not the primary cause of this patient's dehydration. This patient is hyperthermic. Often, patients with DKA have an underlying infection that may be responsible for the temperature elevation. Ketosis results from the formation of ketone bodies with the breakdown of fats for fuel. This promotes acidosis.

4.2 The administration of IV fluids based on estimated fluid volume deficit rehydrates the patient and alone decreases serum glucose levels. Rapid decrease of serum glucose levels can cause insulin shock. Restoring serum potassium to normal is essential in the treatment of the patient in a diabetic crisis, but it is not the initial primary goal. Identifying the precipitating problem is also essential in a patient with HHS. Often, patients have underlying infections as a precipitating cause; however, this, again, is not the initial treatment for this patient.

5.4 The brain has a high requirement for glucose for metabolism. Prolonged hypoglycemia can cause the death of brain cells and result in irreversible brain damage. Insulin results in a decrease of serum glucose levels by allowing glucose to enter the cells. The primary danger of too much insulin is low serum glucose levels and irreversible brain damage. Hyperglycemia results in osmotic diuresis, dehydration, and hypovolemia. Hypoglycemia causes poor concentration, irritability, tremors, and coma.

6.2 Inappropriate secretion of ADH causes increased permeability of the distal tubule of the kidney to water. Extracellular water levels rise, diluting serum sodium. Small increases in BP cause sodium to be lost in the urine through pressure natriuresis, and urine-specific gravity is elevated.

7.4 The most common malignancy associated with SIADH is small-cell lung cancer. Diagnostic evaluation includes urine hyperosmolarity and serum hyponatremia. Muscle cramps are associated with hyponatremia. Although CNS injury and certain medications, including diuretics, can cause SIADH, this is not the best answer. Transient SIADH can result from surgery, but hyponatremia is a clinical manifestation. During pregnancy, women can develop hyponatremia (as low as 130 mEq/L) because of the release of the hormone, relaxin. This is a normal change.

8.4 Hypotension and tachycardia indicate DI. Usually, the patient becomes hypotensive as a result of the loss of fluid. The patient is usually tachycardic, and temperature may be affected. Respiratory rate can vary, depending on the acid-base balance.

9.2 Loss of water in polyuria results in constipation. The patient becomes dehydrated; no extra fluid is available. Hemorrhage and ulcerative colitis do not relate to polyuria and the GI tract in the patient with DI.

10.3 Fluid volume status is directly associated with ADH, and neurologic status changes are clinically indicative of DI. The cardiac rate is important to assess in DI, but the patient's psychological status is not considered crucial at this time. Airway is always an important assessment point, but in DI, the GI loss is not crucial. Pain and pulmonary status are important assessment areas; however, when suspecting DI, these assessment points are also not crucial.

Hematologic System

What You WILL LEARN

After reading this chapter, you will know how to do the following:

- ✔ Differentiate between thrombocytopenia and disseminated intravascular coagulation.
- ✔ Describe the pathophysiologic process associated with thrombocytopenia and disseminated intravascular coagulation.
- ✔ Discuss complications associated with hematologic alterations in a critically ill patient.
- ✔ Identify appropriate nursing interventions for caring for a patient with hematologic alterations.
- ✔ Describe prevention approaches that can be instituted in the critical care environment.
- ✔ Describe relevant patient education topics.

evolve
See http://evolve.elsevier.com/Schumacher/criticalcare for additional NCLEX® review questions.

What IS Thrombocytopenia?

Thrombocytopenia is a decrease (<150,000/μl) in the number of platelets (disk-shaped cells that are formed when mature granular megakaryocytes shed their cytoplasm) that circulate through the body. Platelets function in helping blood to clot, in supplying a phospholipid surface so there can be an interaction between clotting factors in the blood, and in assisting in fibrinolysis, which aids in lysis of fibrin clots and vessel repair. It is unusual for bleeding to occur when the platelet count

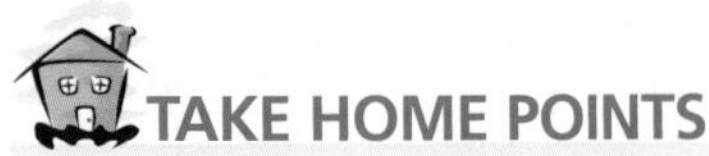

TAKE HOME POINTS

The breakdown, or lysis, of fibrin produces fibrin degradation products (FDP) in the blood.

is greater than 50,000/μl. If patients have counts less than 10,000/μl, they are at high risk for hemorrhage. The two major emergencies associated with thrombocytopenia are (1) hemorrhage and (2) shock (septic or hypovolemic).

What You NEED TO KNOW

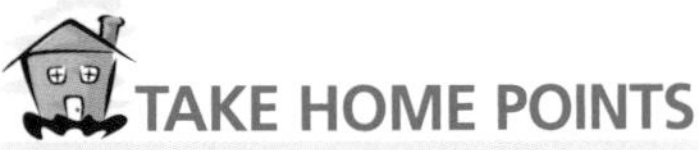

TAKE HOME POINTS

In patients with an enlarged spleen, the platelets become trapped in the spleen and cannot be released into the bloodstream, causing a decrease in the total platelet count on the laboratory report.

Platelets mature in the bone marrow of the pelvis, long bones, ribs, sternum, skull, and spleen and are regulated by the hormone called *thrombopoietin.* Approximately two-thirds of all platelets are then released into the bloodstream, where they aid in the mechanism of clotting, and the remaining one-third are stored in the spleen, where they remain until the body calls for them to be released.

The three main causes of thrombocytopenia are (1) low production of platelets by the body (decreased production of megakaryocytes, called *megakaryocytopoiesis,* because of cancer and its treatment, sex-linked Wiskott-Aldrich syndrome, May-Hegglin anomaly, Fanconi's syndrome, neonatal rubella, and nutritional deficiency of folate or vitamin B_{12}), (2) abnormal distribution of platelets (hypersplenism, liver disease, hypothermia), and (3) increased destruction of platelets or coagulopathy dysfunction as the result of diseases and conditions, medications, or medical treatment.

Causes of Platelet Destruction

Diseases and Conditions	Medications	Medical Treatment
• AIDS/HIV • Cancer • Leukemia • Lymphoma • Hodgkin's disease • Cirrhosis • Cytomegalovirus (CMV) • DIC • Eclampsia • Exanthema subitum • HELLP syndrome • Hepatitis C (chronic)	• Abciximab • Alcohol • Amphotericin B • Aspirin • Beta-lactam antibiotics • Bivalirudin • Cephalosporin antibiotics • Chloramphenicol • Cimetidine • Efalizumab (psoriasis) • Estrogen—large doses • Famotidine • Furosemide	• Alpha-interferon therapy • Bone marrow transplant • Central venous catheters • Chemotherapy (especially platinum-based and alkylating agent therapy) • Post liver transplant • Radiation therapy

Causes of Platelet Destruction—cont'd

Diseases and Conditions	Medications	Medical Treatment
• Hyperthyroidism • Inflammatory bowel disease • ITP • Leptospirosis • Malaria • NAIT or neonatal alloimmune thrombocytopenia • Sepsis • SLE • TIP • Typhoid fever • Vitamin K deficiency	• Gold • H_2 antagonists • Heparin (heparin-induced thrombocytopenia or HIT) • Inamrinone lactate (Amrinone) • Indomethacin • Interferon • Isoniazid • MMR, hepatitis A, or B, DTP, or influenza immunizations • NSAIDs • Oral hypoglycemics • Penicillin • Phenytoin • Procainamide • Proton pump inhibitors or PPIs • Quinidine • Quinine (not available in U. S.) • Ingestion of excessive tonic water • Rifampin • Rituximab • Sulfasalazine (antirheumatic) • Thiazides • Trastuzumab • Tricyclic antidepressants • Trimethoprim sulfamethoxazole • Vaccines • Valproic acid	

AIDS, Acquired immunodeficiency syndrome; *DIC,* disseminated intravascular coagulation; *HELLP,* hemolysis, elevated liver enzymes, low platelets; *HIV,* human immunodeficiency virus; *ITP,* idiopathic thrombocytopenic purpura; *MMR,* measles (rubeola), mumps, rubella; *NSAIDs,* nonsteroidal antiinflammatory drugs; *SLE,* systemic lupus erythematosus; *TTP,* thrombotic thrombocytopenic purpura.

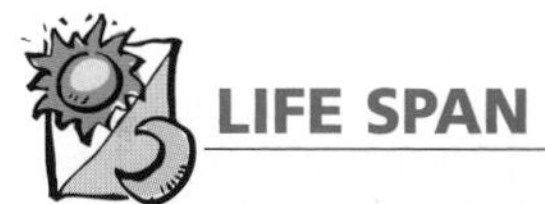

LIFE SPAN

Thrombocytopenia can be seen in children with exanthema subitum who are positive for herpesvirus 2.

Normal total platelet laboratory values for adults range from 150,000 to 400,000 cells/mL or mm^3; cord blood from 100,000 to 290,000 cells/mL or mm^3; newborn from 100,000 to 300,000 cells/mL or mm^3, neonate from 150,000 to 390,000 cells/mL or mm^3; and 3 months to 10 years from 100,000 to 473,000 cells/mL or mm^3.

The most life-threatening condition associated with thrombocytopenia is septic shock, which leads to disseminated intravascular coagulation (DIC), intravascular clotting, and formation of microemboli in the capillaries. Once DIC develops, the body is continuously depleted of clotting factors, leading to hemorrhage. Hemorrhage frequently occurs in the brain, and presentation of intracranial hemorrhage is

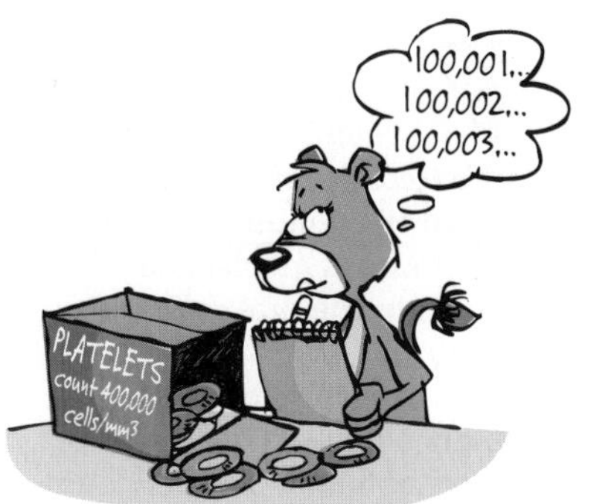

Normal platelet count is more than 100,000 cells/μL.

associated with headache, diplopia, confusion, seizures, and changes in mental state.

What You DO

Care of the patient with potential or actual thrombocytopenia includes physical assessment and laboratory assessment, as well as interventions for prevention, actual hemorrhage, and hypovolemic or septic shock. Hypovolemic shock consists of loss of blood volume, and septic shock consists of increased serum glucose, thrombocytopenia, hypoperfusion, hypotension, hyperglycemia, multisystem organ failure, or a combination of these symptoms.

Physical assessment includes assessment for bleeding from vital organs—brain, lungs, and gastrointestinal tract. Neurologic assessment includes history of recent blow to the head or a fall, headache, blurred vision, papillary changes, confusion, or disorientation. Respiratory assessment includes hemoptysis (coughing up blood), congestion, wet cough, and epistaxis (nosebleed). Gastrointestinal assessment includes hematemesis (vomiting up blood), blood found in stool, or nasogastric (NG) tube drainage with positive occult test. Genitourinary (GU) assessment includes testing for blood in the urine. Vital signs include hypotension and tachycardia. The skin, mucosa, and eyes should be assessed next. Assessment of the skin should include assessing for petechiae, purpura, and easy bruising. The oral mucosa should be assessed for bleeding gums, petechiae, and hemorrhagic blebs on the palate and oral mucosa. Retinas should be assessed for hemorrhage using an ophthalmoscope, and sclera should be observed for bleeding and redness.

Grading system for degree of platelets on laboratory tests:

0 = 100,000/µl or mm^3
1 = 75,000 to 100,000/µl or mm^3
2 = 50,000 to 75,000/µl or mm^3
3 = 25,000 to 50,000/µl or mm^3
4 = <25,000/µl or mm^3

The nurse should assess total platelet counts 1 hour and 24 hours after platelet transfusions. Laboratory values should be assessed as prescribed, and the nurse should know the last two values to make comparisons.

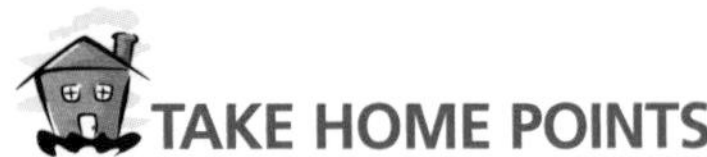

TAKE HOME POINTS

Microliters and mm^3 are the same.

! Heparin-induced thrombocytopenia (HIT) occurs in 5% of patients and typically develops 5 to 14 days after initial heparin administration. These patients have significantly greater risk of thrombosis, renal failure, and mortality in the postoperative setting. Argatroban, danaparoid, or lepirudin provides effective antithrombotic therapy.

TAKE HOME POINTS

- Bone marrow infiltration by tumor cells replaces the normal platelet cells causing thrombocytopenia. Tumor cells also replace red cells, causing anemia, and white blood cells (WBCs), causing granulocytopenia. A decrease in platelets, WBCs, and red blood cells (RBCs) is called *pancytopenia.*
- One 5-grain aspirin tablet can coat platelets, so blood does not clot for 9 to 12 days, the usual lifetime of a platelet.

!

- Panic platelet value is <20,000 cells/µl or mm^3 and exhibition of petechiae of the skin, blood-filled mouth bullae, and mucous membrane bleeding from the oral cavity, nose, uterus, or gastrointestinal, urinary, or respiratory tracts.
- In oncology, no relationship exists between platelet count and risk of hemorrhage; therefore, transfusion support should be aggressive.

Laboratory Assessment for Thrombocytopenia

Test Name	Description	Adult Norm Value	Thrombocytopenia
Platelet count, total	Actual number of circulating platelets per cubic millimeter of blood	150,000-400,000/mm^3	Decreased
PT	Amount of time for clot formation	10-15 seconds	Increased
aPTT	Measures how well the coagulation sequence is functioning for clotting ability	<35 seconds	Increased
INR	Calculated value that monitors response to anticoagulant therapy	≤3.0	Increased or normal
Capillary fragility test	Tourniquet test to measure platelet deficiency	Females ≤ 10 petechiae; Males ≤ 5 petechiae	Increased
FDP	Measures activity of the fibrinolytic system	2-10 μg/ml	Increased
Folic acid, serum	Measures amount of folic acid, folate, in bloodstream	<12 ng/ml or <27.2 nmol/L	Decreased
Vitamin B_{12}	Water soluble vitamin used up in rapid cell turnover	100-1100 ng/ml	Increased in chronic granulocytic leukemia
Platelet antibody, blood	Detect platelet autoantibodies and isoantibodies to transfusion of blood products	Negative or <1000 molecules of IgG per platelet	Positive

aPTT, Activated partial thromboplastin time; *FDP,* fibrin degradation products; *IgG,* immunoglobulin G; *INR,* international normalized ratio; *PT,* prothrombin time.

Nursing Interventions

When treating patients with thrombocytopenia, the nurse should do the following:

- Avoid invasive procedures such as bone marrow biopsies (although this may be necessary for diagnosis), endoscopies, enemas and suppositories, intramuscular or subcutaneous injections, and excessive venipunctures. Obtaining central or peripheral venous access is necessary to infuse platelets and implement hemodynamic monitoring.
- If invasive procedures are necessary, infuse platelets during and after invasive procedures and apply pressure for at least 5 minutes to venipuncture and bone marrow aspiration sites. Use of topical thromboplastin, obtained from a pharmacy, may be necessary to halt bleeding from bone marrow aspiration sites. Insertion of a balloon catheter into the bronchus or nares may also be necessary to create pressure to halt bleeding.
- For intubation with a cuff apparatus, deflate the cuff every 1 to 2 hours to avoid esophageal erosion or trauma that can lead to hemorrhage.
- Remember that constipation, nausea, and vomiting can raise intracranial pressure and should be prevented by use of anticonstipation and antiemetic medications.

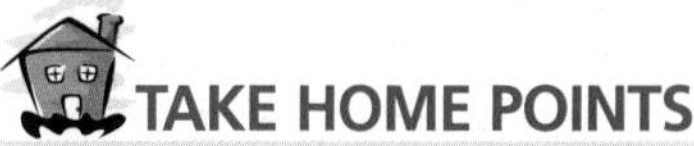

TAKE HOME POINTS

- Platelets, also called *thrombocytes,* are produced in the bone marrow and have an average life span of 10 days.
- The risk of hemorrhage is greater than 50% when the platelet count is <20,000 cells/μl or mm^3.

- Place a person with a nosebleed in high Fowler's position to avoid aspiration and lower anxiety. Apply ice, nasal packing, or topical epinephrine (or a combination of these therapies) to decrease bleeding. Apply direct pressure to the sides of nose just underneath the mid-nose.
- Count the number of menstrual pads used to assess the amount of blood loss in females, and administer hormones to control bleeding if medically necessary.
- Avoid the use of straight razors (use an electric razor instead).
- Avoid use of hard toothbrushes. Instead, use a soft or sponge-type toothbrush.
- Transfuse platelets according to institutional protocol. The usual increase expected is 5000 to 10,000 cells/μl or mm^3 platelets per unit transfused. If the 1-hour posttransfusion platelet count shows less improvement than at least 5000 cells/μl or mm^3 per unit transfused, then the patient is considered to be alloimmunized. This means the patient has developed antibodies against human leukocyte antigens (HLA) transfused with the platelets. In this case, the patient should be given HLA-matched platelets only for transfusion (usually obtained from a family member). If the platelet count continues to decrease 24 hours posttransfusion, then infection, fever, coagulopathy, and hepatosplenomegaly should be considered as causes.
- Administer epinephrine as prescribed to release platelets from the spleen.
- Administer corticosteroids as prescribed to increase platelet production.
- Administer Lepirudin 0.4 mg/kg by intravenous (IV) bolus and follow with 0.15 mg/kg IV per hour to maintain the activated partial thromboplastin time (aPTT) to 1.5 to 2.5 times the median normal.
- Administer immunosuppressive and other medication therapy as prescribed. This can include corticosteroids, vincristine, rituximab (a monoclonal antibody), or alfa-2b interferon with ribavirin.
- Administer lithium carbonate or folate to stimulate production of platelets in the bone marrow.
- Replacement therapy with fresh or frozen plasma transfusions or cryoprecipitate can be effective in augmenting the production of coagulation factors by the liver.

TAKE HOME POINTS

- The platelets found in stored blood lose their effectiveness after 24 hours at the usual storage temperature of 4° C.
- Platelets are stored at room temperature and are effective for up to 5 days. Maximum effectiveness is found in transfusing platelets within 6 hours of obtaining them from a donor.
- All blood products should be exposed to irradiation before transfusion to severely immunocompromised patients, because this limits proliferation of lymphocytes. A label will be found on the transfusion bag saying "Irradiated blood product" or "Irradiated."

- Administer vitamin K (AquaMEPHYTON, Mephyton) intramuscularly in the dose prescribed (usually up to 25 mg for an adult and up to 5 mg for pediatric patients) to assist in hepatic synthesis of factors II, VII, IX, and X that aid in blood clotting.
- Prepare the patient for possible abdominal computed tomography (CT) scan and bone marrow aspiration.
- For septic shock associated with thrombocytopenia, consider these areas for interventions in critical care: hemodynamic monitoring (central venous pressure), pulmonary capillary wedge pressure, pulmonary artery pressure, cardiac output, electrocardiogram; respiratory monitoring (arterial blood gas, breath sounds); fluids and electrolytes; and neurologic (alert, oriented, confused) and hematologic monitoring (complete blood count, platelet count, D-dimer to assess for DIC, FDP, prothrombin time [PT], partial thromboplastin time [PTT], and international normalized ratio [INR]).

- Complications of platelet transfusions include hemolytic and nonhemolytic transfusion reactions, graft-versus-host disease, and transfusion-related acute lung injury.
- The nurse should transfuse whole blood to restore and maintain blood volume during acute hemorrhage.

Do You UNDERSTAND?

DIRECTIONS: Circle the correct answers.

1. Circle all the places in the body where platelets mature.

pelvis	ribs	long bones	bladder
kidneys	sternum	skull	heart

2. Circle all the diseases that can be associated with thrombocytopenia.

AIDS	colitis	cirrhosis
scurvy	leukemia	stroke

DIRECTIONS: Match the body system in Column A with the appropriate nursing assessment in Column B for a patient with thrombocytopenia.

Column A	Column B
_______ 3. Neurologic	a. Blood in the urine
_______ 4. Respiratory	b. Hematemesis
_______ 5. Gastrointestinal	c. Headache
_______ 6. Genitourinary	d. Hemoptysis

DIRECTIONS: Choose the correct answer for each of the following statements from the two italicized options listed in the parentheses.

7. A thrombocytopenic patient with epistaxis should have his or her body placed in high ______________________________ position. *(dorsal recumbent, Fowler's)*
8. Bleeding from the bronchus in a patient with thrombocytopenia can be stopped by the use of ______________________________. *(a balloon catheter, topical dopamine)*
9. The patient has a total platelet count of 4000 cells/mm^3, and the nurse has just discontinued one of the patient's peripheral IV sites. The nurse should apply pressure to this IV site for at least

    ______________________________.

    (1 minute, 5 minutes)
10. The patient is thrombocytopenic and wants to brush his or her teeth. The nurse should offer a ____________________ toothbrush. *(hard bristle, spongelike)*

DIRECTIONS: Match the medication or treatment in Column A with the rationale in Column B associated with a patient with thrombocytopenia.

Column A	Column B
______ 11. Epinephrine	a. Augments coagulation factors in the liver
______ 12. Fresh frozen plasma transfusion	b. Stimulates platelet production in the bone marrow
______ 13. Folate	c. Assists in hepatic synthesis of factors II, VII, IX, and X
______ 14. Vitamin K	d. Releases platelets from the spleen

Answers: 1. pelvis, ribs, long bones, sternum, skull; 2. AIDS, leukemia, cirrhosis; 3. c; 4. d; 5. b; 6. a; 7. Fowler's. 8. a balloon catheter; 9. 5 minutes; 10. spongelike; 11. d; 12. a; 13. b; 14. c.

What IS Disseminated Intravascular Coagulation?

DIC is a condition that clinically ranges from an acute situation in which excessive hemorrhaging and thrombosis occurs to a chronic presentation with minor abnormalities of diffuse bleeding and thrombosis of generalized or local organ infiltration. Stages of microvascular clotting followed by active hemorrhaging characterize DIC because of two important factors: (1) consumption of coagulation factors and platelets and (2) fibrinolysis. Underlying or associative causes for DIC include shock states (sepsis, anaphylactic, circulatory), blood transfusion reactions, neoplasms, vascular and hematopoietic disorders, obstetric complications (retained fetus, eclampsia, septic abortion, abruptio placentae), crush and tissue injury or necrosis, and liver disease.

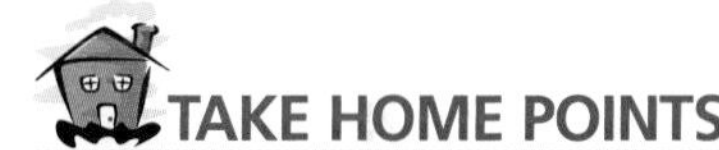

In DIC, diffuse bleeding and clotting occur.

What You NEED TO KNOW

Initiation of DIC results when tissue thromboplastin and tissue factor is liberated by tissue injury (resulting in activation of the extrinsic pathway) or with endothelial damage (thereby instigating the intrinsic pathway). Regardless of the causative and precipitating factor, widespread systemic hypercoagulation results in microvascular and macrovascular thrombosis. Vascular thrombosis interferes with blood flow and potentially results in peripheral ischemia and end-organ destruction. Because organ perfusion is severely hampered, clinical manifestations of multisystem organ dysfunction ultimately result. All organs are involved, but those most at risk include the skin, lungs, and kidneys.

After diffuse microvascular clotting, hemorrhage emerges as the next step in the evolution of DIC. Consumption of the clotting factors and platelets occurs because of systemic coagulation; therefore, activation of the fibrinolytic system arises, producing disseminated fibrinolysis. The normal lysis of clots (fibrinolysis) is produced in the clotting cascade. Because of the overwhelming nature of thrombosis, subsequent lysis of clots is equally intense. (See diagram on the following page.)

Diagnosis

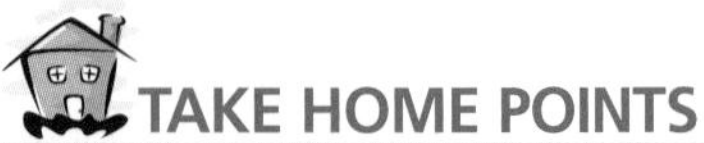

TAKE HOME POINTS

The D-dimer is the most reliable, specific diagnostic test for diagnosing DIC.

Diagnosis of DIC is most reliably based on clinical signs and symptoms. Laboratory evidence is beneficial in confirming clinical manifestations. Often, abnormal clotting profiles in patients with DIC demonstrate thrombocytopenia, prolonged clotting times (PT and aPTT), and suppressed clotting factors. Another diagnostic test is the D-dimer, which is helpful in identifying the activity of thrombin and fibrinolysis, which are integral in the pathophysiology of DIC.

Laboratory Values in Disseminated Intravascular Coagulation

Laboratory Test	Value
Platelet count	Decreased
PT (prothrombin time)	Prolonged
Activated partial thromboplastin time	Prolonged
International normalized ratio	Prolonged
Fibrinogen level	Decreased
D-dimer	Increased
Fibrin degradation products	Increased

Clinical Manifestations

With two separate phases of DIC, clinical manifestations can be widespread, but overall, they signify the lack of tissue perfusion and ultimately poor tissue oxygenation. With the development of microemboli in the vascular circulation, signs and symptoms reflect the lack of tissue oxygenation, which may vary from ischemia to total tissue infarction, ultimately resulting in cellular death. Ischemic changes affect all tissue and organ systems, leading to end-organ failure and possible multisystem organ dysfunction. Because of tissue ischemia and the normal process of clot formation, the body reacts with lysis of clots to increase perfusion to O_2- and nutrient-deprived areas. Because of the extent of lysis of clot formation and consumption of coagulation factors with microemboli development, massive hemorrhage can occur throughout the systemic circulation. Hemorrhaging can

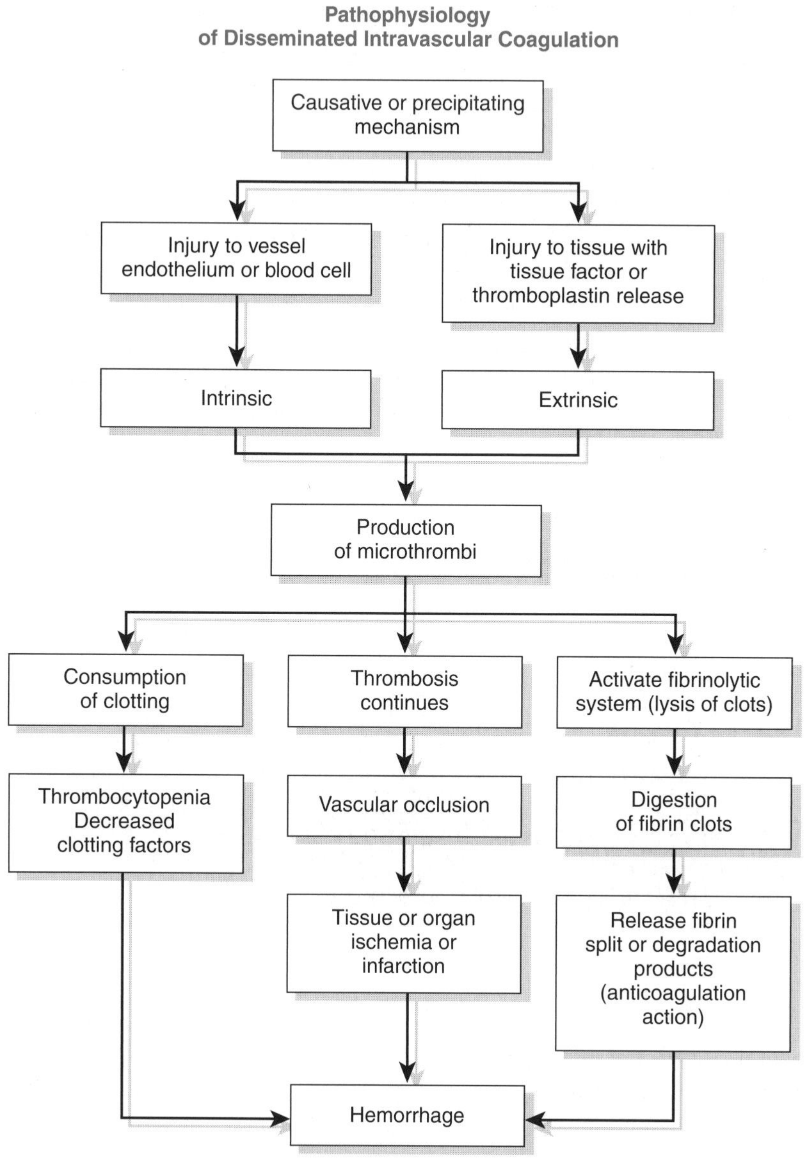

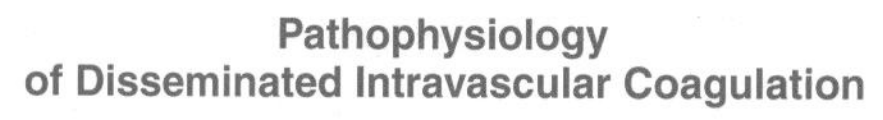

Pathophysiology of Disseminated Intravascular Coagulation

Causative or precipitating mechanism

Injury to vessel endothelium or blood cell

Injury to tissue with tissue factor or thromboplastin release

Intrinsic

Extrinsic

Production of microthrombi

Consumption of clotting

Thrombosis continues

Activate fibrinolytic system (lysis of clots)

Thrombocytopenia Decreased clotting factors

Vascular occlusion

Digestion of fibrin clots

Tissue or organ ischemia or infarction

Release fibrin split or degradation products (anticoagulation action)

Hemorrhage

exacerbate tissue ischemia and worsen possible existing shock states. Circulatory collapse, because of massive bleeding, can necessitate the further use of blood products and vasopressors to maintain tissue perfusion, end-organ perfusion, and oxygenation. Clinical manifestations in organ systems, including ischemic and hemorrhagic changes, are further detailed as follows:

Ischemic and Infarct Changes in Organ Systems in Disseminated Intravascular Coagulation

System	Ischemic	Tissue Infarction
Skin	Pale Cyanosis	Necrosis Gangrene
Central nervous system	Confusion Coma Transient ischemic attacks	Infarct Stroke (CVA)
Renal	Oliguria Azotemia	Acute renal failure Necrosis
Lungs	Hypoxia	Pulmonary embolism Pulmonary infarction
Gastrointestinal	Ulcers Decreased bowel sounds	Bowel necrosis Lack of bowel sounds

CVA, Cerebrovascular accident.

Hemorrhage and Effects on Organ Systems in Disseminated Intravascular Coagulation

System	Effects
Skin	Bruising Bleeding from central lines and puncture sites
Central nervous system	Cerebral bleeding Acute change in level of consciousness
Renal	Hematuria Oliguria
Lungs	Hemoptysis Hypoxia
Gastrointestinal	Distended abdomen Bloody emesis, stool

What You DO

Medical management of DIC is based on its underlying cause and the individual patient's condition. The first step is removal of the underlying pathology if possible. Generally, treatment includes transfusion of blood products, such as packed RBCs, platelets, fresh frozen plasma (to correct clotting factors consumption), and cryoprecipitate (factor VIII) to correct hypofibrinogenemia.

Heparin therapy continues to be a controversial treatment modality. Heparin inhibits the coagulation process by preventing tissue factor from initiating the extrinsic pathway, thus preventing consumption of coagulation factors and fibrin accumulation. However, heparin and other antifibrinolytic agents (especially when used concurrently) are generally contraindicated in patients at risk for severe bleeding dysfunctions and thrombotic complications.

FIRST-LINE AND INITIAL TREATMENT FOR DIC

- Provide supplemental oxygen (O_2).
- Administer IV fluids.
- Collect laboratory (blood) specimens.
- Provide pain relief.

Treatment of DIC Involves:

- Administration of blood products, cryoprecipitate
- Administration of heparin

To ensure optimal tissue and organ perfusion while maintaining blood pressure, CO, and urine output, fluid resuscitation will be required with possible vasopressor therapy. Invasive hemodynamic monitoring may be used to provide further data about intravascular volume and perfusion. Hypoperfusion and organ ischemia necessitate interventions to decrease O_2 demand and increase O_2 delivery. O_2 provision is accomplished through many avenues, which can include mechanical ventilation. Along with providing O_2, decreasing the demand is possible with sedation, decreased temperature (using antipyretics), pain control (using narcotics), and rest. Ensuring that O_2-carrying capacity is optimized requires assessing a patient's blood count and replacing blood products as necessary.

Do You UNDERSTAND?

DIRECTIONS: Provide a short answer to each of the following questions.

1. What are the two distinct stages that characterize DIC?

____

____

____

2. Hemorrhaging within DIC occurs mainly because of what two factors?

3. What are some precipitating mechanisms for DIC?

4. What is the most important step in the medical management of DIC?

5. What is the most reliable, specific laboratory test for diagnosing DIC?

6. What monitoring skills are important to ensure optimal tissue and organ perfusion?

Answers: 1. microvascular clotting followed by active hemorrhaging; 2. consumption of coagulation factors and platelets and fibrinolysis; 3. shock states (septic, anaphylactic, circulatory), blood transfusion reactions, neoplasms, vascular and hematopoietic disorders, obstetric complications (retained fetus, eclampsia, septic abortion, abruptio placentae), crush and tissue injury or necrosis, liver disease; 4. removal of the underlying cause; 5. D-dimer; 6. BP, urine output, capillary refill, skin color and temperature, level of consciousness, O_2 saturation, bowel sounds, abdominal contour, and stool production.

References

Alspach JG: *American Association of Critical Care Nurses core curriculum for critical care nursing,* ed 6, St Louis, 2006, Saunders/Elsevier.

Chernecky CC, Berger BJ: *Laboratory tests and diagnostic procedures,* 2008, St Louis, Elsevier.

Chulay M, Burns SM: *American Association of Critical Care Nurses essentials of critical care nursing,* New York, 2006, *McGraw Hill.*

Gray A, Wallis DE, Hursting MJ, Katz E, Lewis BE: Argatroban therapy for heparin-induced thrombocytopenia in acutely ill patients, *Clinical & Applied Thrombosis/Hemostasis,* 13(4):353-361, 2007.

Kerendi F, Thourani VH, Puskas JD, Kilgo PD, Osgood M, Guyton RA, Lattouf OM: Impact of heparin-induced thrombocytopenia on postoperative outcomes after cardiac surgery, *Annals of Thoracic Surgery,* 85(4):1554-1555, 2007.

Morton PG, Fontaine DK, Hudak CM, Gallo BM: *Critical care nursing: a holistic approach,* ed 8, Philadelphia, 2008, Lippincott Williams & Wilkins.

Sole ML, Klein DG, Moseley MJ: *Introduction to critical care nursing,* ed 4, St Louis, 2005, Elsevier, Saunders.

Urden LD, Stacy KM, Lough ME: *Thelan's critical care nursing diagnosis and management,* ed 5, 2006, St Louis, Elsevier.

Warkentin TE: Heparin-induced thrombocytopenia, *Hematology-Oncology Clinics of North America,* 21(4):589-607, 2007.

NCLEX® Review

1. Which of the following conditions is related to a low production of platelets in the body as a cause of thrombocytopenia?
   1 Vitamin B_{12} deficiency.
   2 Hypersplenism.
   3 Hypothyroidism.
   4 Hydrocephalus.
2. Vital signs for a patient with thrombocytopenia may include:
   1 Hypertension and a low-grade fever.
   2 Pain of 9 on a 1-to-10 scale and fever greater than 102° F.
   3 Hypotension and tachycardia.
   4 Respiratory rate less than 5 breaths/min and bradycardia.
3. What is the rationale for trying to prevent vomiting from occurring in patients with thrombocytopenia?
   1 Vomiting leads to constipation.
   2 Vomiting can rupture the liver, causing release of large amounts of platelets into the bloodstream.
   3 Vomitus can cause aspiration and hypoventilation.
   4 Vomiting raises intracranial pressure (ICP).
4. Your patient's postplatelet transfusion count increases 200 cells/mm^3 per unit of platelet transfused. The advanced practice nurse states the patient has developed antibodies against human leukocyte antigens (HLA). This is called:
   1 Leukocytosis.
   2 Alloimmunization.
   3 Autoregulation.
   4 Red cell lysis syndrome.
5. Your patient's platelet count continues to decrease at 24 hours and again at 36 hours after platelet transfusion. What might be the cause?
   1 Sleep apnea.
   2 Hepatosplenomegaly.
   3 Anxiety.
   4 Chronic scoliosis.
6. When describing the first stages of disseminated intravascular coagulation (DIC), remember that:
   1 DIC is always precipitated by an infectious pathogen.
   2 Profuse bleeding can be immediately expected.
   3 Microthrombi production can be expected.
   4 Heparin and antifibrinolytic therapy should be started without delay.
7. What organ or organs are especially at risk from microemboli during DIC?
   1 Gastrointestinal tract.
   2 Liver.
   3 Kidneys, skin, and lungs.
   4 CNS.
8. The main reason or reasons for the development of hemorrhage late in DIC includes:
   1 Pathogen-releasing endotoxins.
   2 A further spread of microthrombi.
   3 Activation of the fibrinolytic system and consumption of coagulation factors.
   4 A lack of initiation of heparin and antifibrinolytics.
9. The primary approach to consider when treating a patient with DIC is:
   1 Correct the condition, and treat the underlying precipitating mechanism.
   2 Start heparin therapy.
   3 Begin blood products.
   4 Administer excessive IV fluids.

10. When creating a treatment plan to deal with the symptoms of DIC, one would include:
    1 Limiting intravascular fluids.
    2 Administering antibiotic therapy.
    3 Increasing activity.
    4 Preparing possible transfusion of blood products.

NCLEX® Review Answers

1.1 Vitamin B_{12} deficiency causes low production of platelets by the body. Hypersplenism produces abnormal distribution of platelets, not low production of platelets. Hypothyroidism and hydrocephalus have nothing to do with platelets.

2.3 Low BP and increased HR are associated with low amounts of circulating platelets. Extremely low respirations and slow pulse rate are not associated with a low platelet count. A high level of pain is not a factor in thrombocytopenia.

3.4 Increased ICP can lead to bleeding in the brain of patients with thrombocytopenia. Vomiting leads to increased ICP. The spleen can release large amounts of platelets in the bloodstream. Aspiration is not associated with thrombocytopenia or hypoglycemia.

4.2 Alloimmunization is the development of antibodies against HLA antigens from the transfusion of blood products. Leukocytosis is an increase in the number of WBCs. Autoregulation is the control of blood flow through the tissue. Red cell lysis syndrome is the destruction of RBCs.

5.2 Enlargement of spleen can cause thrombocytopenia through abnormal distribution of platelets. Sleep apnea is an alteration in respiratory patterns. Anxiety does not significantly relate to platelet production or destruction. Chronic scoliosis is a curvature of the spine.

6.3 Microthrombi production is noted in the first stage of DIC, which is precipitated by other causes such as cancer. Profuse bleeding is not immediate. Heparin and antifibrinolytic therapy is not an immediate treatment.

7.3 Kidney, skin, and lungs are especially at risk from ischemic damage from microthrombi. Neither the gastrointestinal tract nor the liver is especially at risk for microemboli. CNS is a system, not an organ.

8.3 Hemorrhaging occurs because consumption of coagulation factors and activation of the fibrinolytic system result in lysis of microthrombi. Endotoxins are not associated with hemorrhage. Lysis of microemboli is the main reason. Lack of initiation of heparin and antifibrinolytics is not the main reason for developing hemorrhage.

9.1 Treating the underlying precipitating mechanism is the only way to stop the progression of DIC.

10.4 Blood transfusion is often needed during the hemorrhaging phase of DIC; because coagulation factors are consumed during the first phase of DIC, different factors are often needed to restore homeostasis. Limiting fluids is not a part of symptom treatment. Treatment of infection is not a symptom of DIC. Increasing activity is not a treatment because it can cause bleeding.

Chapter 11

Integumentary System

What You WILL LEARN

After reading this chapter, you will know how to do the following:

- ✔ Describe the types of burns and identify the initial treatment plans for caring for each type of burn patient.
- ✔ Describe the pathophysiologic process associated with the three phases of a burn injury.
- ✔ Discuss complications of inhalation injuries.
- ✔ Identify appropriate nursing interventions for caring for a patient with burn injuries.
- ✔ Describe prevention approaches that can be instituted in the critical care environment.
- ✔ Describe relevant patient education topics.

evolve

See http://evolve.elsevier.com/Schumacher/criticalcare for additional NCLEX® review questions.

What IS a Burn?

Burns are a group of conditions with outcomes that include the removal of skin by thermal (heat or radiation), chemical, or electrical means. Removal of skin can be planned, such as in electrodesiccation of warts or removal of pyogenic granulomas or skin cancers, or unplanned, such as in accidents or infliction by intentional harm (suicide by burning, immolation).

What You NEED TO KNOW

More than 2 million cases of burns, including 440,000 cases in children, are seen in the United States each year. Just over half of all burn fatalities occur at work. In addition, the report of sunburn by adults ages 18 to 29 years is high—57.5%—and the incidence of barbecue and fireworks burns is increasing. Burns in older adults have a high mortality rate—about 59%. In persons older than 65 years, scalding accounts for 41% of burns, flame burns account for 53%, and electrical burns account for 3 %. Assessment of all burns includes the type of burn (thermal, electrical, or chemical) and severity (depth, extent, and co-morbid conditions).

The type of burn indicates the initial care implemented. The severity of the burn includes the depth of the burn (superficial, partial thickness, or full thickness) and the extent of the burn based on percent of body area burned (rule of nines). The figure-of-eight technique is a valid measurement of hand edema and is easier to implement than the water volumetry method.

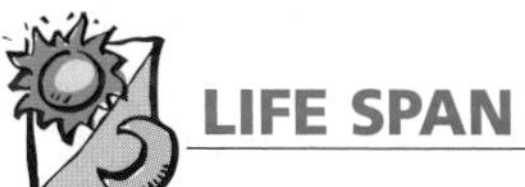

LIFE SPAN

- Burns in children are more severe than in adults because their smaller body surface areas (BSAs) are less able to regulate temperature, their skin is thinner, and they have higher fluid volume needs.
- Causes of burns in older adults include dementia (44%), alcohol use (21%), and cigarette use (10%).
- Chemical burns occur in industries that use MCI/MI (5-chloro-2-methyl-4-4isothizzolin-3-one/ 2-methyl-4-isothaiazolin-3-one), such as in industries that produce textiles, cosmetics, leather, fabric, metal work, latex paints, sunscreens, and moistened towelettes/ wipes.

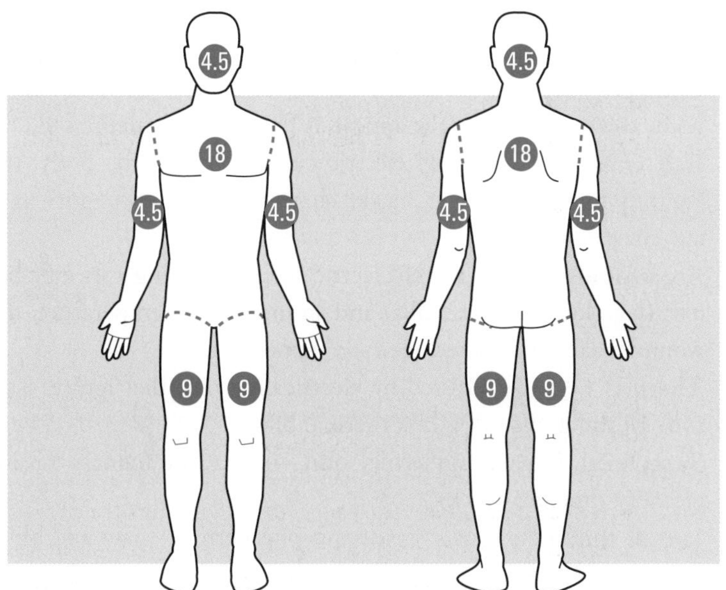

Percent of body burn in an adult. *(From Phipps WJ, et al:* Medical-surgical nursing: health and illness perspectives, *ed 7, St Louis, 2003, Mosby.)*

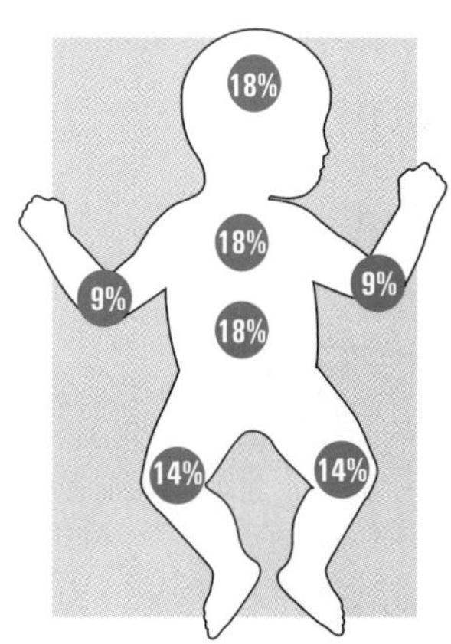

Percent of body burn in an infant. *(From Newberry L:* Sheehy's emergency nursing: principles and practice, *ed 5, St Louis, 2003, Mosby.)*

Hypertrophic scarring (red, hard, raised, itchy, tender, contracted) is disfiguring, with the only effective treatment being reconstructive plastic surgery. Hypertrophic scars are a breeding ground for colonization with an incidence of 88%.

FIRST-LINE AND INITIAL TREATMENTS FOR ENSURING SAFETY AT THE BURN SCENE

- **Thermal.** Ensure scene safety for the nurse and the victim. Remove the victim from the unsafe area only if trained to do so.
- **Electrical.** Ensure scene safety. Do not touch the victim until a person trained to remove the electrical power source does so.
- **Chemical.** Ensure scene safety. A person knowledgeable in chemical fire should determine safety. Wear protective clothing.

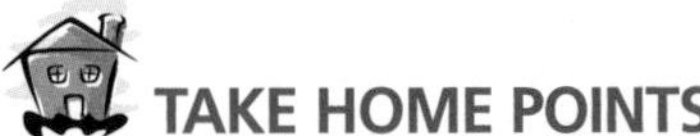

TAKE HOME POINTS

New research shows that for deep dermal burn wounds, the use of polarized light therapy decreases healing time and scarring.

Electrical burns are divided into high- and low-voltage burns. High-voltage electrical burns occur with 1000 volts or greater, and low-voltage electrical burns occur with less than 1000 volts. Tissue injury resulting from electricity is the result of electric energy being converted into heat, and the greatest heat is at the contact points. Four types of injuries are associated with an electrical burn:

- **Entrance wounds.** Caused by entry of electric current into the body, these wounds might appear as flat, black, or depressed.
- **Exit wounds.** Caused by electric current exiting the body, these wounds might appear as black, charred, and "blown out" as the current exits the body.
- **Arc wounds.** Caused by the electric current crossing a specific body part (e.g., knee, elbow, axilla) and an increase in temperature; these wounds take on a "petechiae type" appearance.
- **Thermal wounds.** Caused by electrical current that ignites a person's clothing, resulting in a thermal burn.
- **Superficial burns.** Epidermis only—pain and redness (average recovery time is 1 week).
- **Partial-thickness burns.** Epidermis plus dermis—pain and blistering (average recovery time is 2 months).
- **Full-thickness burns.** All skin layers involved; may include subcutaneous tissue, bones, muscles, and organs (painless if nerves are burnt; average recovery time is 6 months to 1 year).

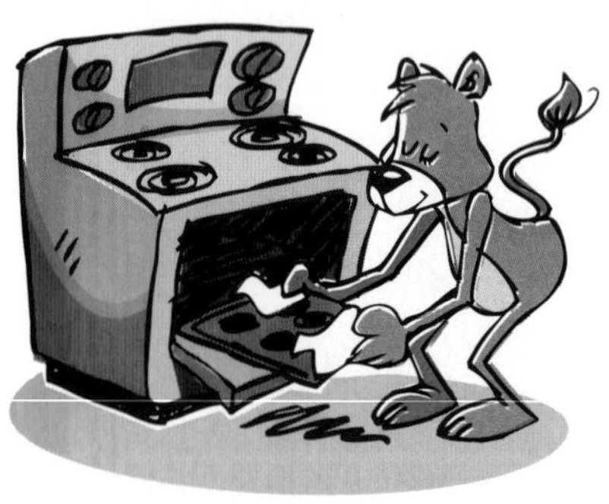

Thermal burn from electric stove.

Depth of Burn Injuries

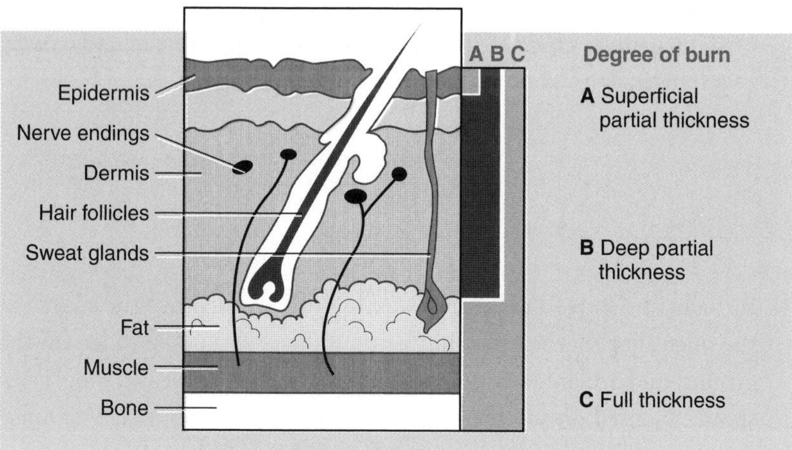

(From Lewis SL, et al: Medical-surgical nursing: assessment and management of clinical problems, *ed 7, St Louis, 2007, Mosby.)*

The co-morbidities to assess for in patients with burns include the following:

- Age younger than 5 years old or older than 55 years old
- Burns to joints, face, genitals, feet, or hands
- Burn encircles body
- Preexisting organ illness: lung disease, heart disease, liver disease, kidney disease
- Preexisting immunosuppression as a result of cancer or acquired immunodeficiency syndrome
- Neurologic trauma such as cervical spine fracture

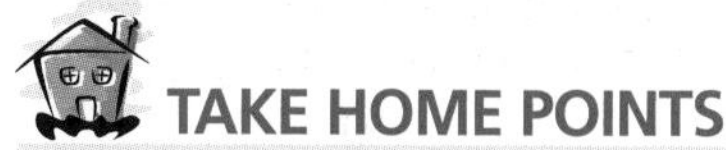

It takes 5 days for edema to decrease in esophageal chemical burns.

The physiologic response of the body to a burn has three phases:

1. During the first phase initially (and up to 48 hours later), a shift of the plasma into the interstitial fluid occurs, causing dehydration, edema, hypotension, decreased cardiac output, increased pulse, oliguria and anuria, hyperkalemia, hyponatremia, increased hematocrit, and a bicarbonate deficit.
2. The second phase is the diuresis that occurs 48 to 72 hours after the burn. A tremendous increase in urinary output occurs, as well as pulmonary edema because of circulatory overload, decreased hematocrit, hyponatremia, hypokalemia, and a bicarbonate deficit.
3. The third and final phase is called *recovery* and begins around the fifth day. In this phase, the patient has hypocalcemia, hyponatremia, hypokalemia, a negative nitrogen balance, and weight loss.

The most serious complication in patients with burns is sepsis, and identifying initial signs in the patient can save his or her life. These signs include changes in sensorium, fever, tachycardia, tachypnea, paralytic ileus, abdominal distention, and oliguria.

What You DO

1. Initially, the nurse should try to extinguish and remove the source of the burn. For thermal heat burns, the subject should be rolled on the ground and a blanket or shirt should be used to cover the fire. Water should be used on smoldering clothes and chemical burns. The nurse should remove objects that can conduct heat, such as clothing, jewelry, eyeglasses, and false limbs, because ischemia could result from swelling because of a tourniquet-like effect. For radiation seed burns, the nurse should remove the radiation source using special forceps and place the source immediately in a lead-lined box. For chemical burns, the chemical should be removed by irrigation with copious amounts of water or known antidote.
2. Assess ABCDEF (**A**irway; **B**reathing; **C**irculation, **C**-spine immobilization, **C**ardiac status; **D**isability—neurologic deficit; **E**xpose body for assessment; **F**luid resuscitation, **F**ahrenheit for assessment of signs of hypothermia).
   - Assess the airway for patency, and note any cyanosis or pharyngeal edema.
   - Assess breathing for shortness of breath, hoarseness, and difficulty swallowing. Be prepared for the possibilities of intubation, suctioning, hemodynamic monitoring, central venous catheter insertion, oxygenation, and mechanical ventilation.
3. Call 911 for emergency assistance.
4. Assess for cervical spine injury; if cervical spine injury is probable, do not move the person.
5. Assess the level of consciousness. Burns will not alter the level of consciousness. Therefore, it is important to collect a detailed history from the patient: How did the burn happen? Did it occur in a closed space? Was there a possibility of smoke inhalation? Were chemicals involved? Was there any related trauma? Were any medications used?
6. Initiate body substance isolation to protect from infectious organisms.

7. Initiate emergency burn management associated with specific type of burn.
   - **Thermal burns:**
     - Evaluate for smoke inhalation and respiratory burn. Maintain the airway.
     - Cool the burn with water for 2 to 5 minutes.
     - Cover the burn with a dry dressing.
   - **Electrical burns:**
     - Assess and monitor vital signs. Anticipate cardiopulmonary arrest. Perform cardiopulmonary resuscitation (CPR) if needed.
     - Assess for entrance and exit sites.
     - Cover burns with dry dressings.
   - **Chemical burns:**
     - Remove all contaminated clothes.
     - Flush with water 20 minutes after brushing off powders.
     - Apply a dry dressing.
8. In general, potential problems should be assessed, such as respiratory distress, sepsis, gastrointestinal (GI) bleeding, pain, anxiety, paralytic ileus, and oliguria.
9. Pain should be relieved.
10. Generally, the priority treatment interventions are focused on ventilation and oxygenation, fluid replacement for hypovolemia and electrolytes with Ringer's lactate, humidity regulation, dressing changes, and skin grafting. Closed dressings for superficial to partial thickness usually include Xeroform-Bacitracin, silver sulfadiazine, or Biobrane followed by a layer of gauze and Flexnet or Ace bandage. Lipidocolloid dressings, such as Urgotul, or mesh grafts treated with polyhexanide and topical oxygen emulsion or TOE help patients with second-degree burns heal faster. Distal limb salvage can occur with the use of dermal substitute Integra (Integra Life Sciences Corp, Plainsbroro, NJ).
11. The use of early nasogastric tube insertion for enteral feeding significantly decreases mortality in 40% to 50% of patients.
12. Use of anabolic steroid oxandrolone (Anavar) increases protein synthesis efficiency in critically ill burned patients.
13. Emotional support should be provided because psychological distress is the most prevalent and enduring secondary complication of burns. Manifestations include sleep disturbances, depression, body image alterations, and posttraumatic distress in 15% to 45% of patients. The nurse should be sensitive to the variable emotions

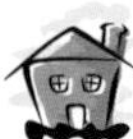

TAKE HOME POINTS

Laboratory tests include: complete blood count (CBC); electrolytes; type and cross match for blood transfusion (each unit of transfused blood increases risk of infection by 13%, so transfuse adults only if hemoglobin < 7 g/dl); PT and INR to assess for heparin-induced thrombocytopenia (HIT); serum creatinine for kidney function; albumin and total protein for nutritional status; and arterial blood gases (ABGs) for respiratory function; and serum glucose, alkaline phosphatase, calcium, phosphorus.

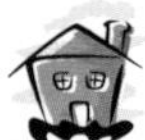

TAKE HOME POINTS

Diagnostic tests include chest radiographs and computed tomography [CT] scans.

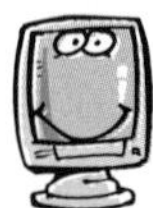

The web site for care of burns can be found at www.burnsurgery.com.

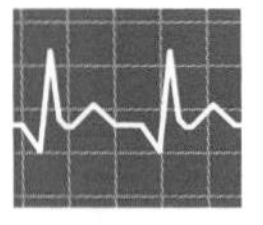

The nurse should assess distal circulation to extremity burns, especially when encircled, because a decreased or absent pulse in a given area can result in limited circulation, ischemia, or cell death and ultimately result in amputation of the extremity for the patient.

that burn patients and their families will experience. Feelings of guilt, fear, anxiety, anger, and depression must be recognized and addressed.

14. Suicide management is important. Self-immolation or other forms of suicide by burning should be considered when a reasonable explanation of the mechanism of the burn is lacking. Self-burning occurs more frequently in females (4.3:1) and in developing countries, and has an 80% death rate. After an unsuccessful suicide attempt, the patient is usually lucid and talkative, either denying the attempt or voluntarily providing information. Pertinent historical information that may facilitate special case management includes the following:
    - Recent onset of problems involving family, marriage, job, finances, or health
    - Expressions of hopelessness
    - History of alcohol or drug abuse
    - History of emotional problems

Immediate management is directed toward protection of the patient from further attempts at self-destruction by controlling agitation, screening for drug and alcohol overdose, and prescribing a mandatory psychiatric consultation.

After emergency treatment is completed, the interventions for the postemergency phase begin. These interventions include ventilator- and respiratory-dependent management, 12-lead electrocardiogram monitoring, hemodynamic monitoring (via central venous pressure [CVP] line, pulmonary artery [PA] catheter, or arterial line), assessment of laboratory and diagnostic tests, nasogastric (NG) tube to low suction for decompression, pain medication as needed, strict intake and output, tetanus toxoid injection to prevent infection from the *Clostridium tetani* organism, antibiotics as prescribed, nutritional management, wound care (including skin grafts with artificial skin such as Integra or with donor skin), and assessment for other injuries (fractures, head injury, chest injuries, and abdominal injury).

FIRST-LINE AND INITIAL TREATMENTS FOR BURNS

- **STOP** the burning process. The type or extent of burn will determine whether this may be implemented in the prehospital setting or in the receiving hospital's emergency department.

Patients with burns have four major systems in which physical complications can occur: (1) the immune system related to infection, (2) GI system related to hemorrhage or paralytic ileus (paralysis of the intestine leading to obstruction), (3) pulmonary system related to respiratory distress syndrome or pneumonia, and (4) musculoskeletal system associated with contractures. Infections are one of the most serious complications, with *Pseudomonas* most commonly occurring within 36 hours after a burn and hemolytic *Staphylococcus aureus* occurring up to 1 week after a burn. Sepsis is the most serious complication, and patients who are more susceptible have impaired production of macrophage inflammatory protein 1 alpha. Contractures are a problematic sequela that can limit mobility and function. The use of such devices as the Watusi® neck collar can improve function, comfort, and mobility.

A need also exists for house assessment, especially for older patients. Does the patient have signs of dementia? Is tap water temperature regulated so that it is not above 43° C? Are ashtrays large enough to use? How much alcohol does the patient consume?

- Insertion of central venous catheter near or overlapping an open wound should be avoided, and the catheter should not be left in place more than 3 days to prevent catheter-related infections.
- The use of intravenous (IV) albumin has been shown to increase the risk of death by 5%; therefore, the rationale for its use needs to be substantiated.
- Electrical wires should only be removed with wood, rubber, or plastic objects (never with metal objects or bare hands).

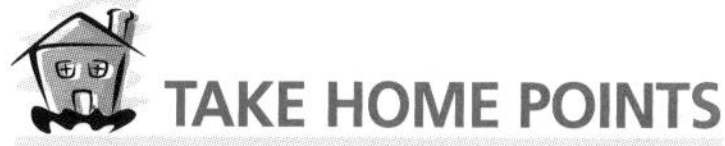

Urinary output greater than 70 mL/hr is beneficial to survival.

What IS Inhalation Injury?

Inhalation injury (INHI) occurs with the aspiration of heated gases or by-products of burned materials. Approximately 20% of patients admitted with burns have some degree of INHI, which results in impaired gas exchange and altered hemodynamics. INHI increases the rate of mortality and treatment requires increased fluid volumes during acute resuscitation.

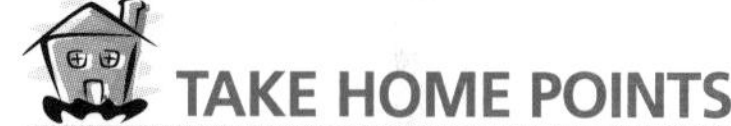

Inhalation injuries have a profound effect on mortality.

What You NEED TO KNOW

The respiratory system from the upper airway to the alveoli can be involved in inhalation injury. The mucosal barrier can be burned, resulting in edema, tissue sloughing, and airway obstruction. Chemicals and irritating gases can trigger bronchospasm. Inhalation injuries result in mucosal edema and loss of airway patency, bronchospasm, intrapulmonary shunting, decreased lung compliance, pneumonias, bronchiectasis, and respiratory failure.

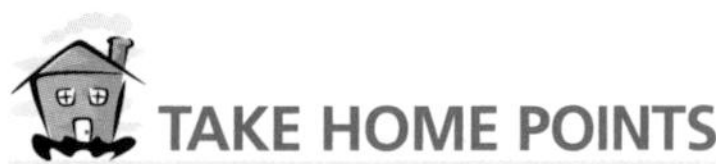

TAKE HOME POINTS

Three types of inhalation injury exist: (1) above the glottis, (2) below the glottis, and (3) carbon monoxide poisoning.

Inhalation injuries are primarily diagnosed through physical assessment data obtained from the patient. On initial presentation, patients may have little or no pulmonary distress and the initial chest radiograph may appear normal. The most useful adjuncts include history, physical examination, and bronchoscopy. Singed nasal hairs, facial burns, carbonaceous material on teeth, and a history of aspiration of hot steam or liquid may indicate the presence of inhalation injuries.

What You DO

Airway patency is essential in the management of patients with inhalation injuries. Change in vocal volume or character of voice, inability to handle secretions, hoarseness, and stridor require intubation. Laryngoscopy or fiberoptic bronchoscopy can be useful in accomplishing intubation in a timely manner before edema becomes advanced.

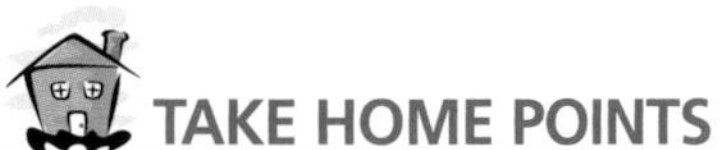

TAKE HOME POINTS

Pulse oximetry will be falsely elevated in carbon monoxide poisoning.

Do You UNDERSTAND?

DIRECTIONS: **Match the types of burn in Column A with the appropriate interventions in Column B.**

Column A	Column B
______ 1. Chemical	a. Use wood to remove source.
______ 2. Electrical	b. Remove source with copious amounts of water.
______ 3. Thermal	c. Use blanket to smother fire.

DIRECTIONS: **Identify the following statements as *true* (T) or *false* (F).**

______ 4. Partial thickness is a co-morbid condition.

______ 5. Superficial burns are never painful.

______ 6. Hypotension is a common physiologic response to an initial burn.

DIRECTIONS: Circle all the criteria for assessing breathing in a patient who has been burnt.

7. hoarseness / pharyngeal edema / finger clubbing / limb flaccidity / difficulty swallowing / color of sclera

DIRECTIONS: Match the laboratory tests in Column A with the associated body systems in the burned patient in Column B.

Column A	Column B
______ 8. Type and cross match	a. Hematologic for blood transfusion
______ 9. Serum creatinine	b. Nutritional status
______ 10. Albumin and total protein	c. Respiratory
______ 11. ABGs	d. Kidney

DIRECTIONS: Fill in the blanks to complete the following statements.

12. The most serious complication of burns is ________________.
13. A CVP line is used for ______________________________ monitoring.
14. A (n) __________________________ tube is inserted to decompress the stomach.
15. The GI complication of burn patients that includes paralysis of the intestines is called ______________________________.

Answers: 1. b; 2. a; 3. c; 4. F; 5. F; 6. T; 7. hoarseness, pharyngeal edema, difficulty swallowing; 8. a; 9. d; 10. b; 11. c; 12. infection; 13. hemodynamic; 14. NG; 15. paralytic ileus.

References

Ahmadi A: Suicide by self-immolation: comprehensive overview, experiences and suggestions, *Journal of Burn Care & Research,* 28(1):30-41, 2007.

Baker RH, et al: Retrospective study of the association between hypertrophic burn scarring and bacterial colonization, *Journal of Burn Care & Research,* 28(1):152-156, 2007.

Bayraktar A., Ozcan M: An unusual case: burn following an accidental exposure to methylchloroisothiazolinone/methylisothiazolinone, *Journal of Burn Care & Research,* 28(1):195-197, 2007.

Bresett J: Would you suspect this skin-eating infection? *Registered Nurse* 69(3):31, 2006.

Centers for Disease Control and Prevention: *Group A streptococcal disease (on-line),* 2008. Available at: www.cdc.gov/ncidod/dbmd/diseaseinfo/groupastreptococcal_g.htm.

Daeschlein G, Assadian O, Bruck JC, Meini C, Kramer A, Koch S: Feasibility and clinical applicability of polihexanide for treatment of second-degree burn wounds. *Skin Pharmacology & Physiology* 20(6):292-296, 2007.

Davis SC, Cazzaniga AL, Ricotti C, Zalesky P, Hsu LC, Creech J, Eaglstein WH, Mertz PM: Topical oxygen emulsion: a novel wound therapy, *Archives of Dermatology,* 143(10):1252-1256, 2007.

Dewey WS, Hedman TL, Chapman TT, Wolf SE, Holcomb JB: The reliability and concurrent validity of the figure-of-eight method for measuring hand edema in patients with burns, *Journal of Burn Care & Research,* 28(1):157-162, 2007.

Ehde DM, Patterson DR, Wiechman SA, Wilson LG: Post-traumatic stress symptoms and distress 1 year after burn injury, *Journal of Burn Care Rehabilitation,* 21:105-111, 2000.

Endorff FW, Gamelli RL: Inhalation injury, pulmonary perturbations, and fluid resuscitation, *Journal of Burn Care & Research,* 28(1):80-83, 2007.

Golger A, et al: Mortality in patients with necrotizing fasciitis, *Journal of Plastic and Reconstructive Surgery,* 119(6):1803, 2007.

Jeng JC, Fidler PE, Sokolich JC, Jaskille AD, Khan S, White PM, et al: Seven years' experience with Integra as a reconstructive tool, *Journal of Burn Care & Research* 28(1):120-126, 2007.

Namias N: Advances in burn care. *Current Opinion in Critical Care,* 13(4):405-410, 2007.

O'Mara MS, Reed NL, Palmieri TL, Greenhalgh DG: Central venous catheter infections in burn patients with scheduled catheter exchange and replacement, *Journal of Surgical Research,* 142(2):341-350, 2007.

Palmieri TL, Caruso DM, Foster KN, et al: Effect of blood transfusion on outcome after major burn injury: a multicenter study, *Critical Care Medicine,* 34:1602-1607, 2006.

Suri MP, Dhingra VJ, Raibagkar SC, Mehta DR: Nutrition in burns: need for an aggressive dynamic approach, *Burns,* 32(7):880-884, 2006.

NCLEX® Review

1. What type of burn occurs when a person's clothes catch on fire as a result of playing with matches?
   1 Chemical.
   2 Electrical.
   3 Ileal.
   4 Thermal.

2. The extent of a burn is based on:
   1 Depth.
   2 Percent of body area burned.
   3 Amount of pain experienced.
   4 Patient's gender.

3. Which type of severity of burn can be painless as a result of nerves being burnt?
   1 Superficial.
   2 Full thickness.
   3 Partial thickness.
   4 Epidermal thickness.

4. A burned patient of what age is most vulnerable based on co-morbidity status?
   1 A 62-year-old.
   2 A 45-year-old.
   3 A 30-year-old.
   4 A 12-year-old.

5. Within 48 hours of a burn, what physiologic responses usually occur?
   1 Hypernatremia, pulmonary edema, paralytic ileus.
   2 Dehydration, edema, oliguria.
   3 Negative nitrogen balance and weight loss.
   4 Tremendous increase in urinary output, hypokalemia, and decreased hematocrit.

6. Which of the following patients has the highest co-morbidity risk for burns?
   1 A 25-year-old with ingrown toenail and fractured wrist.
   2 An 8-year-old with burns to both great toes and history of suicide attempt.
   3 A 70-year-old with chronic obstructive pulmonary disease (COPD) and leukemia with burns to the face and hands.
   4 A 50-year-old with schizophrenia and burns to the left calf.

7. To prevent a burned patient from being infected by the *Clostridium tetani* organism, what injection can be given?
   1 Vitamin K.
   2 Vitamin B_{12}.
   3 Mantoux injection.
   4 Tetanus toxoid.

8. What is the major physical complication associated with the musculoskeletal system that is related to patients who have severe burns?
   1 Loss of pain tolerance.
   2 Contractures.
   3 Fractures.
   4 Muscle spasms.

9. Priority interventions for burns are focused on ventilation, oxygenation, and fluid replacement. Which fluid is best to treat hypovolemia and electrolyte depletion?
   1 Normal saline.
   2 5% Dextrose in water.
   3 5% Dextrose in water with 20 meq (milliequivalents) potassium chloride.
   4 Ringer's lactate.

10. The most serious complication in a person with burns is:
    1 Hypovolemia.
    2 Hypokalemia.
    3 Sepsis.
    4 Retinal hemorrhage.

NCLEX® Review Answers

1.4 Heat or radiation sources are types of thermal burns. Chemical burns are the result of chemical substances. Electrical burns are caused by electricity. Ileal is not a type of burn.

2.2 The rule of 9s is used to determine the percentage or extent of a patient's burns. Depth is a determination of the length of healing. Pain is not an indicator of extent because some burns are not painful. Being either a male or a female patient is not a factor of extent.

3.2 Full-thickness burns may be painless because nerves can be burnt. All the other types of burns listed are painful.

4.1 A co-morbid condition in burns is the age of the patient if the patient is older than 55 years of age.

5.2 Dehydration, edema, and oliguria occur as plasma shifts into interstitial fluid. A generalized edema and no ileus can exist. Edema can cause weight gain with no tremendous output in urine.

6.3 Age, organ illnesses, and burns to the face and hands have the highest co-morbidity risk for burns. The 25-year-old patient is too young and has no comorbidity factors. The 8-year-old is also too young and has a small burned area. The 50-year-old also has too small of a burned area.

7.4 To prevent a burned patient from being infected by the *Clostridium tetani* organism, tetanus toxoid can be given. This injection helps prevent tetanus from occurring. Vitamin K is for clotting problems. Vitamin B_{12} is given for the treatment of pernicious anemia. Mantoux injection tests for tuberculosis.

8.2 Contractures are a major complication of the musculoskeletal system in patients who have severe burns. Severe burns have burnt nerve endings; as a result, no pain is felt. Fractures are associated with the skeletal system and are not major complications. Severe burns are not complicated by muscle spasms.

9.4 Ringer's lactate treats both hypovolemia and electrolyte depletions because it contains sodium, potassium, calcium, chloride, and bicarbonate as lactate. Normal saline and D5W treat hypovolemia and D5W with KCL treats hypovolemia and potassium depletion.

10.3 Sepsis is the most serious because it has the highest mortality and includes multiple symptoms such as fever, tachycardia, paralytic ileus, and oliguria. Hypovolemia and hypokalemia are easy to correct. Retinal hemorrhage is not a complication of burns in general.

Multisystem

Chapter 12

What You WILL LEARN

After reading this chapter, you will know how to do the following:

- ✔ Explain the impact advanced directives have on health care.
- ✔ Compare and contrast the primary and secondary resuscitation management surveys.
- ✔ Identify appropriate interventions for a patient in a cardiopulmonary arrest.
- ✔ Describe the physiologic process of multiple organ system dysfunction.
- ✔ Identify the risk factors that predispose patients to the development of multiple organ system dysfunction.
- ✔ Identify appropriate nursing interventions for caring for a patient with multiple organ system dysfunction.

evolve

See http://evolve.elsevier.com/Schumacher/criticalcare for additional NCLEX® review questions.

What IS Code Management?

Code management is the organization and direction of resuscitation. The American Heart Association (AHA) is a leader in providing guidance for organizing these efforts. When resuscitation is required, many things seem to be happening at once. For resuscitation to be effective, there must be a systematic approach to the delivery of care. The code

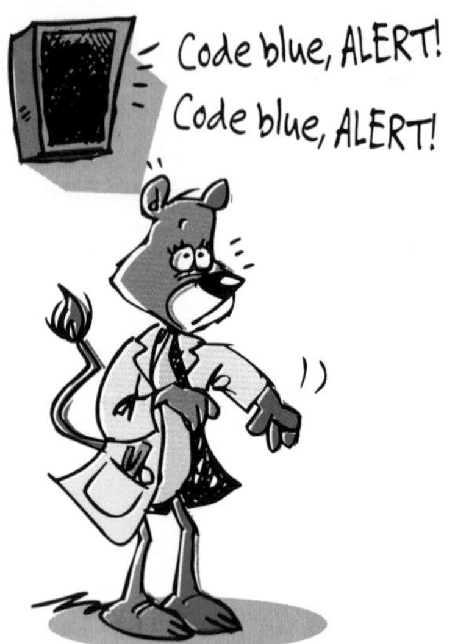

A "code" is an emergency situation and "blue" usually indicates cardiopulmonary arrest.

team must have a captain to lead the efforts, direct, and organize. The team leader should immediately assign one team member to each of the following tasks: managing the airway; providing effective chest compressions; starting an intravenous (IV) line; administering medications; handling the monitor, code cart, and defibrillator; and recording the events of the code. Personnel not involved directly in the resuscitation effort should provide support for the family and control the number of people observing the resuscitation.

A *code* is the commonly used term in the medical community for a cardiopulmonary arrest. Breathing stops, cardiac contractions are absent or ineffective, and little or no cardiac output (CO) occurs. The heart and brain are deprived of oxygenated blood. Clinical death has occurred, and biologic death will quickly follow if appropriate action is not taken.

Currently, many in-hospital settings are using rapid response teams (RRT) or medical emergency teams (MET) whose members are trained to prevent a patient crisis and possibly a cardiopulmonary arrest through prompt intervention. RRTs are usually a nurse-led urgent response team comprised of hospital clinicians with critical care expertise who provide intermediate interventional capability; METs are physician-led teams and have advanced interventional capabilities and often function like a code team. Whether the intervention is performed by an RRT or MET, the goal is to recognize early signs of patient deterioration and intervene promptly to improve patient outcomes and hopefully prevent a cardiopulmonary arrest. The effectiveness of RRTs is currently under investigation. An RRT/MET team can be called into action when any of the following warning signs indicate that a patient's condition is beginning to deteriorate.

- Change in vital signs
  - Unexplained tachycardia ≥ 130/minute
  - Unexplained bradycardia ≤ 50/minute
  - Elevated respiratory rate > 30 breaths/minute
  - Depressed respiratory rate < 8 breaths/minute
  - Low or elevated blood pressure
- Difficulty in breathing (new onset)
- Use of accessory muscles
- Adventitious breath sounds
- Compromised/threatened airway
- Acute decrease in oxygen saturation despite delivery of oxygen
- Change in level of consciousness
- Repeated or prolonged seizures

- Chest pain
- Arrhythmias
- Low urinary output
- Nurse concern about overall deterioration in patient's condition

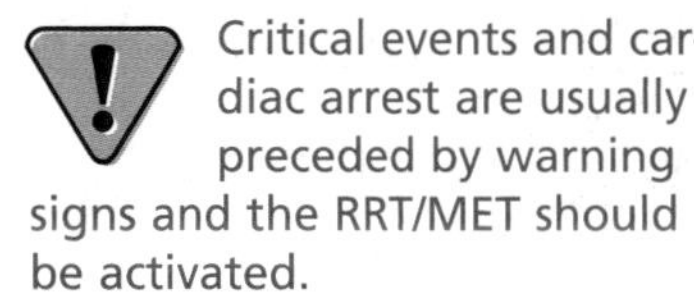
Critical events and cardiac arrest are usually preceded by warning signs and the RRT/MET should be activated.

For the purposes of this text, we will explore adult resuscitation management. Pediatric, infant, and neonatal resuscitation management can vary, because the physiologic cause of the arrest is often different, especially in children.

What IS an Advanced Directive?

Advanced directives are documents that a person writes in anticipation of, at some point, not being able to make his or her wishes known to the health care providers. The Patient Self-Determination Act (PSDA) requires that all health care institutions provide patients with information on advanced directives and to discuss advanced directives with them. Two types of advanced directives are (1) a *living will* and (2) a *durable power of attorney* for health care. A living will describes what kind of health care a person is to receive in the event of certain medical conditions. A durable power of attorney for health care appoints another person to speak for the patient if he or she is no longer able to do so. For purposes of code management, health care professionals are most concerned with the patient's wishes related to the administration of cardiopulmonary resuscitation (CPR) and mechanical ventilation.

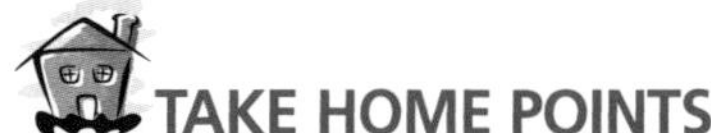

Most often a living will addresses the patient's wishes on such issues as CPR, mechanical ventilation, artificial nutrition or hydration, dialysis, surgery, or antibiotic treatment.

What You NEED TO KNOW

The PSDA allows patients to make decisions about their care. Does the patient have an advanced directive? If the patient has a living will, what does it say? If the patient is unable to verbalize his or her wishes, does he or she have a durable power of attorney for health care?

Patients are permitted to refuse care. Some patients do not want CPR or to be placed on a ventilator. These wishes will affect the patient's *code status.* Most health care institutions have policies concerning the limitation of this type of emergency care. The nurse must follow the policies of the institution where he or she works; however, if a patient refuses CPR, mechanical ventilation, or both, his or her wishes must be respected. Resuscitation should not be started. The challenge for a health care provider is to follow the patient's advanced directives, even if they conflict with the health care provider's own ideas and values.

What You DO

All patients must be asked about advanced directives on admission to the hospital. If a patient has a living will, a copy should be placed in the medical record. If a copy is not available, the nurse should ask the family to bring a copy to the hospital. If the document is not readily available, the nurse should ask the patient about his or her wishes. Health care institutions have policies regarding notification of the health care team regarding the contents of the patient's advanced directives. The nurse must know the status of the advanced directives for any patient in his or her care. It is important to be aware before an emergency arises and to follow the institution's policies.

Do You UNDERSTAND?

DIRECTIONS: **Provide short answers to the following questions.**

1. List the two types of advanced directives.

2. What is the nurse's responsibility related to advanced directives?

Answers: **1. Living will, durable power of attorney for health care; 2. The nurse must always know if a patient has an advanced directive and its contents.**

What ARE the Advanced Cardiac Life Support Guidelines?

The AHA's Advanced Cardiac Life Support (ACLS) guidelines organize resuscitation efforts into a primary (Basic Life Support) and a secondary (ACLS) survey. These eight steps are appropriate for all cardiac emergencies. They are organized in order of priority. Each step involves assessment and management of a problem. By following this approach, the nurse can manage each problem before moving on to the next one.

What You NEED TO KNOW

Before beginning the primary survey, assess the patient for responsiveness. Shake the patient and shout to arouse the patient.

Primary Survey

Assess	Manage
Airway: Is the airway open?	**Airway:** Open the airway.
Breathing: Is the patient breathing?	**Breathing:** If not breathing, provide ventilation.
Circulation: Does the patient have a pulse?	**Circulation:** If there is no pulse, begin chest compressions.
Defibrillation: Does the rhythm require defibrillation?	**Defibrillation:** Is the rhythm VF? Is an AED available?

AED, Automatic external defibrillator; *VF,* ventricular fibrillation.

Secondary Survey

Assess	Manage
Airway: Assess patency of airway.	**Airway:** Is airway management adequate? Provide intubation with an advanced airway (endotracheal tube) if needed.
Breathing: Assess if ventilation is adequate.	**Breathing:** Provide bag-valve ventilations. If advanced airway is placed, confirm tube placement by listening to breath sounds and use an end-tidal carbon dioxide detector.
Circulation: Obtain IV access and determine rhythm.	**Circulation:** Identify the cardiac rhythm. Is IV access available to give medications?
Differential diagnosis: Search for and find reversible causes.	**Differential diagnosis:** What is wrong with this patient? Why did the patient go into cardiac arrest?

Do You UNDERSTAND?

DIRECTIONS: **List the four steps of the primary and secondary surveys.**

Primary Survey

1. ______________________________
2. ______________________________
3. ______________________________
4. ______________________________

Secondary Survey

5. ______________________________
6. ______________________________
7. ______________________________
8. ______________________________

What IS Respiratory Arrest?

A respiratory arrest is defined as *the absence of breathing.* A respiratory arrest is often preceded by progressively worsening respiratory distress or compromise (or both). Patient assessment and intervention are critical to prevent respiratory compromise from becoming arrest. Patients who have a respiratory arrest will have a pulse. If the respiratory arrest is not treated, a cardiac arrest will follow.

What You NEED TO KNOW

Many causes for respiratory compromise and arrest exist. Although the underlying causes are important, emergency treatment is the same no matter what the cause. Adequate oxygenation must be maintained. Slow respiratory rates, shallow respirations, or both do not provide adequate oxygenation and require ventilatory support using a bag-mask. Untreated

Answers: 1. Assess airway; 2. Assess breathing; 3. Assess circulation; 4. Defibrillate; 5. Airway (intubation); 6. Breathing (confirm ventilation); 7. Circulation (IV access); 8. Differential diagnosis.

respiratory compromise may progress to respiratory arrest. Occasional gasping breaths, known as *agonal respiration,* are ineffective. Patients with these symptoms must be treated as if they were in respiratory arrest.

What You DO

If the patient shows any kind of respiratory distress, assessment is critical. The nurse should assess the patient's respiratory rate and quality, assess the work of breathing, and look for use of accessory muscles. Is the patient short of breath? Is the rate too fast or too slow? Does the patient need to sit up or sit in a particular position to breathe? The nurse should auscultate breath sounds. Are they present, absent, abnormal? The patient should be placed on a pulse oximeter if possible. Oxygen saturation below 95% requires attention. The nurse should be prepared to report findings to the physician in charge of the patient's care.

If the patient is not breathing, the nurse must breathe for the patient. Initial ventilation may be provided with mouth-to-mouth, mouth-to-mask, or bag-mask breathing. The nurse may give bag-mask ventilation with or without supplemental oxygen; however, 100% oxygen should be delivered as soon as possible. If continued airway support is needed, the patient should be intubated to provide a secure airway.

TAKE HOME POINTS

- Patients with carbon monoxide poisoning may have a normal pulse oximeter reading, although they require O_2 therapy.
- Avoid hyperventilation. It can be harmful because it increases intrathoracic pressure and thereby diminishes CO and decreases venous return to the heart. Also, hyperventilating a patient can cause vomiting and aspiration.

Do You UNDERSTAND?

DIRECTIONS: Fill in the blanks to complete the following statements.

1. Untreated respiratory compromise may lead to ________________ ____.
2. When assessing respirations, the nurse should assess the ________________________, and ________________________.

Answers: 1. respiratory arrest; 2. rate, quality, breath sounds.

What IS a Cardiac Arrest?

A cardiac arrest is identified by the absence of a palpable pulse. No blood pressure (BP), CO, or breathing is detected. Clinical death has occurred. With prompt action, clinical death is reversible. If pulse and respiration are not promptly restored, biologic death follows.

What You NEED TO KNOW

Three rhythms may be seen in cardiac arrest. The AHA provides algorithms for the treatment of each of the following arrest rhythms:

Ventricular Fibrillation or Pulseless Ventricular Tachycardia

Ventricular fibrillation (VF) or pulseless ventricular tachycardia (PVT) is a chaotic rhythm that does not produce effective contractions. It is by far the most common rhythm in an adult cardiac arrest.

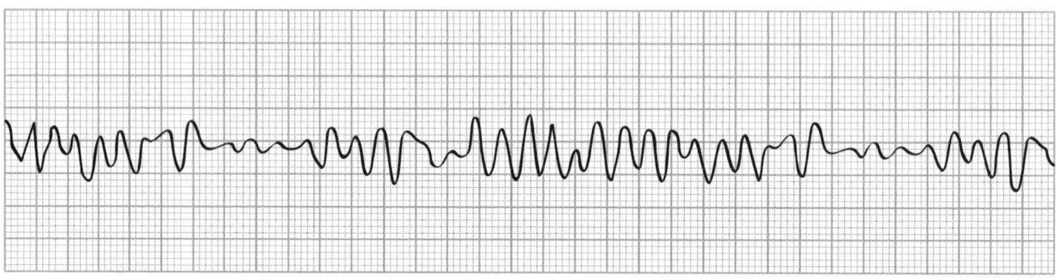

(From Chernecky CC et al: Real-world nursing series: ECGs & the heart, *Philadelphia, 2002, WB Saunders.)*

Pulseless Electrical Activity

In pulseless electrical activity (PEA), any organized electrical activity can be visualized on the cardiac monitor. However, no cardiac contractions or CO are seen. What defines PEA is the fact that the patient is pulseless.

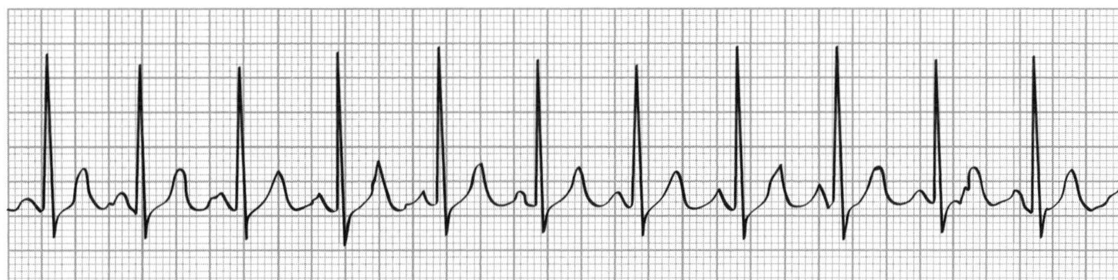

(From Chernecky CC et al: Real-world nursing series: ECGs & the heart, *Philadelphia, 2002, WB Saunders.)*

Asystole

Asystole is the absence of electrical activity in the heart. Asystole is generally considered a terminal rhythm. Very few patients will be resuscitated from asystole.

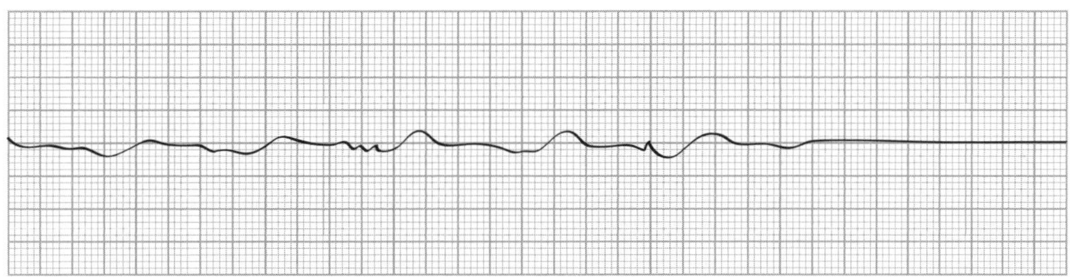

(From Chernecky CC et al: Real-world nursing series: ECGs & the heart, *Philadelphia, 2002, WB Saunders.)*

What You DO

The following is a summary of the main treatment points from the AHA Advanced Cardiac Life Support algorithms based on whether a rhythm is considered shockable or not shockable:

The nurse should always assess and reassess the patient during a code, and he or she should not rely strictly on the monitor.

Shockable Rhythms

VF or PVT heart rhythms are pulseless rhythms that are considered shockable. The nurse should do the following:

- Assess the patient. Complete the primary basic life support (BLS) survey.
- If the patient is not breathing and does not have a pulse, begin CPR.

- If an AED is available, put it on the patient as soon as pulselessness is determined and follow the voice prompts. Electrical defibrillation is the definitive treatment for VF. Do **NOT** delay defibrillation.
- If a monitor defibrillator is available, attach it to the patient and determine the rhythm on the monitor.
- If the patient is in VF or pulseless PVT, prepare to defibrillate. Deliver one shock at 360 joules (J) if using a monophasic defibrillator and 120 to 200 J if using a biphasic defibrillator.
- Immediately resume CPR for 5 cycles.
- Defibrillate patient (monophasic: 360 J; biphasic, same as previous dose or higher).
- Resume CPR for 5 cycles.
- Once IV access is obtained, administer epinephrine (adrenaline) 1 mg or vasopressin (Pitressin) 40 U during CPR before or after defibrillation.
- Remember that epinephrine (adrenaline) is the first-line drug. Administer epinephrine 1 mg IV every 3 to 5 minutes during the resuscitation. No maximum dose of epinephrine exists.
- Remember that vasopressin (Pitressin) 40 U IV **MAY** be given in place of the first or second dose of epinephrine. Only vasopressin may be given as a replacement for epinephrine.
- Defibrillate patient (monophasic: 360 J; biphasic, same as previous dose or higher).
- Resume CPR for 5 cycles.
- Remember that antidysrhythmic drugs are the next drugs to be administered. The antidysrhythmic drugs of choice are amiodarone (Cordarone) 300 mg IV **OR** lidocaine (Xylocaine HCL) 1 to 1.5 mg/kg IV. The physician should choose one, not both.
- Defibrillate patient (monophasic: 360 J; biphasic, same as previous dose or higher).
- Resume CPR for 5 cycles.
- Remember that amiodarone (Cordarone) may be repeated at 150 mg IV **OR** lidocaine (Xylocaine HCL) may be repeated at 0.75 mg/kg, for a maximum of three doses or 3 mg/kg.
- Defibrillate patient (monophasic: 360 J; biphasic, same as previous dose or higher).
- Resume CPR for 5 cycles.

ECG of Torsades de pointes. *(From Chernecky CC et al:* Real-world nursing series: ECGs & the heart, *Philadelphia, 2002, WB Saunders.)*

- Consider administering magnesium sulfate 1 to 2 g IV push, which is generally indicated in two circumstances: (1) in Torsades de pointes (a type of PVT that has both positively and negatively deflected complexes) and (2) in patients with clinical conditions such as alcoholism or malnutrition that lead to low serum magnesium levels.
- When IV access is not available, remember that certain medications can be given via the endotracheal tube. One acronym that can help the nurse remember the drugs is the word *LANE*—lidocaine, atropine, naloxone hydrochloride (Narcan), and epinephrine (adrenaline). Tracheal doses of these drugs should be two to four times the IV dose because of the absorption in the lungs. For example, endotracheal epinephrine should be given at 2.0 to 2.5 times the IV dose.

Vasopressin may only be administered as a one-time dose.

At any time, chest compressions should be minimally interrupted and interruption should not exceed 10 seconds.

Nonshockable Rhythms

When treating patients with nonshockable rhythms such as PEA or asystole, the nurse should do the following:

- Assess the patient. Complete the primary BLS survey.
- If the patient is not breathing and does not have a pulse, begin CPR.
- Complete the secondary survey.
- Check the cardiac rhythm on the monitor. Normal sinus rhythm, bradycardia, or tachycardia may be seen, but the patient will be pulseless.
- Remember that the differential diagnosis is critical in PEA or asystole. One memory aid is to think of the Hs and Ts.
- Once IV access is available, administer epinephrine (adrenaline) 1 mg or vasopressin (Pitressin) 40 U during CPR.
- Remember that epinephrine (adrenaline) is the first-line drug. Administer epinephrine 1 mg IV every 3 to 5 minutes during the resuscitation. No maximum dose of epinephrine exists.

TAKE HOME POINTS

- The nurse should defibrillate VF as soon as possible. He or she should not delay for intubation or obtaining IV access.
- Only one shock is delivered—this is a change from previous guidelines, which recommended three consecutive shocks.
- Know whether your defibrillator discharges using a monophasic or biphasic waveform because the energy delivered varies according to the device.

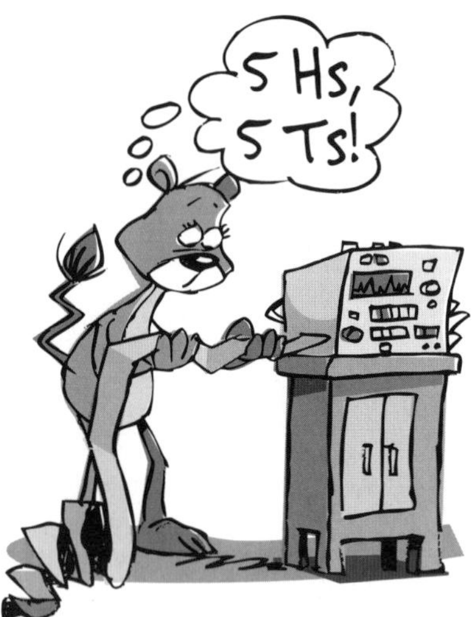

Acronym for pulseless electrical activity (PEA).

The nurse should not treat the monitor! If a patient has normal electrocardiographic activity and is pulseless, this is PEA.

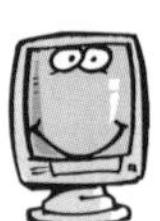

Hypovolemia and hypoxia are the most common causes of PEA that are easily reversed.

Cardiac Rhythm Simulator: www.thehealthcarenet.com/shareware.htm

http://kcsun3.tripod.com/id190.htm

www.skillstat.com/Flash/ECGSim531.html

ACLS self-testing and assessment tool:

www.acls.net/aclsalg.htm

www.mdchoice.com/cyberpt/acls/acls.asp

www.netmedicine.com/cyberpt/acls/al2-001.html

- Remember that vasopressin (Pitressin) 40 U IV **MAY** be given in place of the first or second dose of epinephrine. Vasopressin may only be given once.
- Consider administering atropine 1 mg for asystole or a slow PEA (heart rate [HR] < 60); dose may be repeated every 3 to 5 minutes, up to a total of three doses.
- Because asystole is often a terminal rhythm, consider termination of the code.

Differential Diagnosis for Pulseless Electrical Activity

Causes That Start with H	Treatment
Hypovolemia	Volume infusion
Hypoxia	Oxygenation, ventilation
Hydrogen ion (acidosis)	Sodium bicarbonate, hyperventilation
Hyperkalemia/hypokalemia	Hyperkalemia: sodium bicarbonate, glucose plus insulin, calcium chloride, Kayexalate/sorbitol, dialysis. Hypokalemia: rapid but controlled infusion of potassium.
Hypoglycemia	Administer glucose
Hypothermia	Warm patient
Causes That Start with T	**Treatment**
Toxins (drug overdose)	Drug screen, lavage, activated charcoal, specific antidotes
Tamponade (cardiac)	Pericardiocentesis
Tension pneumothorax	Needle decompression
Thrombosis (coronary)	Thrombolytic agents
Thrombosis (pulmonary)	Thrombolytic agents, surgical embolectomy
Trauma	Identification and treatment of traumatic injury

Do You UNDERSTAND?

DIRECTIONS: **Provide short answers to each of the following questions.**

1. What is the most common rhythm seen in adult cardiac arrest?
____
2. What is the definitive form of treatment for VF? _______________
3. What is the sequence of treatment for VF after the first initial shocks?
____
____

4. What is the first drug of choice in all three cardiac arrest rhythms?

____

5. List at least five Hs and five Ts to be considered in nonshockable rhythms.

____

____

____

____

____

What IS Multiorgan Dysfunction Syndrome?

Multiorgan dysfunction syndrome (MODS) is the progressive dysfunction of more than one organ in patients who are critically ill or injured. It is the leading cause of death in intensive care units (ICUs). The initial insult that stimulates MODS can result from a variety of causes including, but not limited to, extensive burns, trauma, cardiorespiratory failure, multiple blood transfusions, and most commonly, systemic infection.

As health care treatments and procedures become increasingly effective, a greater number of patients are surviving traumatic insults. As a result, ICUs are seeing more cases of MODS.

What You NEED TO KNOW

Pathogenesis

The body is designed to respond to illness and injury by activating compensatory mechanisms to adjust to the insult. These changes include increased HR, contractility, CO, and oxygen consumption. The neurologic and endocrine systems respond by releasing the following mediators to address this insult: catecholamines, cortisol, antidiuretic hormone,

Answers: **1. ventricular fibrillation; 2. defibrillation; 3. CPR, shock, CPR/drug, shock; 4. epinephrine or vasopressin; 5. hypovolemia, hypoxia, hydrogen ion, hyperkalemia or hypokalemia, hypothermia, hypoglycemia; toxins, tamponade, tension pneumothorax, thrombosis (coronary), thrombosis (pulmonary), trauma.**

growth hormone, and glucagons. These changes occur within the first 3 to 5 days after the event and begin to diminish within 7 to 10 days. For some patients, the response does not diminish and tachycardia, fever, and a state of hypermetabolism continue.

Whatever the initial illness or injury, the cause of MODS seems to be an uncontrolled systemic inflammatory response and effects of multiple mediator systems, known as the systemic inflammatory response syndrome (SIRS). Initially, this uncontrolled SIRS response is manifested by two or more of the following conditions:

- Temperature > 100.4° F (38° C); < 96.8° F (36° C)
- HR > 90 beats/minute
- Respiratory rate > 20 breaths/min
- $PaCO_2$ < 32 mm Hg
- White blood cell count > 12,000/mm^3 or < 4,000/mm^3 or more than 10% immature (bands) forms

The by-products of these interactive systems cause effects in the vascular system at an intracellular level, and they eventually affect cell function. Vascular occlusive events disrupt blood flow by enhancing release of thromboxane (a potent vasoconstrictor) and by inhibiting synthesis of prostacyclin (a vasodilating substance). The result is an overall vasoconstrictive effect. Intracellular injury and hyperactivity lead to increased intracellular oxygen demand. Leukocyte activation and other effects that amplify a systemic inflammatory response result in organ distress, organ failure, or both.

Systemic Impact of Multiorgan Dysfunction Syndrome

Organ System	Clinical Manifestations of Failure
CNS	Altered level of consciousness
Heart	HR < 54 or > 100 bpm MAP < 49 mm Hg Mean PA < or >15 mm Hg CO < 4 or > 8 LPM CVP < 2 or > 6 mm Hg Cold, pale skin Weak pulses Urine output < 30 ml/hr Irregular rhythm
Pulmonary	Respiratory rate < 5 or > 49 breaths per minute O_2 saturations < 90 mm Hg pH < 7.35 or > 7.45 $PaCO_2$ < 35 or > 45 mm Hg HCO_3 < 22 or > 26 mEq

Systemic Impact of Multiorgan Dysfunction Syndrome—cont'd

Organ System	Clinical Manifestations of Failure
Kidney	Urine output < 30 ml/hr Serum BUN > 100 mg/dl Serum creatinine > 3.5 mg/dl
GI	Decreased or absent bowel sounds Abdominal distention Diarrhea or constipation Heme-positive stools
Liver	Jaundice Serum bilirubin > 6 mg% PTT > 4 sec over control in the absence of systemic anticoagulation
Hematologic	WBC count < 1000/µl Platelets < 20,000/µl Hematocrit < 20%
Immune system	Generalized immune depression

BUN, Blood urea nitrogen; *CNS,* central nervous system; *CO,* cardiac output; CO_2, carbon dioxide; *CVP,* central venous pressure; *GI,* gastrointestinal; HCO_3, serum bicarbonate; *HR,* heart rate; *LPM,* liters per minute; *MAP,* mean arterial pressure; O_2, oxygen; *PA,* pulmonary artery; $PaCO_2$, arterial platelet level of CO_2; *PTT,* prothrombin time; *WBC,* white blood count.

At-Risk Populations

Patients at greatest risk for developing MODS include the following:

- Patients with systemic infection (particularly, a gram-negative sepsis)
- Extensive burns
- End-organ failure
- Pancreatitis
- Hypovolemia
- Cardiogenic shock
- Human immunodeficiency virus (HIV)
- Aspiration
- Multiple blood transfusions
- Trauma

Prognosis

Although the mortality is high with MODS, patients can recover, even when multiple organs are involved. Potential for recovery depends on the severity of illness or injury, underlying organ reserve, the speed of instituting effective treatment, the adequacy of treatment, and the number and severity of subsequent injuries and complications. If treatment is unsuccessful, death usually occurs between 21 and 28 days after the initial insult.

What You DO

The treatment of MODS is directed toward the following six goals: (1) identifying the underlying cause, (2) maintaining tissue oxygenation, (3) providing nutritional support, (4) avoiding additional complications, (5) preventing infection, and (6) supporting individual organs by means of mechanical ventilation, dialysis, transfusions of blood products, and pharmacologic support as required.

MODS is most commonly associated with systemic infections; therefore, aggressive diagnostics to identify the organism will be performed (i.e., blood, tissue, urine, sputum, and invasive line tips are sent for culture and sensitivity). Tissue oxygenation is maintained by providing adequate airway support, by oxygen administration, and by initiating mechanical ventilation assistance as needed. BP, CO, and fluid volume status may be supported with administration of crystalloids, inotropes such as dobutamine, and vasopressors such as dopamine. Nutritional supplementation of carbohydrates, proteins, and amino acids is provided with IV or enteral feedings to support metabolic demands. Additional complications from nosocomial infections can be prevented by replacing emergently placed lines as soon as possible and by changing central lines every 72 hours. Patients who are intubated should be weaned and extubated as expeditiously as tolerated to reduce the risk of infection. Dialysis may be used as a supportive measure for renal insufficiency and failure. The administration of blood and blood by-products such as albumin, platelets, and fresh frozen plasma may be required to replace those lost as the result of trauma, infection, disseminated intravascular coagulation, or thrombocytopenia. Additional pharmacologic support can include antibiotics to which the organism is sensitive, antioxidants, antiprostaglandins, antihistamines, and corticosteroids. Xigris is a miscellaneous class drug currently being used for the treatment of sepsis in MODS. The mechanism of action is achieved through complex antithrombotic and antiinflammatory effects.

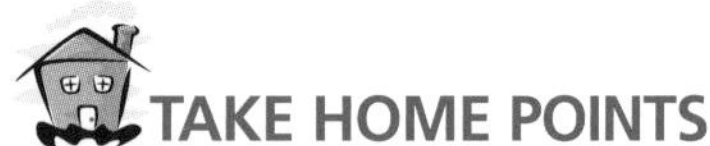

Aggressive support in the ICU is usually required for days or weeks.

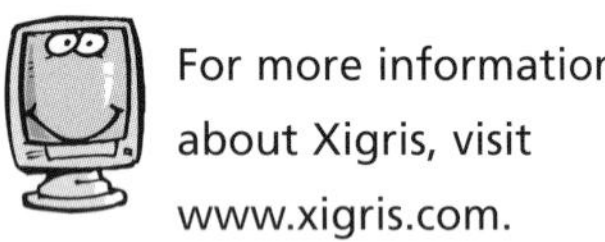

For more information about Xigris, visit www.xigris.com.

Nursing Responsibilities

Clinical Manifestations of Multiorgan Dysfunction Syndrome

System	Nursing Responsibilities
CNS	Assess level of consciousness per Glasgow Coma Scale Observe for respiratory depression Monitor ICP (if indicated)
Pulmonary	Observe for and report: Dyspnea Use of accessory muscles Discolored sputum Wheezes, crackles, rhonchi Poor capillary refill Decreased O_2 saturation Abnormal ABG values Provide emergent airway support as needed
Cardiovascular	Observe for and report changes in: HR BP PAP CO and cardiac index CVP SVR Observe for: Cold, pale skin Diminished pulses Decreased urine output Dysrhythmias Myocardial ischemia Elevated isoenzymes Elevated troponins
GI	Observe for: Decreased bowel sounds Abdominal distention Diarrhea, constipation, or impaction Jaundice Ascites Observe laboratory results for: Increased ammonia Decreased plasma proteins Decreased clotting factors Increased liver enzymes
GU	Observe for any changes in urine output, color, odor Observe laboratory results for increased BUN and creatinine levels

ABG, Arterial blood gas; *BP,* blood pressure; *BUN,* blood urea nitrogen *CNS,* central nervous system; *CO,* cardiac output; *CVP,* central venous pressure; *GI,* gastrointestinal; *GU,* genitourinary; *HR,* heart rate; *ICP,* intracranial pressure; *O_2,* oxygen; *PAP,* pulmonary artery pressure; *SVR,* systemic vascular resistance.

The first line of defense is protection. Hands should be washed properly, and aseptic technique should always be used. Early recognition of symptoms by the vigilant nurse is the first step in providing appropriate treatment. These are most powerful tools in combating MODS in the "at-risk" population.

Do You UNDERSTAND?

DIRECTIONS: **Fill in the blanks to complete each of the following statements.**

1. Name 10 at-risk populations for MODS:

   ____

   ____

   ____

   ____

   ____

2. Tissue oxygenation after an insult is maintained by ensuring adequate ______________, administration of ______________, and initiation of ______________________ support.

DIRECTIONS: **Identify the following statements as *true* (T) or *false* (F).**

_____3. A common clinical sign of MODS is acute respiratory failure.

_____4. Dialysis is a treatment for MODS.

_____5. Nutritional support for the patient in MODS is provided by frequent high-fat feedings.

_____6. Encephalopathy is a clinical manifestation of MODS.

_____7. Fluid volume excess is a problem with MODS.

Answers: **1. patient with systemic infection, extensive burns, end-organ failure, pancreatitis, hypovolemia, cardiogenic shock, HIV, aspiration, multiple blood transfusion, and trauma. 2. airway, oxygen, ventilatory; 3. T; 4. T; 5. F; 6. T; 7. F.**

References

Alspach JG: *American Association of Critical Care Nurses core curriculum for critical care nursing,* ed 6, St Louis, 2006, Saunders/Elsevier.

American Heart Association: *Advanced cardiac life support,* Dallas, 2006, AHA.

American Heart Association: *Guideline* 2005. *for cardiopulmonary resuscitation and emergency cardiovascular care*, Dallas, 2005, AHA.

Baird MS, Keen JH, Swearingen PL: *Manual of critical care nursing: nursing interventions and collaborative management,* ed 5, St Louis, 2006, Elsevier.

Baue AE: MOF, MODS, and SIRS: What is in a name or an acronym? *Shock,* 26(5):438-449, 2006.

Brunkhorst F, Sakr Y, Hager S, Reinhart K: Protein c concentrations correlate with organ dysfunction and predict outcome independent of presence of sepsis, *Anesthesiology,* 107(1):15-23, 2007.

Chulay M, Burns SM:*American Association of Critical Care Nurses essentials of critical care nursing,* New York, 2005, McGraw Hill.

Dacey MJ, Mirza ER, Wilcox V, Doherty M, Mello J, Boyer A, Gates J, Brothers T, Baute R: The effect of a rapid response team on major clinical outcome measures in a community hospital, *Critical Care Medicine,* 35(9):2076-2082, 2007.

DeVita MA, Bellomo R, Hillman K, Kellum J, Rotondi A, Teres D, et al: Findings of the first consensus conference on medical emergency teams, *Critical Care Medicine,* 34(9):2463-2478, 2006.

Jolley J, Holaday B, Harmon C: Rapid response teams: do they make a difference? *Dimensions of Critical Care Nursing,* 26(6):253-260, 2007.

Klein DJ, Derzko A, Foster D, Seely AJ, Brunet F, Romaschin AD, Marshall JC: Daily variation in endotoxin levels is associated with increased organ failure in critically ill patients, *Shock,* 28(5):524-529, 2007.

Later EB, King D: Advance directives: results of a community education symposium, *Critical Care Nurse,* 27(6):31-35, 2007.

Lewis SL, Heitkemper MM, Dirksen SR, O'Brien PG, Bucher L: *Medical-surgical nursing assessment and management of clinical problems,* ed 7, St Louis, 2007, Mosby/Elsevier.

McFarlan SJ, Hensley S: Implementation and outcomes of a rapid response team, *Journal of Nursing Care Quality,* 22(4):307-313, 2007.

Morton PG, Fontaine DK, Hudak CM, Gallo BM: *Critical care nursing: a holistic approach,* ed 8, Philadelphia, 2007, Lippincott Williams & Wilkins.

Scherer Y, Jezewski MA, Graves B, Wu YB, Bu X: Advance directives and end-of-life decision making: survey of critical care nurses' knowledge, attitude, and experience, *Critical Care Nurse,* 26(4):30-40, 2006.

Simkova V, Baumgart K, Radermacher P, Barth E, Calzia E: Year in review 2006. Critical care- multiple organ failure, sepsis, and shock, *Critical Care,* 11(4):221-227, 2007.

Urden LD, Stacy KM, Lough ME: *Thelan's critical care nursing diagnosis and management,* ed 5, St Louis, 2006, Elsevier.

Vincent JL: Metabolic support in sepsis and multiple organ failure: more questions than answers, *Critical Care Medicine,* 35(9):S436-S440, 2007.

Walsh CR: Multiple organ dysfunction syndrome after multiple trauma, *Orthopaedic Nursing,* 24(5):324-333, 2007.

NCLEX® Review

1. You are caring for a patient who is becoming more difficult to arouse. Vital signs are BP 88/42, HR 120, RR 28, and your assessment reveals sternal retractions with crackles. Which nursing action is the most important to perform at this time?
   1 Activate the code team.
   2 Document the change.
   3 Activate the rapid response team.
   4 Continue to monitor the patient.
2. The most common arrest rhythm in adults is:
   1 Asystole.
   2 Pulseless electrical activity (PEA).
   3 Ventricular tachycardia (VT).
   4 Ventricular fibrillation (VF).
3. The most important treatment for VF is:
   1 Defibrillation.
   2 CPR.
   3 Drugs.
   4 Ventilation.
4. When you look at the electrocardiogram, how do you know that the patient is in pulseless electrical activity (PEA)?
   1 You see VF on the monitor.
   2 There is no electrical activity on the monitor.
   3 The rhythm appears normal, but the patient is pulseless.
   4 The monitor shows tachycardia, and the patient has a weak pulse.
5. The first drug to be given in all three arrest rhythms is:
   1 Epinephrine.
   2 Lidocaine.
   3 Atropine.
   4 Amiodarone.
6. Organize the following steps for the patient who is presenting in a cardiac arrest in chronologic order (with 1 being the first step):
   1 Resume CPR.
   2 Ensure the patient has IV access.
   3 Administer amiodarone 150 mg IV.
   4 Initiate CPR.
   5 Defibrillate at 200 joules (biphasic).
   6 Administer vasopressin 40 units IV.
7. Nurses in ICUs are caring for more patients with multiorgan dysfunction syndrome (MODS) because:
   1 Patients with MODS require cardiac monitoring.
   2 Health care treatments and procedures are more effective; therefore, more patients are surviving more traumatic insults.
   3 Only ICUs have adequate isolation facilities.
   4 The primary physicians order a transfer to the ICU on receiving laboratory results positive for MODS.
8. MODS is a progressive dysfunction of more than one organ in patients who are critically ill. A common cause is:
   1 Systemic infection.
   2 West Nile virus.
   3 Angioplasty.
   4 Hypertensive crises.
9. After a serious illness or injury, the critically ill patient may develop an uncontrolled inflammatory response. The by-products eventually cause:
   1 Rapid healing with abundant white blood cells.
   2 Hyperoxygenation to the capillary beds.
   3 Mitral valve prolapse.
   4 Thromboxane, a vasoconstrictor, is released, and the synthesis of prostacyclin, a vasodilator, is inhibited.

10. What could place a patient receiving tube feedings at risk for developing MODS?
 1 The patient already has gastrointestinal failure.
 2 Tube feedings do not provide adequate nutritional support.
 3 Increased potential for aspiration has occurred.
 4 Tube feedings cause diarrhea and dehydration.

NCLEX® Review Answers

1.3 The priority action is to activate the rapid response team because the patient has deteriorated and is more difficult to arouse and is having difficulty breathing. The situation does not warrant a code team activation but soon will. Certainly, the condition does need to be monitored and documented but these are not the priorities.

2.4 VF is the most commonly seen arrest rhythm in adults. Asystole is often a terminal rhythm. PEA is not the first rhythm in most arrests. VT deteriorates into VF.

3.1 Defibrillation is the treatment of choice for VF and is included as the *D* in the primary survey. CPR may help, but defibrillation is the treatment of choice for VF. Drugs may help, but defibrillation is the treatment of choice for VF. Adequate ventilation may help resuscitative efforts, but defibrillation is the treatment of choice for VF.

4.3 The definition of PEA is normal electrical activity on the monitor and the patient is pulseless. VF is different from PEA. No electrical activity on the monitor describes asystole.

5.1 Epinephrine is the first drug to be administered in PEA, asystole, and pulseless VT or VF. Lidocaine is a second-line medication. Atropine is used in PEA and asystole. Amiodarone is a second-line medication.

6.4 The steps for intervening for a patient in cardiac arrest are first to initiate CPR (4); then begin defibrillation (5); resume CPR (1); ensure that IV access exists so medications can be administered (2); establish the IV and administer vasopressin (6); finally, administer amiodarone (3).

7.2 As health care treatments and procedures become increasingly effective, a greater number of patients are surviving traumatic insults. As a result, ICUs are treating more cases of MODS. Although cardiac monitoring is usually part of ICU nursing care, it is not the primary function. The primary reason for the patient to be in the ICU is to receive aggressive support. ICUs are not the only nursing units with isolation capability. Patients with MODS may require isolation, depending on the organism. The patient is admitted to the ICU for aggressive support and does not require a laboratory report for this to be accomplished.

8.1 MODS is defined as the progressive dysfunction of more than one organ in patients who are critically ill or injured; it most commonly results from a systemic infection. Usually, MODS is caused by a bacterial infection, such as a gram-negative organism. Angioplasty and hypertensive crises have nothing directly to do with the cause of MODS.

9.4 Vascular occlusive events disrupt blood flow by enhancing the release of thromboxane, a potent vasoconstrictor, and by inhibiting synthesis of prostacyclin, a vasodilating substance, thus resulting in an overall vasoconstrictive effect. The by-products cause effects in the vascular system. An increased intracellular oxygen demand occurs. The by-products cause effects in the vascular system.

10.3 Patients receiving tube feedings are at risk for aspiration of stomach contents. Aspiration pneumonia may lead to septic infection and potentially MODS. Tube feedings usually help prevent MODS because nutritional demands are being met. Tube feedings do provide adequate nutritional support. Although tube feedings may cause diarrhea and potentially dehydration, they do not directly contribute to the development of MODS.

Index

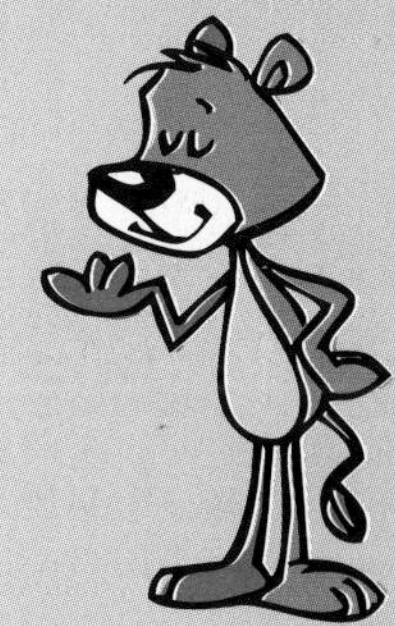

f indicates illustrations, *b* indicates boxes, and *t* indicates tables